VARIETIES OF
DELINQUENT YOUTH

SOCIAL PSYCHIATRY
OF DELINQUENCY

VARIETIES OF
DELINQUENT YOUTH

by

WILLIAM SHELDON, Ph.D., M.D.
DIRECTOR OF THE CONSTITUTION LABORATORY
COLLEGE OF PHYSICIANS & SURGEONS, COLUMBIA UNIVERSITY.

With

EMIL M. HARTL, Ph.D.
DIRECTOR, HAYDEN GOODWILL INN,
BOSTON

and

EUGENE McDERMOTT
CHAIRMAN, GEOPHYSICAL SERVICE, INC.,
DALLAS, TEXAS

VOLUME II

SOCIAL PSYCHIATRY
OF DELINQUENCY

HAFNER PUBLISHING COMPANY
DARIEN, CONN.
1970

Printed and Published by
Hafner Publishing Company, Inc.
260 Heights Road
Darien, Conn. 06820

Library of Congress Catalog Card Number 75-93262

Printed in the U.S.A.

SOCIAL PSYCHIATRY
OF DELINQUENCY

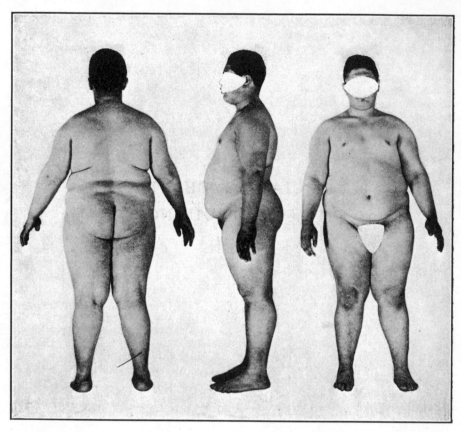

Description: Somatotype 7–3½–1. A 17-year-old extreme endomorph of average stature, with a strong secondary mesomorphy. No particular dysplasia. Primary and secondary $g\pm$. Primary t 2, secondary t 2. Features heavy, coarse, crudely formed. General strength 3, hand strength 3—surprising in this physique. The boy is remarkably strong for an extreme endomorph. Beneath the fat there is heavy muscling. Coordination good despite the knock-kneed appearance, which results from enormous development of the thighs. He has played football, can move with surprising agility, is an excellent swimmer; likes the gymnasium.

Temperament: A very personable youth. He seems a little womanly but in a normal or healthy sense. No trace of the *DAMP RAT* syndrome in any of its aspects. Viscerotonia predominates, with excellent underlying energy and apparently with good cerebrotonic integration. He is relaxed and when once used to the situation is highly socialized and well adapted to people. In a new situation he is at first self-conscious or shy. There are no somatorotic indications—no signs of aggression, no love of gambling or risk, no truculence. The temperamental pattern appears to be a healthy reflection of the somatotype. ψ 1–1–1.

Delinquency: None. Some truancy after 15, also street-corner loafing and staying out late with a gang. Parents and others worried about potential delinquency.

Origins and Family: Only living child, suburban family. Both parents Scandinavian. Father an athletic fellow with great bodily vigor. He has been a successful artisan in this country, establishing a good average home. Mother of about the boy's physique. She comes from substantial stock and has kept the home good and average. Boy reared at home.

Mental History, Achievement: Finished three years of high school. During the third year he failed one or two courses and showed signs of nervousness and maladjustment. IQ reports fall between 110 and 120, here called 115. He talks intelligently, responsively, rather eagerly; gives an impression of excellent latent ability.

No vocational plans or special gifts. The AMI that of a courteous, healthy looking boy, obviously well-bred and likeable.

Medical: Normal birth and early development. No serious illnesses or injuries. He never adapted very well to other boys, never seemed quite able to hold up his end although he always tried hard to do so. PX reveals no significant pathology.

Running Record: In a series of conferences at the Inn it soon developed that the father and several of the father's close friends are not only athletes but devotees of physical culture. Pressure in this direction had been brought to bear on the boy since early childhood. First he was to be a boxer and fighter, then a baseball and soccer player, later a track athlete and football player. He had undergone courses in posture training, muscle development and the like, had suffered humiliation from his failure to develop either muscular strength or athletic prowess. For two years prior to our contact with him he had been under the tutelage of quite a successful young athletic coach and physical educator. There had been a persistent effort to make a football player of him in high school. The boy himself had given his best efforts to the undertaking but clearly he had too much *g* and altogether the wrong somatotype for athletic aspirations. It had been a matter of trying to teach a duck to run with the hounds. The boy took a good look at his somatotype photograph, compared it with a few photographs of athletes—and his education progressed remarkably within a few minutes. He soon adopted an optimistic view of the situation. The parents were easily made cooperative. The idea that there might *really* be constitutional differences in boys was an entirely new one to these people. They had sort of gathered that it was "all a matter of training and conditioning."

The change in this boy's school career was dramatic. He finished high school with good grades, was then inducted into military service. There he made a fine record and after separation from the service addressed himself immediately to college plans. He is doing well and appears to have a good future.

Summary: Endomorphy with conspicuous g and no trace of the *DAMP RAT* syndrome. Mentality college average; excellent health. No delinquency. A problem of misapplied physical education.

ID o–o–o (o)
Insufficiencies:
  IQ ....
  Mop ....
Psychiatric:
  1st order ....
  2nd order ....
  C-phobic ....
  G-phrenic ....
Residual D:
  Primary crim. ....

Comment: Outlook very good although from the standpoint of making an athlete of him the outlook is poor. He is now generally looked upon with favor, is said to have a good personality, and in that comment great interest inheres. Morphologically he is one of the most gynandroid youths in the series. Temperamentally he shows enough of womanly characteristics to make him seem different from most young men.

Yet he cannot be called effeminate in any psychopathic sense of the term, and he seems to be as far from homosexuality or from the *DAMP RAT* syndrome as Jack Dempsey is—which I presume is quite a long way. It is perfectly clear, then, that neither gynandromorphy nor gynandrophrenia should be regarded as pathology per se.

It is interesting to note, too, that I do not recall seeing a homosexual with so much primary g. They usually show a *little* primary g, but not often much of it. Their primary g is often ±. The degree of primary g possessed by this boy appears to be almost as safe a guarantee against homosexuality as the total absence of g. Correlations between primary g and homosexuality have in my experience turned out to be practically zero. I have never tried to run such a correlation with secondary g, for I do not know how to statistify the latter satisfactorily. These considerations point the peculiar difficulties still involved in getting psychology to the point where morons with Monroe calculators and a semester of statistics can take over at the point where the best mentalities find it necessary to leave the product-moment bottom and to try to swim.

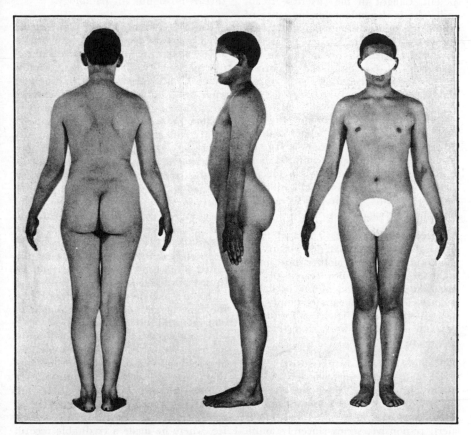

Description: Somatotype 5–3½–3½. An 18-year-old gynandroid endomorph two inches above average stature. Arms fragile with some ectomorphic dysplasia. Primary $g+3$, secondary $g\pm$. General segmental development excellent. Primary t 3, or it would be 3 if he were female. Secondary t 4. Features well formed, cleanly chiseled, and of excellent symmetry. With clothes he is handsome. Hands and feet delicate but well formed. General strength 2, hand strength 2. Coordination excellent. He throws well and is good at minor games but is of course inadequate at athletics in general and is without combative ability. He has first-rate eye-hand coordination. Good at manual dexterity tests, at marble playing, and the like.

Temperament: He is overwhelmingly somatotonic but the somatotonia is for the most part expressed within culturally approved channels. There is no indication of temperamental conflict. He is energetic, direct, athletically competent. Caught in the "exercise treadmill," he is dependent for his sense of well-being upon constant physical activity and exercise. He is assertive in posture and movement; overmature in appearance. This seems to be a normal temperamental expression of the somatotype. ψ 1–1–1.

Delinquency: No record of any formal delinquency. Good school history. Since finishing high school, at 19, he had been vocationally confused and rather bewildered, unable to decide what to do with himself. Question of bad associations, recent poolroom loafing, and drifting.

Origins and Family: Third of four, urban family, both parents Syrian immigrants. Father and mother short, muscular, wiry people. Boy reared in the home and there is no history of delinquency in the immediate family although this family has lived for many years in one of the worst slum districts of the city.

Mental History, Achievement: Finished high school, where he did well at minor athletics and was below average in school subjects. IQ reports range from 99 to 112, here called 105. He is alert, responsive, seems sincerely ambitious to "do something creditable."

No vocational plan except that he knows he is happiest when living wholly for his muscles. He wishes he were twice his size so he could be a heavyweight champion of some kind. The AMI is based on what seems to be a forthright or vigorous sincerity. He has a straightforward manner of social address which is backed by vibrant energy and suggests sincerity. He is no beauty and no sissy.

Medical: Normal growth and developmental history. No serious illnesses or injuries. Never hospitalized although his family belonged to the aristocracy of the poor and could have had unlimited hospitalization for the asking. PX reveals no significant pathology.

Running Record: At the Inn he quickly showed himself to be an intelligent, cooperative youth who despite minor personality difficulties and doubts was seriously interested in finding out what he could about himself, with an eye to a vocational future. In the gymnasium he was at home like a squirrel in his native walnut grove. He already possessed well-developed acrobatic ability along with, for his size, tremendous bodily strength. He readily became interested in a special course in physical education. We were able to give him encouragement and help in carrying out a training program. It was soon found that his acrobatic ability could be perfected to a point where it possessed a market. A few months later he joined a vaudeville troupe, made good in his act, and decided to postpone "for the time being" any further thought of college training.

After two years of this kind of work he was established as a professional in his field and gave up altogether the plan we had originally outlined for helping him through college. He had found his vocation. In the course of time he was inducted into military service, where he made a creditable record. Following the war he has been hampered in his return to acrobatic work because of an unfortunate accident and has been forced to spend many months in idleness. This has been "awful" but he has not yet fallen into the hands of psychiatrists.

Summary: Scrub-oak mesomorphy with great strength and acrobatic agility. Excellent health; normal or average mentality. Vocational problem. No delinquency.

ID o–o–o (o)
   Insufficiencies:
      IQ ....
      Mop ....
   Psychiatric:
      1st order ....
      2nd order ....
      C-phobic ....
      G-phrenic ....
   Residual D:
      Primary crim. ....

Comment: No problem here except vocational guidance, and in this case it would be difficult to make out that any unusual intelligence was needed for a successful solution. This time we did not have to cope with a problem of motivation. The boy needed good advice and a little financial help. The Inn was wonderfully well stocked with the former; was able to supply just a trace of the latter.

One element in the case will be of interest to a student of constitutional psychology. Hurt in an acrobatic accident and recently hospitalized for quite a length of time, this youth has grown very restive and has been most unhappy. He has lived for his muscles, or for one kind of somatotonia. His "somatic demand"—in this case a need for enormous and almost constant muscular exercise—is tremendous. This is like a drug addiction, and the boy may now have to face the problem of finding another *kind* of adaptation. He may eventually have to earn a living in some way other than through the daily satisfaction of his addiction. A change of vocation of such a nature is one of the hardest tests men occasionally must face. In a year it will be known whether or not this youth will have to face that test, and if he does we shall be greatly interested in the outcome.

102. *COMPANY B: THE CHAPLAIN'S UNIT*
No Delinquency: Nos. 101–105

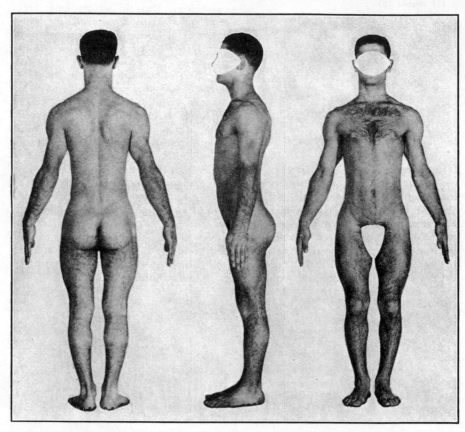

Description: Somatotype 1–6–2. A 21-year-old scrub-oak mesomorph or stunted mesomorph, two inches under average stature. Musculature excellently developed throughout the body except in the distal segments of the legs. Trunk long and narrow. Limbs seem too short, and gnarled or ill-formed. Very small, almost cubical head. This is scrub mesomorphy with superb muscular development. Primary $g\pm$; secondary g, no trace. Primary t 2, secondary t 2. The short limbs and gnarled appearance mark a contrast with the classical conception of thoroughbred mesomorphy. Features coarse, irregularly molded, expression lowering. Hands and feet crude but strong. General strength 5, hand strength 4. He scores 148 on our physical fitness test, and this is exceptionally high. Superb coordination suggesting that of a fox terrier—a natural acrobat.

Temperament: He is essentially so-matotonic and energetic both posturally and in general behavior. He loves physical activity, delights in competitive athletics, yet is refreshingly relaxed at all times. No indication of cerebrotonic interference or of temperamental conflict of any kind. Probably a normal temperament, but if any pathology is present it would lie in cerebropenia. He is a sleek, well-fed Russian bear. ψ 1–1–1.

Delinquency: No history of truancy. Minor stealing, particularly in association with a gang, between 10 and 12. From 12 to 15 or thereabouts he was known to associate closely with a street-corner gang which progressed gradually from fruit-stand and notion-store pilfering to well-organized stealing. At 17, caught at breaking and entering with several other boys. This was shortly before our contact with him.

Origins and Family: Third, of four, slum-district family. Father a stout, rugged immigrant from the Ukraine. He has a good employment history and was never known to be delinquent. He seems solid, level-headed. Mother a powerfully built immigrant from Poland who also has done well in this country and has kept out of trouble. Both parents have worked regularly. Social agencies have raised the question of neglect of children. The very few voluntary agency contacts of the family appear to represent legitimate financial difficulty during depression years. On the whole it is a solid, law-abiding Russian family —not a delinquent family.

Mental History, Achievement: Finished three years of high school with a fair record. IQ reports cluster at about 100. He gives the impression of slow or plodding mentality, but also of being rather sure of himself. He has shown good mechanical ability.

No vocational plan and no gifts except the general one of vigorous health and good coordination. The AMI is that of sturdy solidness. He suggests dependability and sincerity.

Medical: Normal birth and early development. No illnesses other than childhood diseases. Excellent medical history. PX reveals no significant pathology.

Running Record: From the beginning he made a favorable impression. We gave him the best opportunities we could and he made good, accepting responsibility and in general reflecting credit on the Inn. After his initial probationary period a school program was started and a series of psychological consultations was held with him. He seemed genuinely astonished to discover his own relative strength. Comparison of his physical foundation with that of other youths of his age appeared to give him a new picture of himself.

On the school program he made a creditable although not brilliant record; graduated from high school, spent an additional year at a technical school, then got a job and held it successfully for several months until drafted into military service. In the war he did well, and almost immediately following discharge from the service he picked up where he had left off, got a job, appears to be making good.

Summary: Sturdy ursine mesomorphy of great strength and weight, with an excellent medical history. Average mentality. Long-standing juvenile identification with minor delinquency but abrupt cessation of delinquency at 18.

ID 0–0–0 (0)
  Insufficiencies:
    IQ . . . .
    Mop . . . .
  Psychiatric:
    1st order . . . .
    2nd order . . . .
    C-phobic . . . .

G-phrenic ....
Residual D:
Primary crim. ....

Comment: Outlook considered excellent. The delinquency appears to have been a transitory by-product of a total situation in which the constitutional factors were essentially good. He "got over" the delinquency as one gets over the measles. If the view is taken that delinquent social behavior is comparable to physiological ineptitude when the organism fails to maintain immunity to pathogenic invaders, then he recovered from delinquency because of an essentially sound constitution which in the end was capable of throwing off the disease. Such a view is too simple, although in this one case the essential soundness of the constitution is demonstrable. As an organism the youth is a pretty good specimen of normality —and perhaps of a kind of Russian normality with which we in this country will in the course of time have an opportunity to enjoy a more intimate acquaintanceship.

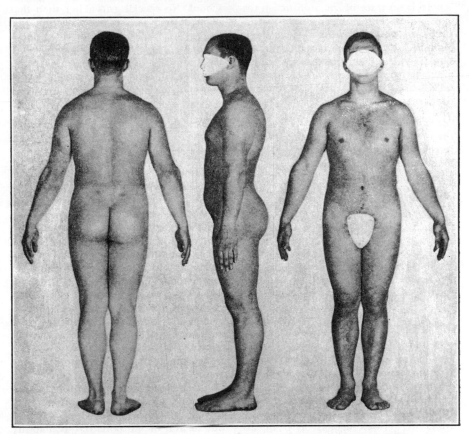

Description: Somatotype 4–6–1. An 18-year-old endomorphic meso-morph an inch above average stature, and almost an extreme mesomorph. One of the sturdiest of physical patterns—built both for comfort and for durability. This physique suggests a well-inflated balloon tire and it can flourish under great punishment. Only the distal segments of the arms and legs fall away from extreme mesomorphy. A centrotonic physique having most of the strength and mass in the trunk and proximal segments; yet the distal segments are by no means weak. Primary and secondary $g\pm$. Primary t 3, secondary t 3. Features symmetrical and well formed but lacking in any suggestion of fine modeling. General strength 5, hand strength 4—a tre-mendously strong youth. Good coordination although he is too slow and lumbering for first-rate athletic competition. An ursine physical personality.

Temperament: The pattern is that of readiness for action. He is direct, a little overmature in appearance, energetic. Yet he is quiet and self-possessed. There is no trace of somatorotic aggression and no indication of cerebrotic apprehensiveness. He has a hard steely look in his face and gives the impression of mental and physical alertness. The temperamental pattern appears to be a healthy, well-energized reflection of the somatotype. ψ 1–1–1.

Delinquency: No court record, although he lived throughout childhood in the very thick of delinquency. He attended the public schools and spent his formative period in what is regarded by social ' agencies as the most delinquent section of the city. Many of his acquaintances and early companions were involved in delinquent gangs, some of them in major delinquency. There was a murder in which some of his streetmates were involved and this incident was the direct precipitant of his contact with the Inn. His record shows truancy from school but no stealing and no violence.

Origins and Family: Youngest of four, Scandinavian family. The father, a vigorous and healthy young man, was killed in an accident when the boy was 2. The mother, thrifty and self-reliant, applied herself to such jobs as were available, refused agency help of all kinds, raised her family as best she could in the midst of poverty and almost universal delinquency. The family remained together except as the older boys grew up and emerged from the home.

Mental History, Achievement: He had finished three years of high school with a good record. IQ reports range narrowly around 120, and he gives the impression of about this degree of intelligence. Far from the genius level, he is at least college average and is practical in outlook.

The vocational plan had been simply that of wanting to go to work and to earn money. The question was whether to go to work or to stay longer in school. No special gifts other than that of a rather prepossessing personality. The AMI based on somewhat precocious manliness or sense of responsibility, and on a suggestion of quiet competence. He is a tall, well-built lad with mesomorphic steadiness in his eyes.

Medical: Normal birth and early history; no serious illnesses or injuries. PX reveals no significant pathology. Never referred to a hospital.

Running Record: In this case the problem was not one of correcting delinquency but of helping to direct and encourage a better than average personality to raise its sights and to make the best of an apparently good endowment. He was cooperative from the beginning and counseling contacts with him were satisfactory. At first he wanted to get money as soon as possible. He had little sentiment and no sentimentalism. However, the Inn was able to interest him gradually in the idea that there were at least two professional fields which might in the long run offer him more, in one way or another, than a commercial job. He seemed well fitted, according to aptitude tests and our impressions of him, for either of these fields. Hope was held out to him of the potential availability of scholarship help in getting through college and through professional school if he could go that far.

He has made good beyond the original expectation. During the past seven years he has graduated from high school and from college, on scholarship, and is now far advanced in a good professional school, also on scholarship and with good standing. He seems successfully to have lifted his sights without overshooting.

Summary: Moderate mesomorphy with high primary and secondary t. College level mentality; excellent health; intimate contact with, but no record of participation in delinquency. Good vocational adaptation.

ID o–o–o (o)
Insufficiencies:
IQ ....
Mop ....
Psychiatric:
1st order ....
2nd order ....
C-phobic ....
G-phrenic ....
Residual D:
Primary crim. ....

Comment: An excellent case in a delinquency series because he seems to define a good contrast with delinquency. A normal, healthy youth, perhaps a little hardened and "realistic" because of his early associations, but with an apparent immunity to the virus of delinquency which has been well tested and may be considered well established. Fatherless at two, he grew up with future drunkards, criminals, and social agency parasites almost without number. Yet neither he nor any of his siblings was ever known to commit a seriously delinquent act, and when an opportunity to raise his sights was offered he was ready to make the most of it. Why?

Wise choice of parents? He did choose good parents. Good early ideals? The mother did her best to protect her children from all sorts of superstition, and to teach them responsibility. Anyhow here is a personality which, coming from sound stock and blessed with a responsible parent, reaffirmed its soundness in the face of adversity and corruption.

COMPANY B: THE CHAPLAIN'S UNIT
No Delinquency: Nos. 101–105

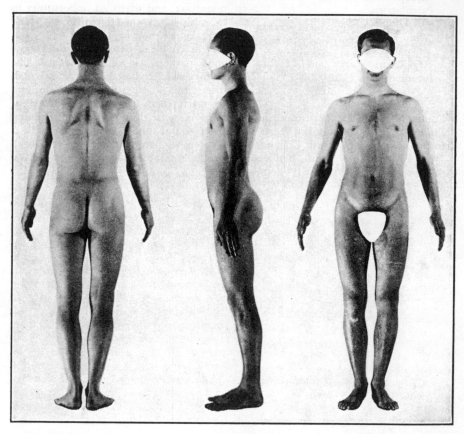

Description: Somatotype 2½–4½–3½. An 18-year-old moderate meso-morph four inches above average stature. No dysplasias. Primary and secondary $g\pm$. Primary t 4, secondary t 4. Features strong, cleanly modeled, and sharply chiseled. An entirely masculine face—he is not a "pretty boy." General strength 3, hand strength 4. Coordination excellent. He moves as if all parts of the body belonged together, although he is not a very powerful youth and is too brittle for successful fighting or for professional or collegiate athletics.

Temperament: Somatotonia predominates. He is essentially direct, fond of risk, seems mature for his age. He is mainly a boy of action, physically well poised; yet there is constant evidence of cerebrotonic modulation of the tendency to action. He is tight-lipped, a little intent, abrupt or sharp-cornered in his decisions and in some of his bodily movements. No somatorotic tendency and no indication of temperamental pathology of any kind. ψ 1–1–1.

Delinquency: History of recalcitrancy in foster homes, especially at age 12 and 13. Good behavior before that. At 16, involved with a group of previous foster home associates in one serious theft. No other history of stealing and no delinquency of violence.

Origins and Family: Only child, suburban family, Old American stock on both sides. Father described as a rather weak descendant of a well-known family. He was never delinquent, had a good health history, but left the family shortly after the birth of this child. The mother then turned the boy over to foster homes. He "did well" and never caused trouble until about age 12.

Mental History, Achievement: Graduated from high school with a good record. Admitted to a university but unable to enter because of lack of money. It was during the following autumn that all of his delinquency of record occurred. IQ reports range from 115 to 120, which is just about average college level. A bright, alert youth with excellent verbalization but manifesting a certain impatience, particularly with academic institutions. Attitude toward college a strongly rationalized negative one. "Colleges are impractical. They teach you a lot of outdated nonsense."

No specific vocational plan. He would like to do some sort of technical work. The AMI rests on a rather quiet directness or manliness. He has the mesomorphic way of looking steadily into a person's eyes and thus inspiring confidence. Generally regarded as a handsome, attractive boy.

Medical: Normal birth. Walked and talked at 10–12 months. No serious illnesses or injuries. Medical history entirely negative except for childhood diseases. PX reveals no significant pathology.

Running Record: At the Inn he gave early and constant evidence of trustworthiness, and his general response was good. He participated in a series of consultations; seemed to show quick insight into his own physical, social, and psychological history. Our relationship with him was largely a contest in which we undertook to overcome his prejudice against returning to school. We wanted to send him to college, but he demurred vigorously and in the end successfully. Throughout his stay he exerted a good influence in the House, and so far as we know there was no identification with delinquency of any kind. At camp he made a good record, was considered a superior camper. On the work program he not only did well but carried responsibility well. We felt that he was a promising youth who ought to be encouraged to get a good educational foundation, but we failed to steer him to that trail. In the end his possibly myopic view of the situation prevailed over our perhaps hyperopic view.

After severing his relations with the Inn he entered upon a course in technical training, did well in it for a few months, and then was inducted into military service. There he acquitted himself with honor, received at least one citation, and shortly before the end of the war was killed in action.

Summary: Ectomorphic mesomorph reflecting good blood or good breeding,

with high primary and secondary *t*.
College level mentality; excellent
health. No psychopathy. Transitory
juvenile delinquency only.

ID o–o–o (o)
  Insufficiencies:
    IQ ....
    Mop ....
  Psychiatric:
    1st order ....
    2nd order ....
    C-phobic ....
    C-phrenic ....

Residual D:
  Primary crim. ....

Comment: This youth's association
with delinquency seems obviously cir-
cumstantial or accidental. His story
demonstrates a need for the utmost cau-
tion in making generalizations
about delinquency, for it seems reasonable to suppose that if he could once
have been regarded as delinquent, then
almost anybody under certain unfavorable circumstances could be delinquent.
In studying delinquency the job is
clearly to describe people—not "criminal types."

105. *COMPANY B: THE CHAPLAIN'S UNIT*
No Delinquency: Nos. 101–105

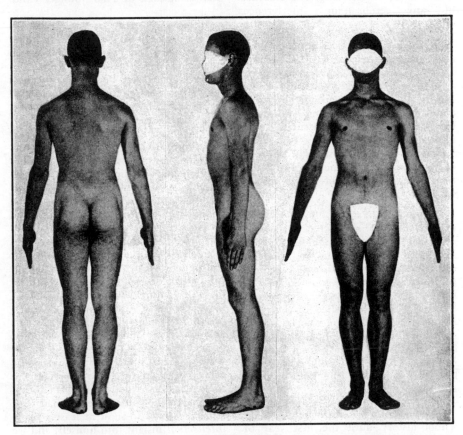

Description: Somatotype 2½–4½–4. A 17-year-old ectomorphic mesomorph two inches above average stature. Excellent general and segmental development. No dysplasias. Primary and secondary $g\pm$. Primary and secondary t 4. An almost perfectly proportioned body for the somatotype. Features strongly developed, well molded, cleanly chiseled. General strength 3, hand strength 4. Coordination excellent. He moves gracefully and lightly, dances well. Good at minor athletics, too light for successful competition at the body contact games.

Temperament: An overenergized, enormously overblown, romantically imaginative boy who seems in mental outlook about nine. He did not become adolescent until 15. The temperamental pattern seems to be that of viscerotonic extraversion complicated by excessive energy or by a dycrastically heavy endowment of somatotonia. No evidence of any cerebrotonic interference. ψ 4–1–1.

Delinquency: No delinquency until after the mother's death, when he was 15. At 16 he seems to have embarked on a delinquency binge, prowling about the neighborhood at night, breaking and entering, and joining two other boys of established delinquent status in systematic looting. He set a barn afire, was involved in at least eight episodes of breaking and entering, tried to wreck a railroad train—all of this within a span of a few weeks.

Origins and Family: First of two, urban family. The father a tall and at one time professionally athletic Swedish immigrant. He has done well in this country, having established a successful business and kept a good home. The mother was a tall and heavily built Swedish woman who died of cancer at about 40 when the boy was 15. Latter continued to live at home with his father who is said to have been "uneven in his discipline" as well as more or less disappointed in the boy's nonathletic propensities.

Mental History, Achievement: Good school history until the first year of high school, which was the year his mother died—and also the year he became adolescent. He then appeared to lose interest in school. Early records indicate that he was considered rather bright. IQ reports place him at about 120. There is no question as to his basic intelligence. His mind seems alert, comprehensive, and accurate. He is of at least average college mentality.

No vocational plans or special gifts. He hates athletics but loves swimming. The AMI that of a stupendous hulk of a youth who is friendly and viscerotonic, seems a little hypomanic, tends to sweep you off your feet with a torrential flow of language. He is bright but somehow gives the impression of possessing the mental outlook of a far younger child.

Medical: Normal birth and early development. Not a very large baby although he gained weight like a bear cub during the first three years. No serious illnesses or injuries. Periodic heavy chest colds. PX reveals no further pathology of significance. He might be called well nourished.

Running Record: His conduct at the Inn was that of a gracious and friendly but loquaciously breezy guest. On the second day after he arrived one of our jokesters appeared with his arm inside his coat, leaving an empty sleeve. The jokester explained that "that new boy" had talked his arm off. The latter committed no delinquency in the House, did willingly what he was asked to do, in the end made himself popular both by his entertaining yarns and by his willingness to assist other boys to write letters and the like—especially love letters. He was at the time favorably disposed toward love—said he believed in it. After a short stay here for diagnostic study he was returned to the referring agency and everybody was sorry to see him go. In the conferences we had with him he seemed to show at least a ready *intellectual* insight into himself, and we had a feeling that his delinquency could be considered episodic.

From here he went to a farm, where he immediately resumed the pattern of delinquency. He was then sent to one of the correctional schools and there he seems at once to have settled down. Upon release, or graduation, he had a perfect record and was described as a model boy at the school. An effort was then made to return him to high school but at this he rebelled and would have none of it. He wanted to go to work, was finally permitted to do so. For three years he has been an excellent workman, with no further signs of delinquency.

Summary: Extreme endomorphy with too much energy. Superior mentality and good health. History of quite a vigorous episodic binge of delinquency, following the death of the mother and a late adolescence.

ID 0–2–0 (2)

Insufficiencies:

IQ ....

Mop ....

Psychiatric:

1st order .... (?)

2nd order 2

Episodic Dionysian outburst (4–1–1)

C-phobic ....

G-phrenic ....

Residual D:

Primary crim. ....

Comment: Outlook very good. He is no criminal. His postadolescent binge may turn out to be the one fling in an otherwise humdrum life. Possibly this was his cosmic protest against his burden—the extreme endomorphy. Since he did no serious damage and stole nothing of any particular value, perhaps the view can be taken that we are glad the boy had a little fun. People of his somatotype are reputed to be jolly, but perhaps they need to be jolly to keep up their spirits. Everybody loves a fat man but nobody loves him *much*. Fortunately people of this kind of physical endowment usually have little sexuality to worry about. However, they do have some, and this youth may have been washed off his feet by a wave of it without altogether knowing what hit him. Constitutionally estranged from his father and therefore a disappointment to the latter, he had been emotionally close to his mother and the shock of her death probably affected him profoundly. Because we do not in most cases put this kind of consideration forward as the one factor of foremost importance in shaping personality, it does not follow that we think it should be ignored. In the present instance loss of the mother almost certainly played a part in the boy's failure to continue in school. Compared with this failure the delinquency was an inconsequential episode, for his one real chance lay in the development of a mind, and having missed that chance he is at best wasted ammunition.

His behavior during the acute episode seems to have been almost disorientational, although from what we can gather it was never quite disorientational. Despite the unusual provocation of a late and sudden adolescence reenforced by an emotional tragedy, such behavior reveals the latent presence of at least second-order psychopathy, and it *may* point to first-order psychopathy. The Dionysian episode could be a forerunner of a later cycloid psychosis. This is another youth who should be watched with interest.

106. COMPANY B, PLATOON 1, SECTION 1
Second-Order Psychopathy; Bordering on First-Order
Psychopathy: Nos. 106–114

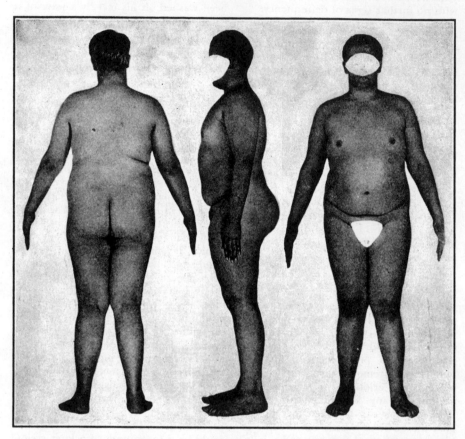

Description: Somatotype 7–3–1½. A 16-year-old extreme endomorph four inches above average stature. Strong secondary mesomorphy throughout the body except in the arms, which are comparatively poor in muscle and a little flaccid. There is solid muscling in the neck, trunk, and thighs. Primary $g+1$, secondary $g\pm$. He is hypogenital but normally so for extreme endomorphy. Not a Froelich physique, although perhaps a second or third cousin to it. Primary t 3, secondary t 2. General segmental development good. Features small, badly shaped, and poorly formed. General strength 3, which is very high for the somatotype; hand strength 1. Coordination good. He moves about spryly and can run like a bear. He cannot walk on the water but might be able to sit on it.

Temperament: The hallmark is a slow, persistent stubbornness, with infrequent episodes of temper. One of our staff describes his behavior as "exactly like that of a tame she bear." He is nearly always relaxed, almost impossible to persuade to do anything, free from cerebrotonic restraint or tenseness. He has been called paranoid and also hypochondriac, since he is obsessed with somatic complaints. He is as earnestly humorless as a haberdashery salesman. When contradicted or crossed he usually ignores the incident, but occasionally will break out in a tantrum of feminine somatorotic fury. Violent names are called, gestures of annihilation agitate the air, furniture may be broken, but there is no destruction of human flesh. He cannot fight or hit, and if bullied cannot defend himself. Most of the time he manifests what has been aptly called a stubborn lethargy. ψ 2–2–1.

Delinquency: Mainly the delinquency of disappointing performance. History of loafing, living principally off social agencies, complaining of numerous aches and pains, of dizziness, "head trouble," and so on for four or five years. Referred to various medical clinics and to nearly all the psychiatric clinics of the city, with no pathology found. The usual diagnoses of *psychoneurotic, psychopathic personality,* and *prepsychotic* have been collected. Refusal to work, insistence upon spending all his time in search of "the right psychiatrist." No stealing or violence.

Origins and Family: Youngest of four, urban Negro family. Father of medium build, considered "not strong," died in his early fifties of unknown cause (he "just up and died") when this boy was 10. Mother of medium heavy build, described as "a dazed, forgetful woman." She struggled along with much agency help and raised her children at home. The family as a whole is described as slow, stubborn, ineffectual; on the edge of delinquency but not actively delinquent. Each of the other siblings has found a niche and is getting along.

Mental History, Achievement: Finished high school with barely passing grades but with a good deportment record. During the final two years he confined himself largely to courses in music, typing, and the like. A grade school teacher described him as a good boy, "whose mind seemed to wander." IQ reports vary widely from 80 to 110, the latter figure achieved in a test which he had taken many times previously. IQ here placed at 90. He gives the impression of being dull and slow, although earnest.

His own vocational plan is to play in an orchestra, but he has long been subjected to pressure from social workers, and in this rather Negrophilic city has frequently been offered financial inducements to go to college. He plays several musical instruments, seems to be happy only when doing so. The AMI that of an extraordinarily sincere, serious, and bewildered youth who has been overcaseworked, overbabied, and overprodded in the direction of higher education.

Medical: Odd and aloof as a child, never mixing with other children. No record of serious illness or injury, and no complaints until about the middle of his high school career. He experienced academic difficulty during the last two years of high school, and as various college programs were offered he became worried, confused. Many somatic complaints appeared. He seemed to become dazed and "forgetful like his mother." His "mind jumped" or "seemed to skip." Almost endless clinical referral revealed nothing but an array of psychiatric diagnoses attached like a cluster of grapes around the terms "psychoneurotic" and "hypochondriac."

PX reveals no significant pathology of any kind.

Running Record: Throughout a series of brief stays at the Inn he behaved well and carried out work assignments faithfully except for the periodic episodes of temper already described. Here he was not encouraged to go to college but was tried on several jobs which, if carried through, would have led to clerical work or white collar work. Always after a few days he developed severe somatic symptoms and "had to quit." For some reason of his own he did not, when with us, desire to go directly into musical work. He was still under pressure or in conflict over going to college, wanted to be a "leader of his race," and had accepted a compromise of working for a year or two in order to get his bearings and to "recover from his mental confusion." Several months of life at the Inn seemed to accomplish no overtly manifest good results, and he left still unhappy at not finding the right psychiatrist.

After trying the Merchant Marine and two or three other enterprises at which he quickly became "psychoneurotic," he was inducted into military service. There he spent more than three years, apparently following much the same pattern he had followed in civilian life. Many times hospitalized and tried at a number of jobs, he did well and was happy only at orchestral work. His commanding officers appear to have had the good sense, during the latter part of his military career, to keep him in that kind of work. After discharge from the service he drifted unhappily for upwards of a year and at last report was again in conflict about going to college. Now in addition to the pressure from social workers he has the GI Bill of Rights bait to worry about.

Summary: Mesomorphic Negro with gynandroid complications. Normal subaverage mentality; good health. Path-

ological lack of humor which in this case probably stems from cerebropenia. Hypochondriasis. Suggestion of second-order psychopathy and a weak epileptoid characteristic.

ID 0–4–0 (4)
Insufficiencies:
  IQ ....
  Mop ....
Psychiatric:
  1st order .... (?)
  2nd order 3
  (2–2–1)
  C-phobic ....
  G-phrenic 1
Residual D:
  Primary crim. ....

Comment: Outlook probably good, when he forgets about higher education. Whether the psychopathy in this case is of first or second order is a question that lies beyond any diagnostic technique known to me. There is just enough indication of early attentional difficulty, and of queerness or oddness as a child, to leave a lurking impression that the trouble may stem from a mild psychotic component rather than merely from "psychoneurosis with hypochondriac ruminations," as one psychiatrist has diagnosed him. Diagnostically it is rather a delicate case, and the youth probably belongs to that narrow border of population for whom minor exigencies of environmental pressure will determine whether or not he goes over into psychosis. He seems already to have progressed a little further in school than the mental endowment would quite warrant, and it may be that the pressure which has been put upon him to go to college is an immediate cause of the symptoms of psychopathy. The army saved him from college once. Perhaps time will rescue him again. If he does have a psychotic component it is a mixed one. The guess here ventured is that his psychopathy will remain of the second order—that he is not psychotic.

COMPANY B, PLATOON 1, SECTION 1
Second-Order Psychopathy; Bordering on First-Order Psychopathy: Nos. 106–114

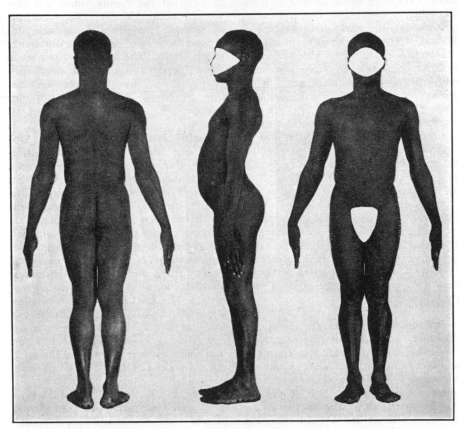

Description: Somatotype 4–4½–3. A 21-year-old Negro. An endomorphic mesomorph an inch under average stature. Arms and legs show the ectomorphic dysplasia of the distal segments usually seen in Negroes of Nilotic ancestry (see p. 19). In this instance the dysplasia of the forearms is more pronounced than that of the legs. The arms are brittle below the elbows. Primary g+1, secondary g+1. There is a somewhat soft, expansible look about the whole body and he will become heavy in later life. Primary t 3 despite the lordotic posture, which is a common Negro characteristic. Secondary t 3 or average for the racial stock. Features wholly Negro and possibly a little finer or more delicate than usual. Hands almost fragile. General strength 3, hand strength 2. Coordination good although he moves with a slow or lazy shuffle. Bodily locomotion seems feline or ursine. He has poor mechanical ability, throws like a girl, is no fighter or athlete.

Temperament: The sense of having too much energy is the outstanding characteristic. Somatotonia and viscerotonia seem both to be present in overwhelming strength and they appear to get continuously entangled, like playful kittens. He is enthusiastic, impulsive, unrestrained. Inclined toward alcoholism, he becomes even more Dionysian with that drug. He overflows with affection, or with a viscerotonic engulfing warmth both for people and for the world at large. He is sociophilic to an extreme degree; is a great sharer and an unbosomer. There are frequent episodes of extraversional emotionality which suggest manic disturbance. This is an off-the-deep-end personality, subject to enthusiasms that are like waves of religious conversion. There is no manifest trace of cerebrotonia. He is an extreme viscerotonic extravert and at the same time an extreme somatotonic extravert. He lives a hypomanic pattern although that does not necessarily imply a psychotic pattern. ψ 5–1–1.

Delinquency: From childhood he presented a psychiatric problem with conflicting diagnoses. Unable to adapt to other boys or to get along with contemporaries of either sex. Considered queer or peculiar in high school although there his vast energy was triumphant and he had a good time. He twice started college but in each instance had a "serious breakdown" followed by amnesia and by wandering about the country. Hospitalized on three different occasions for psychiatric observation, between 18 and 22. During this same period he was known to start thirty different jobs but could not carry through on any of them. Auditory hallucinations reported at 20. Numerous rumors of and furors over homosexuality, although there have been no arrests on that count.

Origins and Family: Third of four, urban family. Father Old American and of heavy build. "Emotionally unstable" as a youth, he later developed a manic tendency along with alcoholism and has been intermittently hospitalized. He left or deserted the family when this boy was an infant. Mother Old American of heavy, gynandroid build and described in agency records as unreliable and hysterical. She has been a persistent agency person and has rather unadroitly attempted to use different agencies simultaneously. Boy reared with the mother.

Mental History, Achievement: Finished one year of college with passing grades although with interruptive psychiatric difficulties. IQ reports range between 98 and 120, here called 110. He appears to have a quick mentality which has been poorly disciplined.

Many divergent vocational plans. He has alternated between the desire to be a great religious reformer or saviour of society, and a multimillionaire businessman who would save the world by economics. The AMI that of an overwhelming youth who is manifestly intelligent and has a call. He is by nature an evangelist or missionary, but has run into difficulty in trying to find the modern equivalent of Christian evangelism.

Medical: Birth and early development called normal. As a young child he was "very serious and very nervous." Enuretic at least until age 12. At least four serious infections—in each case septicemia following minor scratches. Many hospital referrals for somatic complaints, dizziness, supposed metabolic and cardiac disturbances. A long list of psychiatric referrals with the following diagnoses: *Simple behavior disorder; psychopathic personality, manic tendency; psychopathic personality, homosexual trends; religious disturbance; dementia praecox, hebephrenic; dementia praecox, other types; prepsychotic, manic-depressive, mixed type.* PX reveals no significant pathology other than moderate flaccidity of the arms, general bodily oversensitivity, defective vision, and a continual coarse tremor of the hands.

Running Record: His behavior at the Inn was that of a gentlemanly and Promethean *DAMP RAT*. He was an impulsive dilettante, had effeminate mannerisms with arty, affected speech, yet was a good worker and was sincerely enthusiastic about saving the world. He gave his time and energy generously to all sorts of projects, and was meanwhile embroiled in a Laocoön-like struggle with his three great problems—religion, economics, and sexuality. He was driven by the idea of saving the world, was frantically trying to find a way to get rich, and sexually seemed in a state of prolonged adolescent flush. Each of the three problems was a full-time job with him. Within a winter he played with half a dozen wild religions, explored and rejected a score of jobs, was adventurously exploratory in the field of sexuality. In the latter field he seemed caught halfway between homosexual and heterosexual leanings, appeared to be making at least verbal progress toward the latter pole. The real problem seemed to be that he was overenergized and could find no channels for adequate expression of his energy. There was still warfare in his mind over going back to college and in the course of his stay at the Inn he reached a decision to give up on this ambition. After that he seemed to feel much better, and soon left for a job.

The job lasted for more than two years, or until he was inducted into military service. He was given a discharge from the service within a few months, then returned to work, and now for another three years has got along. There has been no delinquency of record. He has grown heavier, is considered "a queer one" but has been a satisfactory employee. He seems to have settled back to a more reasonable level of energy expenditure. If he is now homosexual, he has it under excellent control.

Summary: A massive, overenergized gynandroid youth who is physically ineffectual. Mentality above average but probably not quite college level. Enuresis and many infections. *DAMP RAT* syndrome. Psychiatric delinquency.

ID 2–4–0 (6)
  Insufficiencies:
    IQ ....
    Mop 2
  Psychiatric:
    1st order .... (?)
    2nd order 3
      (5–1–1)
    C-phobic ....
    G-phrenic 1
      DAMP RAT
  Residual D:
    Primary crim. ....

Comments: Prognosis guarded although doubtless improving. He was called psychotic or prepsychotic at three different clinics; in at least one of them has since been referred to as "recovered." Whether or not he does actually have some first-order psychopathy is a question of great interest but one which I think nobody is yet in a position to answer. His psychopathy now looks more like a second-order problem which was intensified by excessive energy and by the *DAMP RAT* complication. The college business was the last straw but the camel's back may not have been broken. The boy had the good fortune to fall under the influence of one psychiatrist who appears to have seen this picture clearly and advised strongly against a second return to college. This may have saved him from going over into psychosis. He appears to be about as close to the border between first- and second-order psychopathy as anyone in the series. Certainly many, perhaps all of the alleged recoveries from psychosis dwell near this border, and it is possible that all of the true recoveries came in the first place from the right side of the tracks.

COMPANY B, PLATOON 1, SECTION 1
Second-Order Psychopathy; Bordering on First-Order Psychopathy: Nos. 106–114

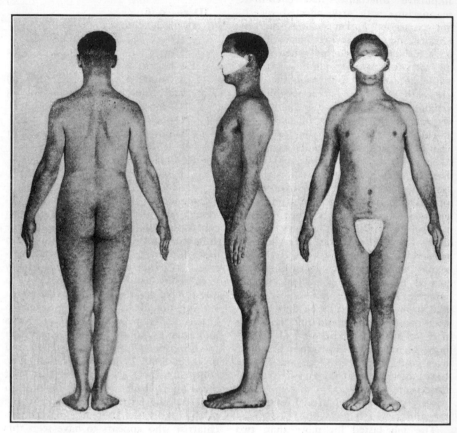

Description: Somatotype 5–4½–2. A 22-year-old mesomorphic endomorph two inches above average stature. Soft, heavily built youth, massive and solid through the trunk and neck, with a trace of ectomorphic dysplasia in the distal segments of arms and legs. He has the neck of a Roman emperor but is otherwise not dangerous looking. Primary $g+2$, secondary $g+1$. Primary t 3, secondary t 3. Features strongly formed but a little blobby and asymmetrical. Hands fragile and weak, feet well formed. General strength 3, hand strength 2. Coordination poor. He handles himself like a floundering woman, and is physically ineffectual in spite of abundant energy.

Temperament: He gives a first impression of shyness. As acquaintanceship progresses, however, the impression is corrected. He tends to become too familiar, expressing both viscerotonic and somatotonic extraversion. He laughs and cries easily, is loquacious and effusive when at ease. Toward some people he seems stubborn, hostile; but he expresses his hostility, as some women do, by a kind of snubbing superciliousness. There is no pugnacity or physical effectuality in him. He likes alcohol and with a small amount of it indulges in rollicking profanity, becomes for the time being quite a cut-up. He has long periods of aloof quiescence. Twice at psychiatric clinics the question of *catatonic schizophrenia* has been raised, and once he was called (with a question mark) *prepsychotic, manic tendency*. He does show some schizoid traits and also a cycloid trend, but the manifest psychopathy seems clearly of the second, not of the first order. ψ 3–2–3.

Delinquency: Persistent truancy during early school years and minor stealing between 10 and 14. All of his stealing was done alone. No identification with gangs, few associations of any kind with other boys. Larceny at 15. At 16 he was a source of concern to social workers, with resultant psychiatric referrals. In some quarters he is considered prepsychotic.

Origins and Family: Seventh of twelve, urban family. Father "a tall and weak French-Canadian" who as a young man was called unreliable, immature. Many court appearances for alcoholism, indigence, and quarreling. Now a chronic alcoholic. Paternal grandfather was a chronic alcoholic. A paternal aunt is feebleminded and obese, with a family of children on agency support. Mother Irish and tuberculous. An agency report describes her as "always in a chronic state of general debility." Hospitalized about a quarter of the time during twenty years, she has meanwhile given birth to twelve children, seven of whom survived infancy. Of the living siblings one is called defective, three have delinquent records. Boy lived at home throughout his childhood.

Mental History, Achievement: Finished grade school, although regarded as a "weak, unsatisfactory pupil." At 8, reported as being "smart but unteachable." IQ records fall between 85 and 95, here put at 90. He gives the impression of possessing a sensitive, responsive mentality, but he seems unable to cope with the objectivity of ordinary human relations.

No vocational identifications or plans, and no particular abilities. The AMI that of an oddly shy, confiding youth who presents at least second-order psychopathy and clearly needs something.

Medical: Birth and early development called "not unusual." No history of serious illnesses or injuries. The actual medical history is good although he has been repeatedly referred to psychiatrists because of low energy, temper tantrums, lack of school efficiency, "introversion," and so on. Aloof, queer, unpredictable at 10 and later. Diagnosed by one psychiatrist *psychopathic personality*, by another as *prepsychotic*. PX reveals no significant pathology of any kind.

Running Record: At the Inn and at camp he remained an ineffectual, odd youth so far as the general group was concerned, but continued to manifest minor floods of viscerotonic conviviality when individually encouraged. He was like a St. Bernard puppy in this respect, showing the same clumsy loose-jointedness and the promise of a vast endomorphy to blossom in the future. Decidedly unhappy in the presence of noise, confusion, and the inevitable somatotonic competitiveness which characterizes boys' gatherings, he hated group activities of all sorts. He seemed to do well when permitted to wander off on nature-study jaunts with one or two companions. However, he took advantage of every opportunity to imbibe alcoholic beverages and seemed to get drunk with the utmost ease. Under alcohol he was flamboyantly aggressive and vulgarly profane; he seemed to present an unfavorable preview of things to come.

Exempted from military service, he has drifted and has seemed to go downhill during the years following his contact with us. He has been involved in larceny, has become decidedly more alcoholic, and repeated referral to psychiatric clinics has yielded such diagnoses as: *primary behavior disorder; simple adult maladjustment; state of deterioration; psychopathic personality; inadequate emotional response.* The first component has blossomed. He has put on 40 or more pounds and the suggestion of schizoid shyness has superficially disappeared. He now seems hearty and Dionysian. Already called a confirmed alcoholic.

Summary: Gangling physique of midrange or slightly ectomorphic somatotype. Mentality in the lower normal range; good health. Second-order psychopathy, alcoholism, and gynandrophrenic confusion.

ID 0–7–0 (7)
Insufficiencies:
  IQ ....
  Mop ....
Psychiatric:
  1st order .... (?)
  2nd order 3
    (3–2–3)
  C-phobic 2
  G-phrenic 2
Residual D:
  Primary crim. ....

Comment: Outlook dark gray, although he may be having a good time. He is probably as good an example of what might be called borderline psychosis as any in the series. With early indications of schizoid isolation and with postadolescent indications of a schizoid temperament, there is doubtless reason to suspect the presence of some degree of first-order psychopathy. Yet he seemed *almost* to get along, and through the late teens gave some promise of making an acceptable adaptation. Alcohol was entirely too much for him. It seemed to tip a finely balanced scale. If the youth could have been kept away from that drug for life he probably could have been a little more nearly self-supportive than he will be. But life might then have been more unpleasant for him. Would you give him the drug, or would you take it away from him?

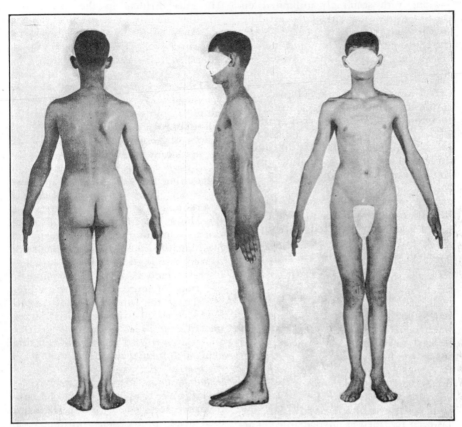

Description: Somatotype 4–3½–4½. A 16-year-old immature youth four inches above average stature, with a gangling, loose-jointed midrange physique. He may well cross 200 pounds before he reaches 30. Arms and legs ectomorphic. Head and neck mesomorphic. Trunk midrange. Primary g+1, secondary g+2. He is soft, with feminoid subcutaneous finish, long eyelashes, and feminine features. He has large brown eyes like those of a deer. Primary t 3, with all segments of the body harmoniously developed. No asthenia here. Secondary t 3. Features delicate and soft, mouth small but viscerotonic and overly relaxed. He is almost pretty. Hands and feet crude, weak. General strength 2, hand strength 2. Coordination fair, although he moves in a loose, floppy manner. Ineffectual at all athletic games and displeased by the gymnasium. He walks like a girl.

Temperament: The pattern is that of astonishingly well sustained Dionysian extraversion. He has both kinds of extraversion, viscerotonic and somatotonic —along with seemingly unlimited energy. He appears ruthless, overriding, psychologically callous. There is no trace of manifest cerebrotonic interference. He has been called hypomanic. ψ 6–1–1.

Delinquency: Quarrelsomeness throughout childhood. Long history of somatorotic altercations with parents, school teachers, siblings, and others. Described by local police as "an uncontrollable boy and a community problem" at about age 8. Known to be alcoholic as early as 14. No court delinquency until 16, when he frequently was in trouble because of unbridled sexual aggression. Arrested twice in his eighteenth year for stealing. Repeatedly alcoholic at 17 and 18.

Origins and Family: Third of five, rural village. Father Old American and Irish, described as a "husky, handsome man with keen eyes and a brusque manner." He did well at farming and at small-town business, enjoyed vigorous health, became "alcoholic and wild" at about 40—then squandered his money and left his family. This was when the boy was about 16. He has not been under psychiatric observation but has been regarded as "hypomanic." The mother, Old American and of average physique, is a quietly relaxed woman, described as "religious." Before 15, the boy was reared in what passed as a good American home.

Mental History, Achievement: Finished a year of high school, quit in the second year after a series of somatorotic upheavals. IQ reports range widely between 92 and 133, here called 110. He is mentally alert, imaginative; almost professionally mendacious, he rarely contradicts himself even in the most extravagant yarns.

No vocational plans or special gifts. The AMI that of a breezy and overtalkative youth who is obviously but interestingly pulling the social worker leg. He tells thrillers in the first person singular, mainly of criminal adventure, and they hold you enthralled whoever you may be. His nickname in the House: The Great North Wind.

Medical: Normal birth and early development. No serious illnesses or injuries. Coming as he does from the self-supportive middle class, there is no history of hospital referral. PX reveals no significant pathology.

Running Record: With his incessant and colorful yarns he was a source of entertainment and friendly interest at the House. Several programs of educational rehabilitation were set up for him, but these quickly fell through. He seemed unable to hold to any sustained interest, could never keep his mind on one trail for more than a few minutes. His stay at the Inn was virtually a prolonged orgy of vocal grandeur, interspersed with brief periods of inaction and recovery. The question of a manic-depressive tendency was raised by a psychiatric clinic to which he was referred, but we did not feel that his behavior quite indicated first-order psychopathy. He seemed to keep his manic tendencies pretty well within vocal boundaries. It was impossible, however, to handle him satisfactorily either on the work program or on a job placement program, and we failed to prevent him from drinking. He finally left for one of the government construction projects with plans for reorganizing and redirecting the project.

He remained on the new job for a day and a half, then disappeared and was not heard from for six months. Shortly after this he was inducted into military service, where he stayed for nearly three years, although with numerous episodes of AWOL. He was finally given a medical discharge. Almost immediately he was involved in a series of robberies and then spent two years under detention. Shortly after his release he was again apprehended at robbery; at the present writing is again under detention.

Summary: A physique approaching extreme endomorphy, with too much energy. Dionysian temperament; mentality above average; good health history. Troublesome from early childhood, delinquent after adolescence. Alcoholism, somatorotic irresponsibility, and later delinquency of appropriation.

ID 0–5–2 (7)
  Insufficiencies:
    IQ ....
    Mop ....
  Psychiatric:
    1st order .... (?)
    2nd order 3
      (6–1–1)
    C-phobic 2
    G-phrenic ....
  Residual D:
    Primary crim. 2

Comment: Prognosis guarded. In some quarters he is now looked upon as a confirmed criminal, although the number of actual charges against him is still comparatively small. What he *is* confirmed in is Dionysian somatorosis and the question as to whether or not he has a psychotic component is one of great interest. He certainly has more energy than he can handle, and although we took the view six years ago that he was not psychotic we may have been wrong. I was able to find no evidence of disorientation in his early history. He is undoubtedly close to the psychotic borderline and to follow him through the decade to come ought to constitute a valuable exercise in psychiatry.

This is a case on which the Army failed, although for a while he seemed to do well there. He is reported to have said that he liked the Army fine until he found out "how much everybody got away with." His history presents still another factor of interest. The court delinquency about corresponds in time with his father's climactic departure. Yet before putting all the explanatory eggs into one basket of this nature, it should be recalled that from age 8 the boy was known to local police as uncontrollable and a community problem. His shortcomings may be related to his father's shortcomings through biological as well as through sociological ties.

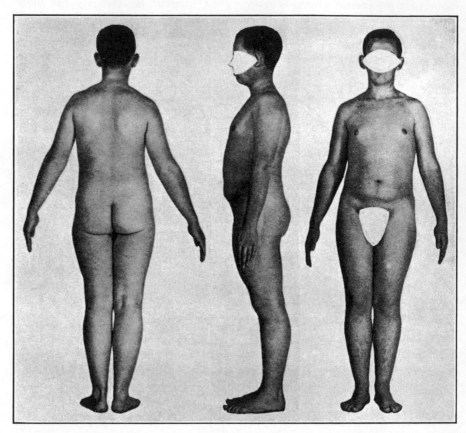

Description: Somatotype 6–3–1½. An 18-year-old endomorph two inches above average stature. Heavy mesomorphic as well as endomorphic reinforcement below the diaphragm, and there is a trace of mesomorphic dysplasia in the first region. He is a very large youth, weighing nearly 200 pounds. Primary $g+1$, secondary g, no trace. The facial expression is ward-boss hard. Primary t 3, secondary t 3. Features regular and even although too hard and too prominent for the somatotype. Mouth strikingly straight and firm for this degree of endomorphy. General strength 3, which is good for the somatotype. Hand strength 3. Coordination good. He moves with springy alacrity, like a fat panther or a thin bear. A good swimmer, but no other athletic ability. His fighting punch is a roundhouse slap.

Temperament: He is dependent on people, greedy for approval, easily communicative of feelings. Viscerotonia is predominant. Yet in many of his moods he is harshly critical and suspicious. He has a loud, strident voice. One member of the staff says "That boy always speaks in the accusative." Psychiatrists have for years referred to him as paranoid. At times he is somatorotic; loves to take long chances and is incessantly into things. Several times he ran away from correctional schools and led police on a merry chase. He is courageous, although because of the weak arms is unable to fight. There seems to be overloading in the second component, with manifestations which are sometimes Dionysian, sometimes paranoid. On one referral to a psychiatric clinic he was called *hypomanic, probably prepsychotic;* at another clinic, a few weeks later, the report was *paranoid tendency, not psychotic.* ψ 4–3–2.

Delinquency: Early truancy and long history of stealing, beginning at least as early as age 8. Five court appearances before 13 for breaking and entering. Three times sent to state correctional school between 13 and 16, always for stealing. Dishonorable discharge from CCC, same reason. Sent twice more to correctional school between 16 and 18, ran away each time. Several episodes of automophilia, although never formally charged with automobile stealing. Twice he wrecked "borrowed" automobiles.

Origins and Family: Second of five, urban family. The father was a short, husky Old American who never had a regular vocation but lived by odd jobs. He died of apoplexy at about 40 when the boy was 6. The mother, French-Irish and short, weighed 170 pounds and died of an undiagnosed malignancy in her thirties when the boy was 7. Before marriage she had a court history as a "wayward girl" and had an illegitimate child. She was one of a large family which may be described as medically delinquent. Of her eleven siblings, all but one died between 4 and 40. That one has long been institutionalized for delinquency. Many other near relatives are on agency support. After the death of the mother the boy was reared in foster homes under agency management. Of his four brothers and sisters two died in childhood. The other two, both congenital luetics, have police records and one has produced illegitimate children.

Mental History, Achievement: Finished two years of high school with passing grades. IQ reports fall between 85 and 96; here called 90. He gives a first impression of somewhat better mentality; talks rapidly and well, but it is soon noted that the flow of ideas is not cogently consecutive.

No vocational plans and no special gifts. The AMI that of a large dumpy youth, slow and overly serious, who is sociophilic and yet displeased with all environments.

Medical: Good example of what has been called the infectious diathesis (p. 255). He has had seven or eight serious infections of record, with septicemia and high temperature. At least three have required surgical intervention and two others resulted in hospitalization. Several hospital referrals for abscesses and the like. History of heavy chest colds, with question of pneumonia occasionally raised. PX reveals no significant pathology except badly formed extremities and rather high blood pressure.

Running Record: He gave an early impression of serious intent and was placed on the school program. He soon failed or lost interest in school and quit that program, but remained at the Inn for many months. His relations with the staff were at times good, at times poor. He was always paranoid and harsh in outlook, a chronic complainer or castigator, yet as a worker he was competent and comparatively reliable. When feeling especially well or high, perhaps with a bit of alcohol in his blood stream, he seemed to enjoy mild delusions of grandeur and for the moment would be faintly Dionysian. Then he "could not be bothered." But with him the uncomplicated Dionysian mood was rare and in the more common paranoid mood he was a good worker. He did well at what might be called orderly work, poorly at clerical and personnel work. We tried him on several outside job placements but the only work he really liked was that of hospital orderly.

He went from the Inn almost directly into military service, where for four years he made an adaptation and got along although with much hospitalization. From brief contacts that the staff had with him during this period, when he was on furlough, it was learned that the Army had shockingly poor officer material. After the war he tried civilian life for a time, found it distasteful and reenlisted. During the six months prior to the present writing he has been under hospital care for about half the time. There is no delinquency of record since our first contact with him.

Summary: Heavy mesomorphic endomorph with both Dionysian and paranoid tendencies. Mentality within normal limits; infectious syndrome. Early persistent delinquency. Short-lived stock.

ID 2–4–0 (6)
Insufficiencies:
  IQ ....

Mop 2
Psychiatric:
  1st order .... (?)
  2nd order 4
  (4–3–2)
  C-phobic ....
  G-phrenic ....
Residual D:
  Primary crim. ....

Comment: Outlook uncertain. A degree of first-order psychopathy may be present, although we have placed the guess in the other direction. There is no record of any behavior indicating disorientation, but the second-order psychopathy is sufficiently remarkable to raise the question of an ultimate need for institutional help. Also he comes from short-lived stock and is likely soon to run into serious medical difficulties. Through a decade of observation of more or less delinquent youths I have sometimes fancied that a relationship may exist between delinquency and the outlook for longevity. Youngsters *of physical vigor* who come from short-lived stock and have a poor outlook for longevity seem more often inclined toward juvenile delinquency than youngsters of greater life expectancy. But such a problem is too complex for any statistical approach with which I am acquainted. Too many factors enter into both sides of the equation, and it is too difficult to statistify a definition either of short-lived stock or of inclination to delinquency. Yet such a relationship may exist, and may have entered into the etiology of this youth's early delinquent fling.

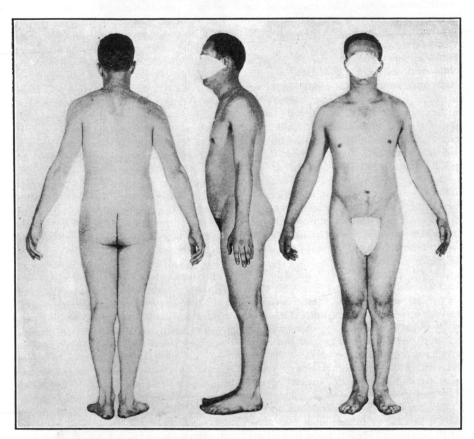

Description: Somatotype 5–4–2. A 20-year-old mesomorphic endomorph an inch above average stature. A heavy, solid physique which a little later may be much heavier. Asthenic or underdeveloped arms with distal segments short and budlike, not ectomorphic. Heavily muscled neck, trunk, and thighs. Primary $g+1$, secondary $g\pm$. Primary t 2—the body as a whole has a dumpy appearance. Secondary t 2—features coarse and badly molded. Hands and feet crudely weak. General strength 3, hand strength 2. Coordination rather poor. He moves in an elephantine, lumbering manner and has no athletic abilities except in the water. Good swimmer.

Temperament: He seems weakly viscerotonic, with intermittent lack or failure of expression of all primary components. He is slow and dependent on others for cues to action as well as for ideas. He is indiscriminately amiable, cries easily—sometimes without outward provocation. The emotional extraversion is perhaps the primary characteristic. The only evidence of manifest somatotonia we saw was a mulish stubbornness about work. He resisted the work program vigorously but that may have been only a reflection of the attitude then predominant in the environment. He is quiet to a fault, speaking in a nearly inaudible voice, but there is no indication of active or cerebrotonic restraint. No apparent strain, no hyperattentionality or sign of self-consciousness. The temperamental pattern seems to be that of underloading or falling away from the somatotype in the second and third component. Such a picture suggests what has been called *hebephrenic schizophrenia,* but this boy is not quite schizophrenic. ψ 2–2–3.

Delinquency: Early truancy or failure to arrive at school. A long series of minor episodes of stealing. He stole milk from back doors "because he was hungry." On other occasions he stole groceries for the same reason. At 16, larceny, breaking and entering, possession of burglary tools.

Origins and Family: Oldest of five, urban family. Father a large and obese Irish bartender. He has been irregularly employed, is said to be moderately alcoholic, and has been frequently hospitalized with various illnesses. He served one sentence for incest. Mother Irish and of average physique. As a girl, called "neurotic or neurasthenic." She left the father when this boy was 6. Her only sibling is institutionalized as feebleminded and she has repeatedly been under observation in local psychiatric clinics; question of *schizophrenia.* Boy

grew up in the home and the family as a whole show thirty-eight agency contacts within a period of twenty years. One of the siblings died of congenital lues.

Mental History, Achievement: Finished a year of high school after a long history of failure and low grades. IQ reports fall between 78 and 96, here called 85. He gives the impression of mental incompetence, has no positive ideas, seems literally weak-minded— rather than lacking in mind.

No vocational plans or special gifts. The AMI that of a soggy dumpling-like youth who for years has been coached by social agencies to tell a heart-warming Freudian story. He guesses he has fears and guilt feelings and he surely has a castration complex as big as a cow. But he tells the story without sure command of the language and without insight into the magic inherent within the various benedictions and maledictions he has learned to mumble.

Medical: Birth history and early development not known. No serious illnesses of record, but often referred to clinics for minor ailments. Called "unhealthy child" at 13. Always peculiar or "schizoid," but no good description of his early behavior is available. First referred to a psychiatric clinic at 12; no diagnosis. PX reveals no significant pathology except flat feet, sluggishness of deep reflexes, and general muscular flaccidity. He has the hebephrenic inability to innervate the extensor muscles —especially those of the arms.

Running Record: At the Inn he showed consistently a hebephrenic trend but because of his emotional extraversion and his fairly well oriented viscerotonia did not impress us as schizophrenic. "Rejected" by nearly all the other boys, he had a tendency to agglutinate with the very young and the very weak. He liked to play the games of little boys and to behave in general as a seven- or eight-year-old. He did poorly on the work program but in this seemed merely to follow his close associates. After he had been around a couple of months he attached himself as a sort of flunky or arms bearer to one of our toughest youths. The staff tried to break up this attachment; finally expelled the older boy because of it. However, the attachment continued even after both boys had left the House, and the two lived together for a time outside. Soon both were picked up on various counts of breaking and entering, larceny and robbery. The other boy complained bitterly and with reason that his apprehension was a result of the stupidity of his flunky. He philosophized that your best friends are "the ones ya hafta watch out fer."

For two more years our boy drifted in the community, living mainly by agency symbiosis, but there was no more delinquency of record. Finally he was inducted into military service where he stayed for another two years, did menial work and got along, although with much medical attention. After discharge he picked up where he had left off and has again drifted, with temporary jobs and handouts. There has been no more delinquency of record and he has shown no indication of "breaking over" into psychosis.

Summary: Flaccid endomorph with a hebephrenic suggestion in both the morphological and the temperamental picture. Mentality dull normal; health history only fair. Delinquency incidental to indiscriminate agglutination.

ID 2–4–0 (6)
Insufficiencies:
    IQ 1
    Mop 1
  Psychiatric:
    1st order .... (?)
    2nd order 4
      Hebephrenic, probably not
      schizophrenic (2–2–3)
    C-phobic ....
    G-phrenic ....
  Residual D:
    Primary crim. ....

Comment: Outlook in doubt. From the standpoint of psychiatric understanding this is one of the most important cases in the series. Psychiatrists generally use the adjective hebephrenic only in association with the noun schizophrenia. Yet hebephrenia, like schizophrenia, is a name for a continuum, not for an all-or-none occurrence, and these two continua are not coincident. There are many schizophrenes who are not hebephrenic, and there may be many hebephrenes who are not schizophrenic. Here seems to be one.

112.

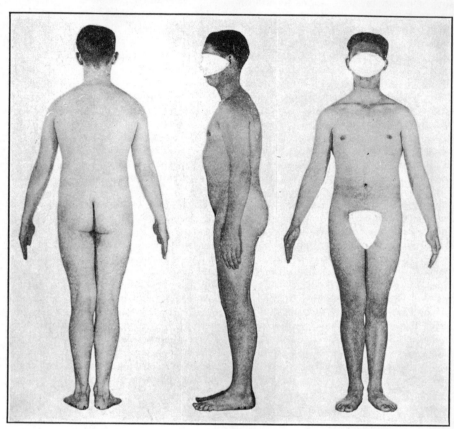

Description: Somatotype 5–4–2½. A 16-year-old endomorph an inch above average stature. Mesomorphic increment in the neck and chest. Arms flaccid, underdeveloped, weak. He cannot or will not extend the arms—a characteristic strongly suggestive of hebephrenia. Primary $g+1$, secondary $g\pm$. Primary t 2, secondary t 2. The body as a whole is dumpy and flaccid. Features seem carelessly made, doughy, and there is no "character" in the broad flabby face. Hands soft, atonic, poorly formed. Feet extraordinarily flat. General strength 2, hand strength 1. Coordination poor. He moves with a listless shuffle and is helpless at anything that involves effective use of the body.

Temperament: Epileptoid. For the most part he is relaxed, very like a tame bear; but at frequent intervals and usually without apparent provocation there is a violent eruption of rage. On these occasions the boy screams out hate and fury, rushes about, threatens to kill somebody; seems for the time being berserk. On close observation the episodes appear to be preceded by more or less circumscribed prodromal periods in which his behavior seems paranoid. For half a day before an outburst he is surly, suspicious, abrupt. Although his behavior appears to have shown this characteristic pattern all his life he has never yet injured anybody. No indications of cerebrotonia. Except when the tantrum is on he seems viscerotonic, greedy for approval, childish, and overpleased by attention. ψ 4–2–1.

Delinquency: School and psychiatric delinquency only. Much intermittent truancy, and between 12 and 16 there were especially violent outbursts of temper in school. Teachers were afraid of the boy and he in turn reported being afraid of teachers, dogs, the water, ghosts, death, and many other things. Several referrals to psychiatric clinics yielded such diagnoses as *psychoneurotic; psychopathic personality; prepsychotic.*

Origins and Family: Fourth of six, urban Negro family. The father was a competent although irritable and quick-tempered ("paranoid") full-blood Negro who did well for his family and died suddenly in his late forties, presumably of apoplexy. This was a year or two after our first contact with the boy. The mother, an enormously powerful Negress weighing well over 250 pounds, is a healthy example of the very black West Coast Negro stock which when maximally fed produces what are probably the heaviest human beings. Boy reared at home under good circumstances. The other siblings have all done well.

Mental History, Achievement: He had finished the seventh grade, was encountering difficulty in the eighth. IQ reports range from 65 to 90, here put at 80. The first impression is that of infantile mentality or of some sort of arrested development.

No vocational plan, no special abilities. The AMI that of extreme mesomorphy in awkward or bewildering circumstances. He appeals to us common mortals as the lion in the hunter's net appealed to the mouse.

Medical: Very large 12-pound baby. Slow development. Walked at 2½ years, talked at 2 years. Medical history negative except for violent tantrums beginning in infancy and continuing to the present. Congenitally defective vision. Always regarded as a strange or problem child. Never got along with other children. On psychiatric referral, called *schizoid* at 8, *psychopathic personality* at 12. He never liked any other children, seemed to have prolonged daydreams as a boy of 6 and older. Sometimes lethargic and unresponsive, at other times aggressively insistent with infantile questions, even to the present time.

Running Record: When closely supervised he did well on work programs. He found that he liked kitchen work and announced an ambition to be the greatest dishwasher in the world. This was serious—he did not mean it jokingly. At camp he disliked group activities, insisted on wandering around alone. There he had his tantrums regularly and at the height of one of these would chase certain boys in very much the way a muscle-bound bulldog chases the neighbor's tomcat. He would emit sounds of annihilative rage but never caught his victim or did any serious damage. In the end he was regarded by other boys with friendly amusement but also with a certain underlying respect—the sort of respect you have for a bear while laughing at him through the bars. While with us he always arose punctually at five in the morning; could never understand why others wouldn't do the same. We made no progress with him in the direction of vocational training but did persuade him to return to school and try to graduate.

Five years later we find that he graduated not only from grade school but also from high school. During the interim the pattern has remained almost the same. He is now a huge youth crowding 200 pounds, still aloof and childlike, still epileptoid, still considered psychopathic or prepsychotic. His appearance begins to suggest acromegaly. Through high school he received poor grades, repeated many courses. Now very sex conscious, he seems more paranoid, and it is said that the tantrums are less overt. His recently stated ambition is to "lead his race out of the wilderness." He has become religious.

Summary: Enormously powerful Negro mesomorph, not athletic. Mentality close to borderline; general health good. Psychopathy suggestive of the first order; childlike outlook; epileptoid. No identification with criminality. Feared, regarded as dangerous.

ID 1–5–0 (6)
  Insufficiencies:
    IQ 1
    Mop ....
  Psychiatric:
    1st order .... (?)

  2nd order 4
    Epileptoid—considered
    dangerous (4–2–1)
  C-phobic ....
  G-phrenic 1
  Residual D:
  Primary crim. ....

Comment: Outlook doubtful but it may be good. If not good, likely to be very bad. He seems to border on psychosis, has the physical power of two ordinary men, and appears to have no understanding that he is not still a child. No knowledge of his own strength, and loaded with energy. Subject to regular outbursts of fury. Although he has been hitherto harmless, there is probably danger of his "tasting blood" some day and if he does he may wallow in it. He presents a difficult problem from the standpoint of crime control. There is no ground on which he could be regarded as a criminal or detained as a psychotic, yet he is dangerous as dynamite. Such a case once more emphasizes the need for a bureau of human records which would be more than a list of crimes committed and of dates of births and marriages. If the idea of developing a social science ever should be taken seriously one of the major functions of such a science would be to keep records not only of what people do but also of what they are. Only through the use of such records could psychology ever become a realistic praxis, and until psychology *is* a realistic praxis all talk of social science is hogwash.

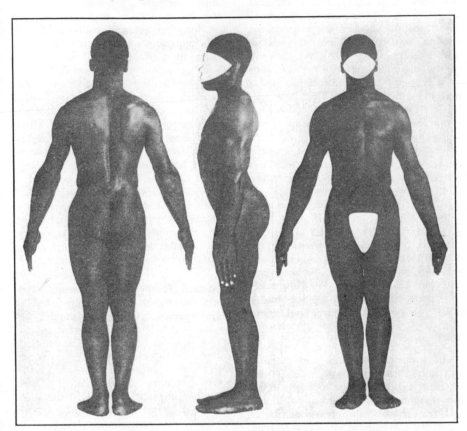

Description: Somatotype 3½–6½–1. A 16-year-old extremely meso-morphic Negro two inches above average stature. A tremendously power-ful physique with all segments heavily developed. Primary $g+1$ and this introduces what amounts to a dramatic disharmony or dysmorphy in the presence of extreme mesomorphy. Secondary $g\pm$. Primary t 3 despite the g. Secondary t 1 by any standards. Coarse, primitive features. Mouth 3½ inches wide, with lower lip protruding a full inch. One local clinic calls him "a throwback to aboriginal ancestors." General strength 5, hand strength 3—possibly the strongest boy in the series. Coordination like that of a bear. He gets around actively with a lumbering or ambling shuffle, and although school coaches have tried for years to make an athlete of him the only conventionalized game to which he seems to be adapted is wrestling. Repeated attempts to teach him to box have been fruitless.

Temperament: He is somatorotic without an adequate underlying somatotonia. He presses in the role of bad boy and tough fellow, but when challenged gives a poor account of himself even against smaller boys. One of our loudest youngsters. When he has an audience he struts and plays the role of the bold racketeer. When the audience is gone he tends to collapse and to become a divan draper. He is a wild boaster and a very excitable fellow, but the active phase is poorly sustained and when fatigued he falls back to a pattern of childish dependency. Then he cries easily and pours out his feeling like water. Both of his phases are extravertive; one of them somatotonic, one viscerotonic. Being tough, he always goes to bed nude; but being soft and a little gynandroid, he gets up after a while in the dark and puts on pajamas. In the dormitory that was a regular ceremony with him. A confused, somatorotic youth with just the trace of a cycloid tendency and poor fighting ability. He has a pinch of gynandrophrenia but leans over backward *away from* the *DAMP RAT* pattern. ψ 4–2–2.

Delinquency: Persistent early truancy and minor stealing, before 10. Between 10 and 15, identification with delinquent and mischievous groups, although as a fringer and follower, not as one of the active ingredients. He seems to have been always a little peripheral, and to have fallen short of nuclear requirements. Picked up twice at 15 for larceny, at 16 for assault and battery (with three other boys). Later he ran away with two of these same boys, was then involved in minor delinquency in another city and was sent back by social agencies. Regarded by police as "a good kid to watch," on the theory that he is agglutinative with more dangerous delinquents, and that his easily followed trail will lead to mischief.

Origins and Family: Youngest of four, urban family. Father Irish, heavy, and rather soft; long regarded as a borderline psychotic. In and out of mental hospitals a number of times, diagnosed *manic-depressive psychosis, depressed type*. Never able to maintain a home and long an agency problem. Mother Irish, muscular, stocky. Confined permanently in a state mental hospital at about 45, when this boy was 6. Diagnosis, *paranoia and paranoid conditions*. She is described by agencies as having been from childhood "a most difficult and uncertain person." At one clinic called *manic-depressive*. All five of her own siblings have been confined in mental hospitals. Of the three siblings of this boy, one is dead, one considered prepsychotic and confined as a delinquent, one hospitalized with tuberculosis and a parent of several children who are under agency management. Boy at home until age 6, then to foster homes under agency management.

Mental History, Achievement: Finished the eighth grade. Considered of about average brightness although a behavior problem and a persistent truant. IQ reports fall between 80 and 96, here called 90. His reactions or responses are quick but superficial. He knows how to recite his story rapidly with the best Freudian implications and in the most approved agency manner, but once this is done his mental muscles are exhausted.

No vocational plan. He plays several musical instruments and likes orchestras but has declined to undergo the discipline necessary to commercialize the talent. The AMI rests on his well-drilled story of parental difficulties, guilt feelings, fears, and so on. He sublimates his homosexuality by hating all of women teachers; can apply nearly all of the common Freudian clichés to his own history with the offhandedness of an earlier generation reciting the catechism.

Medical: Infancy history not known. No record of serious illnesses or injuries.

PX reveals no significant pathology beyond severe dental caries and flat feet.

Running Record: Through two years of intermittent association at the Inn he remained a sort of minor agitator and a haunter of delinquent fringes. He seemed to try hard to get in on major delinquency but never succeeded. When the real toughs went out on serious business they left him home, although his homage was welcome enough on off days. From our point of view he was like butter that is about ready to turn— a little rancid but not quite spoiled. His *persona* was that of exploiter and racketeer. On the work program life was a game at which to work was to lose a trick. On outside jobs he would regularly quit after the first payday. Late in his stay here, in a series of conferences with him, one of us got him interested in his physical constitution. He *seemed* to see a great light when it was pointed out why he could not fight, and why his prospects at big-league crime were poor. In this seemingly conversional mood he left for military service.

Three years later he was discharged from the service with a fair record. On returning to visit the Inn, he gave us viscerotic credit for conducting him to a great awakening. We reached for the salt. He then expressed high ambition of an academic nature and set forth directly on an educational program under the GI bill. However, after a few weeks of noninstitutional life he fell back into his old irresponsible pattern, quit school, and was again adrift. After a minor brush with authorities, he re-enlisted in military service where again he appears to be "all right."

Summary: A large, imperfectly developed mesomorph with poor coordination and gynandroid interference. Mentality within the normal range; good general health. Psychotic parentage on both sides. No clearly psychotic manifestations yet. The psychopathy seems to be of the second order—somatorotic and cycloid. A fringer in delinquency.

ID o–6–o (6)
  Insufficiencies:
    IQ ....
    Mop ....
  Psychiatric:
    1st order .... (?)
    2nd order 5
    (4–2–2)
    C-phobic ....
    G-phrenic 1
  Residual D:
    Primary crim. ....

Comment: Prognosis guarded, and the outcome is still far from settled. His history to date is very similar to that of his father, whom we have not seen but whose story sounds as if he might be a second- rather than a first-order psychopath. In the light of the paternal and maternal heredity it will be wise to wait at least another couple of decades before going to press with an enthusiastic prognosis. Both of the parents began to come to serious psychiatric attention after they had passed their thirtieth birthdays, although of course both had shown psychopathy long before. This is a good case for counselors and guidance people to meditate upon. With his enthusiastic, one-directional pattern of mentality this youth is easily "converted" to things. When we first knew him he talked Freudian theology with easy reverence. Later we converted him to a constitutional "religion." He might then have been heralded as a success for a particular brand of treatment. But a little reflection will reveal that he remains what he is, and that the task of describing or diagnosing him is still far from completed.

114.

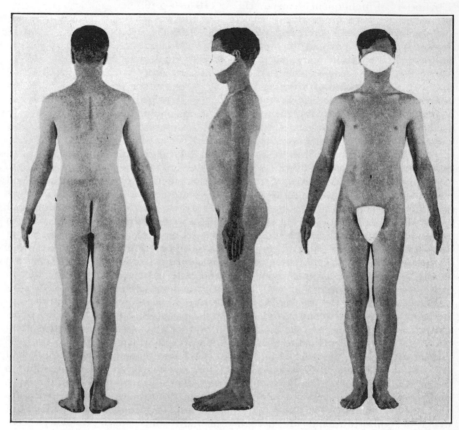

Description: Somatotype 3½–4½–3. A 17-year-old moderately mesomorphic youth three inches above average stature. Chest and arms show a
trace of the arrested or incomplete mesomorphic development so often
seen in this series. Head and neck, especially the latter, are decidely mesomorphic. Primary *g*+1, secondary *g*±. Primary *t* 3, secondary *t* 3. Individual
features of the face unusually well formed but imperfectly harmonized.
Hands and feet coarse; feet flat, poorly arched. General strength 3, hand
strength 3. Coordination imperfect. He is spry and gets about rapidly but
his movements are jerky and ineffectual. Barely fair at minor games. Poor
at fighting.

Temperament: He has a remarkable supply of energy. Seems tireless but not somatorotic. He is quiet, both in moving about and in speech. Walks as silently as a shadow, has overly fast reactions, is hyperattentional, agoraphobic, intent with a birdlike alertness. He is as watchful as a chipmunk of whatever is going on. All this is normal cerebrotonia for a well-energized extreme ectomorph. But his posture is usually somatotonic—upright and straight. He is up early in the morning, rarely seems fatigued, vigorously carries out his own idea of intrigue or circumvention; is aggressive in an indirect way. All this seems to constitute somatotonic dyscrasia. The boy is different from the first impression given by his ectomorphy. Temperamental pattern: Perhaps a nearly normal expression of cerebrotonia complicated by a dysplastic increment of the second component. ψ 1–2–1.

Delinquency. Excessive truancy and running away during the early school years. Persistent stealing in foster homes between 7 and 13. Larceny from stores, automobiles, and individuals between 10 and 13. Persistent identification with street gangs during this same period. Sent to state correctional schools nine times. Three charges of automobile stealing at 17 and 18. A remarkable record for such a somatotype.

Origins and Family: First of two, urban family. The father was a tall, elderly businessman of Old American extraction who advertised for a wife and died of cause unknown shortly after finding one. The mother is described as "a tall and gynandroid Irish girl with a history of some obscure mental disorder." She attempted to support this child, and also another that arrived extramaritally a couple of years later, from her slender income as a migrant waitress. After five years she was committed to a mental hospital: Diagnosis, *paranoia*. The children were turned over to foster homes under agency management. The second child was feebleminded.

Mental History, Achievement: Finished a year of high school with low grades. A long series of IQ reports range from 79 to 113, here called 95. He gives an impression of potentially better mentality than this. He is polite and courteous, but it is soon noted that he does not possess any enduring mental interests.

No vocational plans or special gifts. The AMI that of an alert, hatchet-faced youth who seems slender and delicate but bright.

Medical: Birth history and early development not known. No serious illnesses or injuries of record. PX reveals no significant pathology. Heart seems large to percussion and all externally observable blood vessels are large for the somatotype. He gives the impression of possessing a mesomorphic dysplasia in his cardiovascular system. This may account for, or may be associated with his apparent overendowment in energy for the somatotype.

Running Record: At the Inn he was quiet and inconspicuous. He succeeded in keeping out of sight most of the time; had a nearly uncanny ability to be absent or to be doing something else when scheduled for work. He was never involved in overt delinquency in the House and did not get into trouble while with us. He was an enigma to everybody. By some he was darkly suspected of all the stealing and underhanded trickery that went on during his stay—by others he was regarded as a promising and interesting youth. For a time he toyed with the school program which we offered, but the clouds of war were gathering fast and the idea of school was not able to hold his attention for long. One day he left abruptly, "headed West."

During the succeeding two years inquiries concerning him were received from half a dozen western states. He was apparently involved in numerous episodes of vagrancy and stealing. Finally he was inducted into military service. There he seems to have found himself and to have straightened out altogether. He stayed in until the end of the war, gained nearly 30 pounds, and was discharged with a good record, meanwhile accumulating a wife and family. After separation from the service he almost immediately settled down to a job which he has now held for two years. He *seems* to be a prosperous, happy, and forward-looking young man.

Summary: Ectomorphy with minor mesomorphic dysplasias and apparently a mesomorphic increment in the cardiovascular system. Seemingly overendowed with energy. Mentality about average; excellent health. Persistent juvenile and later delinquency which stopped abruptly with military service.

ID 0–1–0 (1)
  Insufficiencies:
    IQ . . . .
    Mop . . . .
  Psychiatric:
    1st order . . . .
    2nd order   1
    Somatorotic (1–2–1)
    C-phobic . . . .
    G-phrenic . . . .
  Residual D:
    Primary crim. . . . . (?)

Comment: Outlook apparently good. He is well regarded by the company for which he is now working, has an apartment home, and pays his bills. His excess energy now appears to be applied to his job instead of to delinquency. The change has been a dramatic one but I regret to have to report that he attributes it to the Army, not to the Inn. Perhaps it took the Army to convince him that he was an ectomorph. We tried hard enough.

This is a physique worth studying. At the time when the photograph was taken the boy weighed 120 pounds. Now, at 25, he weighs 150 and to superficial observation looks mesomorphic, although a *careful* look will reveal the somatotype readily enough. It cannot be too often pointed out that the human physique is a dynamic, not a static entity, and that the somatotype is a prediction, or a course through time along which the physique may be expected to travel (see p. 34). To predict the probable characteristics of the fully adult body from the immature body is not very difficult after you have observed and followed a few thousands, but dramatic changes occur. It is the same in botany. When once you have learned to predict the leaf from the bud, for a few score of trees and plants, it is easy enough, but to your mother-in-law they may still be "just leaves" or "just buds." Moreover, give her some religious or emotional reason for believing that one kind of leaf changes readily to another, under slightly varying circumstances, and she will perhaps believe it easily enough.

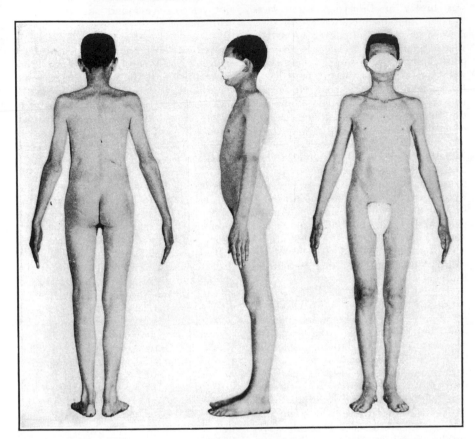

Description: Somatotype 2–2½–6½. An 18-year-old ectomorphic youth four inches above average stature. The arms, chest, and legs show extreme ectomorphy. In later life this trunk will broaden out and such a physique can take on goodly weight. Primary $g\pm$; secondary g, no trace. Primary t 3. All segments fully and rather harmoniously developed. Secondary t 4. Features clean-cut, well molded, a little too strong or prominent for the somatotype (local mesomorphic dysplasia). He is generally called good looking—with clothes. General strength 4 and remarkably high for the physique. Hand strength also 4. Coordination excellent. He moves with graceful economy of effort. With such arms he of course cannot fight, but he is good at tennis and at long- or middle-distance running; fairly good at baseball. For the physique, he is an outstanding athlete. This case defines a good contrast to the asthenic characteristic and well illustrates the ambiguity of Kretschmer's term *asthenic* when used in place of *ectomorphic*.

Temperament: When we first knew him he had grown six inches in two years and the outstanding characteristic was breezy or Dionysian carelessness. He was an offhanded waster—of time, money, property. Whatever he sat on was in grave danger. He was an energetic lounger, very sloppy and floppy, with a tendency to thrash about like a fish in the bottom of a boat. He seemed to have growing pains. Somatotonia was the dominant component and he was overendowed with energy. ψ 2–2–1.

Delinquency: His delinquency had consisted in a too-vigorous participation in warfare with the mother. The two were in the habit of indulging routinely in violent altercation. They had made extraordinary accusations against one another and the mother had three times had the boy arrested on "stubborn child" complaints. No other formal delinquency.

Origins and Family: Only child, rural family. The parents were married but a few months, separating before the boy was born. The father was a tall, lean New Englander who had been a motorman and later died in his mid-thirties of "some kind of malignancy." The mother, a large mesomorphic woman of Irish extraction, is described as "energetic, confused." Through early childhood the boy lived with his mother, who moved many times. When the boy was 7 his support was taken over largely by agencies and he spent the succeeding nine years intermittently with his mother and in foster homes.

Mental History, Achievement: Finished the eighth grade. No school failure and no history of truancy. IQ reports fall between 91 and 100, here called 95. He seems confused and bewildered, but there are evidences of a certain energetic competence and he has a wide diversity of interests.

No vocational plan except that he wants to be an aviator. No special gifts. The AMI that of a tall, awkward youth who is loaded with energy and seems not yet to have found out what to do with it.

Medical: Normal birth and early development. No serious illnesses or injuries. He was always big and throughout childhood was regarded as unusually awkward. Was unable to participate in games or to play happily with other boys. No gynandroid or "sissy" tendencies. PX reveals no significant pathology other than poorly formed feet.

Running Record: He came to the Inn after a series of skirmishes in force with the mother, and after a large amount of psychiatric consultation and agency manipulation. Previous sorties with the mother, dating back half a dozen years, had resulted in one of the agencies subsidizing the latter to a house so that she and the boy could live together happily. This had resulted in real warfare, in police interference, and in extensive psychiatric study of the youth; the latter had been called paranoid, although there had been no particular diagnosis. At the Inn the boy was somatorotic, but in his Dionysian destructiveness he appeared to be having a good time. This was the first time that he had been to any extent on his own. After a month we tried to return him to school. That didn't work. He would have none of it. On the work program he was just a puppy who seemed to pretend not to understand. We got no work out of him at all. He appeared to need "breaking." After another two months we concurred in a recommendation that he be sent to one of the state correctional schools.

He was sent to the correctional school and there, after the first few weeks, he did well and made a good record. Within a few months after leaving the school he was inducted into military service where he did very well, emerging from the war with a good record and with 30 pounds of added weight. He has since settled down to a job, seems to be a normal citizen. Now, eight years after our first contact with him, he weighs 180 pounds, has the general atmosphere of a relaxed big man. He likes to drink and celebrate "of an occasion—but nothing out of bounds."

Summary: Tall, awkward mesomorph who was a late developer. Dionysian temperament and history of warfare with the mother. Mentality about average; excellent health. No real delinquency. Normal citizen, with a Dionysian trend.

ID 0–1–0 (1)
  Insufficiencies:
    IQ . . . .
    Mop . . . .
  Psychiatric:
    1st order . . . .
    2nd order 1
      Dionysian (2–2–1)
    C-phobic . . . .
    G-phrenic . . . .
  Residual D:
    Primary crim. . . . .

Comment: Outlook apparently good. He has become a towering, imposing figure although he will never be an athlete and any fighting that he may do will be an affair of slapping, not hitting. He is still no doubt subject to somatorotic confusion, but the somatorosis now sleeps beneath a softer endomorphic blanket and is no longer the predominant trait in his behavior. Much of the confusion was very likely a result of his late development, or of the late development of his full mesomorphic power. When he began the warfare with the mother he was in fact overmatched, as children usually are. The situation did not—and generally does not—become absurd until the child had unknowingly drifted across the bar between childhood and maturity. We accomplished nothing for this youth and if anything was "done for" him, it was the correctional school and the Army that did it. The case illustrates one fairly good generalization in constitutional psychology. Dionysian carelessness or flamboyancy in children is usually a sign of future physical vigor and bigness. The youngster seems to feel the rising tide of energy and in a sense is cashing his future. Perhaps this applies particularly to children reared under poor discipline.

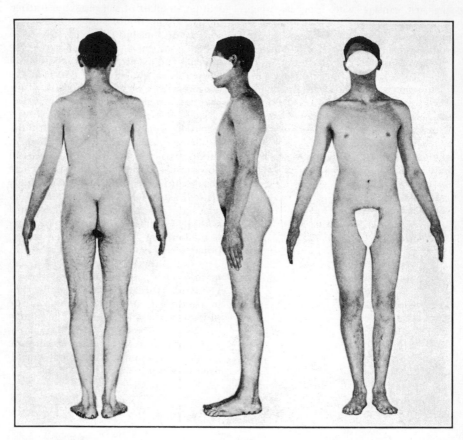

Description: Somatotype 3–4½–4. A 17-year-old slightly mesomorphic youth five inches above average stature, with a fairly strong endowment of both the other primary components. He is comparatively ectomorphic in the arms and legs, more mesomorphic in the trunk and neck. All segments well developed—no asthenic characteristics. Waist high but no other sign of *g*. Primary *g*±; secondary *g*, no trace. Primary *t* 3, secondary *t* 3. Features well formed and bold but a little on the coarse or heavy side. Hands strong and well formed. Feet flat. General strength 3, hand strength 3. Coordination rather poor. He moves awkwardly, seems to be all hands and feet, dislikes the gymnasium. When he hits he slaps. This is a slow or late developing physique and in the photograph he is not fully mature. Later he will be much heavier, and possibly less awkward.

Temperament: Tremendous push and energy, with frequent emotional outbursts and spasms of excited truculence. However, the latter rarely progress beyond vocal somatorosis. He strives vigorously but deviously to dominate and control his environment. He is aggressive, shrewd and mentally active, always has irons in the fire and plots brewing; loves to manipulate people. He has no stomach—or other equipment—for personal combat but is overriding and psychologically callous. He is noisy and coarse, yet warmly sociophilic. The world is an oyster for him to consume. He has good relaxation, easy extraversion of feeling, and a wide-open channel of emotional flow. There is the usual Jewish "paranoid" alertness of the eyes and the quick head movements. The voice is loud and strident. ψ 3–2–1.

Delinquency: A few episodes of minor stealing before age 14, although no court sentence. Never considered particularly delinquent. At 19 he got into trouble with federal authorities for tampering with his draft card, and for "employment of a ruse for evading the draft." About this time he went on what he later called a delinquency binge, turning up at several psychiatric clinics, getting himself diagnosed *psychoneurotic, psychopathic personality,* and the like. He later explained that all this had been part of a program to avoid the draft.

Origins and Family: First of two, urban family. Both parents Assyrian-Jewish. Father a muscular man of average physique described as having been nervous and excitable but never delinquent. He died in his forties of cardiorenal complications when the boy was 15. Mother a short, muscular woman of great energy and high blood pressure, described as alert and ambitious. Both parents came to this country in their teens and on the whole did well here. They "used the agencies" but progressed and made money. Boy reared with the family although at times hazardously.

Mental History, Achievement: Finished three years of high school with good standing. IQ reports range from 103 to 121, here called 115. He gives the impression of possessing first-rate practical intelligence; seems to know how to get what he wants and his relations with people are good in that he sizes them up well and proceeds accordingly. This boy is nobody's fool.

Vocational plan: To go to college and get into some profession. He is straightforwardly and realistically ambitious. The AMI that of an obviously intelligent, aggressive, demanding youth.

Medical: Normal birth and early development. Always a vigorous child although he never got along smoothly with other children. Long list of minor medical complaints with many hospital referrals; no serious illnesses. Psychiatric referrals as mentioned. PX reveals no significant pathology except weak, flat feet and moderate impairment of vision.

Running Record: At the Inn he was a canny opportunist but a refreshing one because he was going somewhere. He was disliked by the boys and rather respected by the staff. He never took the work program seriously, indeed would not work at all unless a staff member stood over him and directed his movements. He always had too many things to do and too much big business going on to be bothered by menialities. He would undertake unusual or special assignments and would either leave them at loose ends or would find a way of cajoling some weaker boy to do the work. There was an odd sadistic element in his make-up. He was a wrist twister, a finger bender, and a biter, apparently deriving a kind of ecstatic pleasure from inflicting pain on weaker boys. We three times treated small boys for such injuries. He once explained that during such episodes he had the feeling of "doing valiant battle with the universe." Despite these minor matters we were able to place him on a school program and he finished high school with good standing.

Through further scholarships and with the help of other agencies he went on to college and has since done well, although with minor interruptions for defense jobs and the like. Exempted from military service on psychiatric or medical grounds, he made progress steadily through the war years, now seems to be in a good position and gives promise of going ahead successfully with a professional training.

Summary: Chunky, massive youth with a vigorous body but with comparatively weak extremities. Mentality college average; good health. Ambitious and successfully so. Some minor incidental delinquency.

ID 0–1–0 (1)
Insufficiencies:
  IQ ....
  Mop ....
Psychiatric:
  1st order ....
  2nd order 1
    C-penic. Feebly inhibited
    (3–2–1)
  C-phobic ....
  G-phrenic ....
Residual D:
  Primary crim. ....

Comment: Outlook good. He has the situation in hand; probably has always had it in hand. He is no idealist but a practical man of affairs and his concern is with results, not methods. The "delinquency" was merely a bit of practical business that went wrong, although in the end it worked all right anyway. His lack of inhibition, or lack of scruple, is not necessarily pathological. From his point of view it is his best asset and is the thing that will make him rich and successful.

117. COMPANY B, PLATOON 1, SECTION 2
Second-Order Psychopathy; with Minor Somatoroses: Nos. 115–132

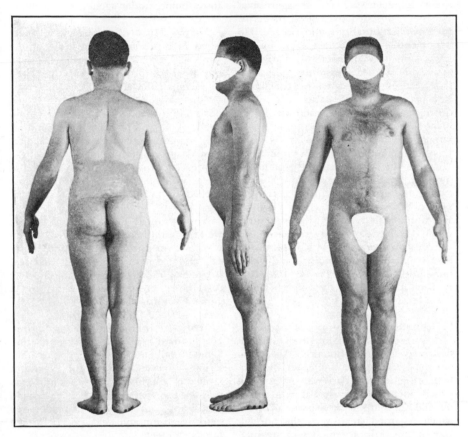

Description: Somatotype 5–4½–1½. A 19-year-old mesomorphic endomorph of average stature. All segments heavily and about equally developed except the distal segments of the legs, which in this stock are usually asthenic or underdeveloped. Both a heavily endormorphic and a strongly mesomorphic physique. Primary $g+1$, secondary $g\pm$. Primary t 3, secondary t 2. Features coarsely prominent, crude. Hands and feet weak. General strength 3, hand strength 2. He shows the pattern of central massing of strength with comparatively weak extremities, but is not an extreme example of it. Coordination rather good in that he moves efficiently. Too gynandroid for athletics or for fighting. Good swimmer. If he were to fight, he would slap.

Temperament: Somatotonia predominates overwhelmingly, although with his weakness in the hands and feet the common pugnacious expression of somatotonia is not seen. An easy extraversion, especially of affect, is the predominant characteristic. He is aggressive, persistent, obsessed by a need or desire to dominate situations and people. He is outwardly lazy like a bear but his energy is in fact tremendous. Fatiguing activity is needed constantly, although this need is complicated by the weakness of the extremities and by a consequent lack of athletic interests. There is no indication of cerebrotonic interference of any kind. The voice is as relaxed and full as that of a violincello. He lacks the usual steady eye of mesomorphy, has instead a tic-like habit of casting the eyes about during a conversation. He is a schemer and a planner. His thinking is radical, ruthless, courageous. He has the bodily relaxation of the great cats together with viscerotonic love of comfort, sociophilia, and good orientation to people. He has frequently been called a "paranoid schemer." ψ 2–2–1.

Delinquency: History of stealing, but no record of truancy and none of destructiveness or violence. Always a vigorously aggressive youngster, he ran with a delinquent juvenile gang, was closely identified with what was going on and grew up with a point of view which regarded stealing as the normal way of life. Minor episodes of stealing between 15 and 20 but none of much magnitude or importance. At 20 he expanded too far and was involved in a carefully planned but too extensive swindle which went awry. He was apprehended by federal agents and was given a long sentence which was later suspended.

Origins and Family: Born extramaritally, urban setting, father unknown. The mother was a young immigrant from Poland who is said also to be part Austrian. She is described as "a sturdy, healthy-appearing girl who was easily imposed on by men." Later she married and raised a family, with agency contacts; but this boy was reared mainly in foster homes under agency management.

Mental History, Achievement: Finished high school. At the time of the Inn's first contact with him he had been out of school for several years, had lived in various cities, and had made his way by the judicious use of his wits. IQ reports fall consistently in the neighborhood of 115. The first impression of him would about support this indication. As acquaintanceship progresses the impression grows that he possesses also a certain toughness of mental fabric backed by persistence and physical energy.

No vocational plan, although before we knew him he had manifested an omnivorous curiosity, had a radical political and economic ideology, and expressed opinions on many subjects. The AMI based on alertness, energy, and a general ambitiousness.

Medical: Infancy history not known. Hospitalized briefly at 20 with an undiagnosed pulmonary disorder. No other serious illnesses. History of persistent "somatic" complaints of pain and weakness in the extremities. PX reveals no significant pathology except moderately defective vision and weak, poorly formed hands and feet.

Running Record: He revealed intelligence and industry in his early associations at the Inn, and was soon placed on the school program, at first for high school postgraduate work in order to gain credits for college entrance; later on a college program. Throughout his stay he was a lusty schemer and an ambitious politician around whom deep currents and eddies swirled. He had the energy and the desire to keep a finger in everything. In time he seemed to become convinced that there are better and safer rackets than stealing, and then he turned his energy prodigiously to school. The transition seemed to take place abruptly from a fairly successful delinquent pattern to an equally successful academic pattern—perhaps that wasn't much of a transition after all.

In the course of several years he graduated from a local college and at the outbreak of war was inducted into military service. There he got along, but after two years developed an incapacitating medical disorder and was given a medical discharge. Immediately he resumed academic ambitions and, taking advantage of the GI bill, started graduate work. Two years later the report is that he is "getting along fine."

Summary: An endomorphic mesomorph with asthenic extremities. Fair general health and above average mentality. Great energy with a somatorotic lust to dominate. Early close identification with delinquency. Later development of mental interests and academic ambition—he found a better game.

ID 1–1–0 (2)
Insufficiencies:
    IQ ....
    Mop 1
Psychiatric:
    1st order ....
    2nd order 1
    Lust for power (2–2–1)
    C-phobic ....
    G-phrenic ....
Residual D:
    Primary crim. ....

Comment: Outlook probably good. Certainly there is no fatal insufficiency or crippling psychopathy. His lust to dominate people and situations seems at one time to have supplied the incentive for criminal activity and scheming. The same motive appears now to be at work within a legitimate or noncriminal field of activity. He still wants to be a big shot and if short cuts can be found perhaps he will take them. But that is not criminality. From the present perspective this looks like one of the rare cases where a youth who was quite heavily involved in delinquency has been able to take advantage of an opportunity to transfer to a better and safer interest. The wonder would seem to be not that he should have done it but that so many do not. He of course may not yet have had time to show his true colors. Some of those who know him point out that he has not yet done anything to prove that he isn't the same opportunist as of old. They point out that he may still be at heart a milker of agencies and a watcher for the main chance; that he went through college on funds and a living provided by the Inn, and is now pursuing further work on funds and a living provided by the government; that as yet he may have been merely following the path of least resistance, doing the easiest and pleasantest thing at no cost or sacrifice on his part. This may be the correct view of the case and he may in the end turn out to be merely a *better educated* opportunist than the average run. Even at that, he might in some fields be a better than average professor, and whatever else may be said of him he never can be called a bore.

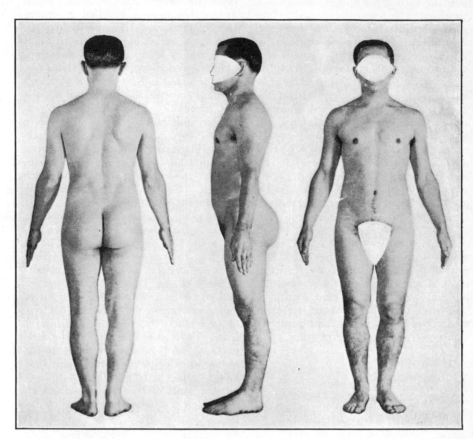

Description: Somatotype 4–5½–1½. A 21-year-old chunky mesomorph, four inches under average stature. Trunk heavily and fully developed, approaching extreme mesomorphy. The distal segments of both extremities— arms and legs—show asthenic characteristics or underdevelopment with weak musculature, and these segments are short. Head massive but irregularly shaped. Hands and feet strikingly small and weak for the degree of mesomorphy of the body as a whole. Except that he is not known to be a Jew, this is a fine example of a common Jewish physique. Primary and secondary g±, or just a trace. Primary t 3, secondary t 3. Features strongly developed and the texture of the body as a whole, except in the extremities, is fine. General strength 4, hand strength 1. Coordination good in the sense that he moves smoothly, with feline grace. He detests athletics and of course cannot fight, but is a good swimmer.

Temperament: Predominantly somatotonic and of enormously high energy. He is lusty, direct, courageous. He loves risk and action, is generous, sociophilic; at his best in a crowd where there is plenty of noise and confusion. This is the complete extravert in both the viscerotonic and the somatotonic sense. There is no trace of cerebrotonic restraint. He defines a good antithesis to the schizoid temperament and also he is free from any suggestion of a cycloid tendency. He is sustainedly Dionysian. His physical constitution seems fully up to carrying the load which the extreme somatotonia puts on it. If there is pathology in this temperament it is pathological cerebropenia. ψ 3–1–1.

Delinquency: Persistent early truancy and history of minor stealing between 6 and 15. Frequent bouts of drunken brawling between 15 and 17, with charges of disorderly conduct. At 18 and 19, sexual aggression accompanied by boisterous brawling resulting in police action. Called irresponsible in the handling of money and the paying of debts. Considered by police a potential major delinquent but never such in fact.

Origins and Family: Second of four, both parents immigrant Poles. Father called violent, irresponsible, and alcoholic. He was a very muscular man who deserted the family when this boy was 2 and later died at about 40 of apoplexy. Mother powerfully built and called "violent, abusive." She died of hypertension and complications in her forties when the boy was about 15. The home was intermittently under police supervision and our boy was transferred to foster homes under agency management at 12. Of the three other siblings one is feebleminded, one a major delinquent, and one has got along normally.

Mental History, Achievement: Finished the eighth grade after many difficulties of a disciplinary nature. IQ reports fall uniformly between 90 and 100, here put at 95.

No vocational plan and no special gifts except that of mesomorphy. The AMI based on joviality, buoyancy, and high health. He has a richly ribald personality which carries a fraternal appeal wherever a drop of well-oxygenated blood may flow. His presence was especially welcome to us, working as we were with so many weaklings. With his sustained Dionysian irresponsibility he had a mesomorphy which fully supported the role, and this rendered him in a psychological sense honest.

Medical: No early data. Since age 3, at least, always of vigorous good health. Moderately defective vision. PX reveals no other significant pathology. This is a hearty, healthy physical constitution with slightly high blood pressure. To age 40 or 45 the prognosis is good. Beyond that it grows rapidly doubtful.

Running Record: A rollicking extraversional influence in the House through a period of nearly two years, he put a strain on the staff at times but on the whole his behavior could be called good. He was never maliciously destructive, could usually be depended on to keep his word, and during the latter part of his stay established himself as a sort of champion of the downtrodden and a punisher of bullies. He took a most active part in athletics, was responsible for much of the success of various teams during the time of his stay. The main problem with him was alcohol. Never quite a drunkard, he loved to have a few beers under his belt and these tended to elevate the extraversional somatotonia to nearly volcanic proportions. He was hard on our gynandrophrenes and *DAMP RATs*, rode herd on them very much as the old family dog does on the neighbors' cats. He was occasionally in trouble with police for ribald rough-housing but after several abortive attempts he made good on a trade school program and then seemed to settle down somewhat.

Rejected for military service because of imperfect vision—they took some of our asthenic weaklings who could scarcely see at all—he has kept out of trouble during the half dozen years since leaving the Inn, has held a job with one firm for four years now, and is looked upon by police and other authorities as a successfully "reformed" youth. He is heavier, even more relaxed, now says he requires three quarts of beer a day and is worried about the rising cost—of beer.

Summary: Extreme mesomorphy with excellent general health and good athletic ability. Mentality about average. Perhaps a trace of pathological cerebropenia. Mild alcoholism. Early incidental delinquency of a Dionysian nature.

ID 0–2–0 (2)
Insufficiencies:
    IQ ....
    Mop ....
Psychiatric:
    1st order ....
    2nd order 1
    C-penia. Dionysian (3–1–1)

C-phobic 1
G-phrenic ....
Residual D:
    Primary crim. ....

Comment: The outlook must be called good. He has kept out of trouble and has been self-supporting since his days at the Inn. He seems to grow a little more alcoholic but he also grows fatter, and as a generalization somatorosis tends to recede with the advance of the endomorphic tide. Extreme mesomorphy usually presents a good prognosis or a very bad one. This youth appears to have about passed the danger of the latter alternative. He is well liked and except for his chronic complaint on the rapid advance of old age appears to enjoy life richly. Most people *want* to like and to be liked by extreme mesomorphs. There are few of us who do not know subconsciously that it is a good thing to have friends among them, rationalize the attitude as we may. We are usually inclined to express overt friendliness for Belgian police dogs and mastiffs too, when in territory patrolled by the latter. It would be the same with lions if lions were to roam about among us on anything like equal terms.

COMPANY B, PLATOON 1, SECTION 2
Second-Order Psychopathy; with Minor Somatoroses:
Nos. 115–132

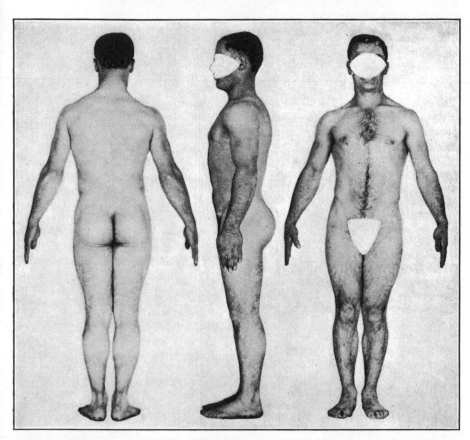

Description: Somatotype 3–7–1. A 19-year-old extreme mesomorph an inch under average stature. No dramatic dyplasia. Legs less muscular than the rest of the physique but everywhere above the hips he is a 7 in mesomorphy. Primary $g\pm$—there is a distinct trace of g below the waist. It is enough to block the boy from professional athletics or successful pugilism but not enough to be called $+1$ on the scale we are using here. Secondary g, no trace. Primary t 4, secondary t 2. Rather a magnificent mesomorphic body but the facial features are heavy, coarse, and stubby. Polish peasant physique. General strength 5, hand strength 3—one of our strongest boys. Coordination excellent. He moves as a compact unit and with feline efficiency. An effective fighter and very hard to stop although he does not quite have the legs for professional pugilism.

Temperament: The pattern is that of breezy, overbearing somatotonia. He seems overloaded with energy and always in a hurry, as if responsible for matters of the utmost importance. His bearing is that of a topflight politician. There is an urbane brusqueness about him along with a faint suggestion of big business. A confident, well-poised youth of easy social grace when pleased, and of sneering or overbearing superiority when displeased. There are no manifest signs of cerebrotonia. Temperamental pattern: Highly energized somatotonia well buffered with viscerotonic relaxation. The temperament seems nearly normal to the somatotype, although there is a Dionysian flavor and a faintly manic suggestion. ψ 2–1–1.

Delinquency: Extensive truancy during the first few years of school. Early vandalism, destructiveness, and rowdyism. Between 10 and 15 he ran with a wild gang and competed with the leaders at all sorts of minor delinquency, such as petty stealing and general trouble-making. At 15 he was a flamboyant breaker of rules, defier of authorities, and outwardly a tough boy. He drank a little and advertised it a lot. Also he let it be known that he had the "highest connections" among the aristocracy of big-city gangdom. He associated with really tough characters, was involved in many minor scrapes; was never caught at any major delinquency. This was the picture at age 18, when we first knew him.

Origins and Family: Second of three, respectable suburban family. The father was a large, handsome young Irishman who married "above his level." After marriage he never altogether settled down, was more or less alcoholic, got involved in minor delinquency. As a boy he had been "wild, unstable, a frequent runaway." He finally deserted the family. The mother, described as an accomplished although impetuous woman

of good Old American family, raised her children without outside help. Only the present boy became involved in any delinquent episodes.

Mental History, Achievement: Finished grade school and entered high school but soon dropped out after a history of maladjustment and low grades. IQ reports cluster at 100 with only slight variation. He gives a first impression of better mentality than that, but the impression fades with further acquaintanceship. He is sophisticated, overbearing, mentally superficial.

No vocational plans or special abilities. He was never athletic and this has been a source of great perplexity to teachers and family advisers. The problem of gynandromorphy does not yet seem to be popularly understood in child development and vocational guidance centers. Much pressure was brought on the boy, during his developmental years, to participate in athletic and physical education programs. It may have been against this pressure that he particularly rebelled. At any rate he carried for years a violent hatred for things athletic. The AMI that of a big, exuberant, excellently proportioned youth with a ready smile and a breezy air.

Medical: Normal birth and early development. Walked and talked at about 12 months. No serious illnesses or injuries. PX reveals no significant pathology. An excellently nourished, healthy body, but one which may become enormous in middle age.

Running Record: For a time at the Inn this boy found life an excellent joke. He overrode other boys and staff alike, was alcoholic, and regaled the neighbors with roistering pranks. He sloughed off work programs, laughed at jobs, was an altogether untamed fellow. He was sexually somatorotic, entangled himself in a number of local alley intrigues, was two or three times badly beaten by combative mesomorphs who were hunting in the same jungle. After a series of mainly unsatisfactory conferences some progress seemed to be achieved in leading this boy to understand both his overendowment in "blood and energy," and the gynandroid reason for his essential inadequacy at combat. One morning, following a severe beating by a much smaller mesomorph who appears elsewhere in this series, the youth seemed particularly full of insight.

Shortly after the episode mentioned he left the Inn and within a few months entered the Merchant Marine. There he soon gained 40 or 50 pounds and seemed to calm down to a remarkable degree. There has been no more delinquency of record. During the succeeding five years he has married, now looks prosperous, and weighs, we would estimate, about an eighth of a ton.

Summary: Endomorphic mesomorph with high health and with a somatorotic plethora of energy. Enough gynandromorphy to incapacitate him for fighting and to present him with a problem. Normal mentality. Early hobby of delinquency.

ID 0–2–0 (2)
  Insufficiencies:
    IQ ....
    Mop ....
  Psychiatric:
    1st order ....

    2nd order 1
      Dionysian (2–1–1)
    C-phobic ....
    G-phrenic 1
  Residual D:
    Primary crim. ....

Comment: Outlook presumably good, so far as criminality is concerned. He will never read cuneiform and probably will not make a scientific advance, but neither is he a criminal. He might be regarded simply as an overenergized youth who liked sowing wild oats so well that he put in a multiple crop. Also he could be presented as an instance of successful "guidance," although it is a good idea to be skeptical of all instances of successful guidance. The weight of the impingement of one personality among the thousands to which a growing youth gets exposed is not often likely to be such as to change the course of a life radically.

From the standpoint of diagnosis and psychological understanding, this is a case of great interest. We often make the statement, in the privacy of the Constitution Laboratory, that all medical or psychological interviews should be preceded by standardized photography of the subject. This boy presents a case in point. Without such a photograph it would have been impossible to detect objectively what was really going on.

120.

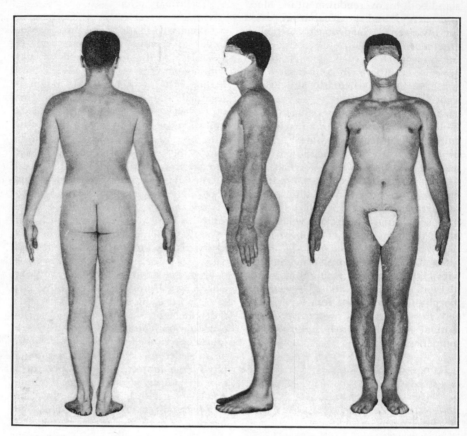

Description: Somatotype 4½–5–2½. An 18-year-old endomorphic meso-morph, four inches above average stature. A large, well-developed youth with wide chest, broad shoulders, and good harmonious development in all segments of the body. High, gynandroid waist, moderately gynandroid hips, and a generalized softness throughout the body. Broad, healthy looking face with high color and a plethoric flush. Primary $g+1$, secondary $g\pm$. Primary t 4, despite the gynandroid interference. Secondary t 3. Features strongly developed but heavy and a little coarse. General strength 3, hand strength 3. Coordination good in a feminoid sense. He moves smoothly and gracefully but is not good at fighting and not good at any of the standardized group games.

Temperament: Well-sustained and well-relaxed somatotonia, although somatorotically belligerent under alcohol. When not alcoholized he is a well-adapted extreme mesomorph with no somatorotic straining in the role. He walks about with the confidence and poise of the king of beasts in his native jungle. Interests all center in muscular expression or in athletic activity. At need he can summon tremendous energy and endurance. He ran the athletic contests at the Inn and captained the teams with poise and success. Superficial observers of personality might not rate him as aggressive or pugnacious, since he rarely has to *parade* his pugnacity in order to establish his place at the top of the "peck order." He is poised, is usually seen smiling; but in the only biologically meaningful sense of the term he is of the highest aggressiveness, as the lion is—at need. Note: On the first face of things, the barking mongrel may seem more aggressive than the lion, but in psychology we have to penetrate beyond that level of observation. This is why rating scales, and for that matter psychological observations on personality in general, *unless made by people trained to think through to the operative pattern of the underlying structure itself,* are inclined to be worthless. Constitutional psychology is really no more than *persistent* operational analysis. ψ 2–1–1.

Delinquency: Early truancy and stubborn behavior in school. Called incorrigible and unmanageable by one teacher, at 8. Minor stealing and running with a street gang, between 10 and 15. Later, considered to be "the brains" of a highly delinquent gang and known to be associated with boys caught at serious mischief; but he himself was never caught at anything serious, and except for five or six episodes of drunkenness and brawling there are no charges against him after 16. His real delinquency, in the literal sense, has been

sexual. Eschewing contraception and unhampered by inhibitions, he has freely exercised his great power over girls, producing "trouble" in a number of quarters. This has been his principal expression of the first psychiatric component.

Origins and Family: Second of two, urban family. Father Irish and Old American, considered a fairly competent man but somewhat unreliable and improvident. Mother Irish-Old American, of stout athletic physique and high blood pressure, called quarrelsome and unstable; also called "hypomanic." The family has had many contacts with agencies and has been called exploitative. Boy reared in the home. The sibling has a court record for major delinquency.

Mental History, Achievement: Finished a year of high school with unsatisfactory grades. IQ reports fall uniformly between 90 and 100, here called 95. He seems mentally dull, but it is hard to gauge the mentality of extreme mesomorphs. They don't have to show their hands, or what they know.

No vocational plan although he has "talked about" physical education as a profession, with hearty encouragement. The AMI that of the composed security of a muscular aristocrat. Social workers love to *touch* him, as we like to touch a really healthy looking tomcat.

Medical: Large baby. Walked and talked at 12 months. No serious illnesses or injuries. He has always been robust to an extreme degree. PX reveals no significant pathology although blood pressure is 150/80—high for a youth under 20 even though an extreme mesomorph. He is of the *apoplectic habitus* and will be old indeed at 50. He is a splendid risk for today, but would be a poor life insurance risk after 45.

Running Record: At the Inn he was an outstanding personality and was probably on the whole a good influence. He "took hold of" the athletic program and the gymnasium almost on arrival, and for more than a year dominated that phase of life. He came to be regarded by younger boys as a symbol of uprightness and virility; had boxing classes, coached teams, played the role of leader in physical education work. He blossomed in such a role and during his stay not only avoided participation in active delinquency but seemed to break off his associations with it. However, he had periodic bouts with alcohol and when partially drunk was an ugly customer. When alcoholized he tended to forget, or to remember—which way it is put matters little —just how strong he was. Several of the *semi*-extreme mesomorphs took up his challenge at these times, but were no match for his speed and hitting power. Two of them got sufficiently "educated" to require hospital attention. When it finally was settled beyond every doubt that he was the champion and the boss, his belligerence under alcohol ceased to result in casualties; he was then king and unofficial redresser of wrongs. His unrestrained sexual aggression caused the House more embarrassment than his drinking or his fighting. But we grew philosophical about such matters. If you want the advantages of having a champion around you must be ready to tolerate some of the disadvantages. Moreover, even though he was a little overly inclined toward bastardy he seemed to transmit a fairly good physical stock.

We tried to get him to carry through on a school program which would lead him to college on the physical education racket. Several colleges were decidedly interested in him. Three times he started to attend high school with this in mind, but there were too many distractions. Finally he was inducted into military service and there he made a fine record, coming back from the war a hero with decorations—earned and deserved ones too. For another two years now he has drifted. He seems relaxed, healthy, free from any disturbing ambition. He likes life as he finds it and guesses he won't work any more. He is more alcoholic than when he lived with us.

Summary: Extreme mesomorphy with superb strength and fighting power. Good health; about average mentality. Moderate alcoholism and a degree of irresponsibility which may approach criminality.

ID 0–2–1 (3)
  Insufficiencies:
    IQ ....
    Mop ....
  Psychiatric:
    1st order ....
    2nd order 1
      C-penia (2–1–1)
    C-phobic 1
    G-phrenic ....
  Residual D:
    Primary crim. 1

Comment: Outlook good, although the president of the W.T.C.U. might not think so. In a sense he is one of the aristocrats of the earth. Fearless, strong, and manly in the most basic or primitive sense, he has perhaps as good a birthright to recognition and honor as has the youth with outstandingly high IQ. In war he proved his mettle as naturally and routinely as on athletic fields. Here was no parasite in time of need; no weakling living off the military institution. This boy is a man. Delinquent by some criteria, he carries a superior physical and in some sense a superior temperamental endowment. It is a kind of endowment which cannot be ignored in any realistic view of the future. There are many who believe that superior mental qualities are incompatible with this kind of physical superiority. They may be right, but how are we to find out? There is no way to prove or disprove it except by accurately describing and following a few thousand people. This is a job which statistical machines cannot be trained to do for us. Too many variables are involved.

COMPANY B, PLATOON 1, SECTION 2
Second-Order Psychopathy; with Minor Somatoroses:
Nos. 115–132

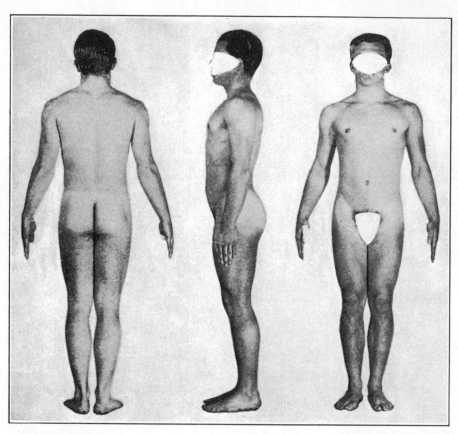

Description: Somatotype 2½–7–1. A 17-year-old extreme mesomorph an inch above average stature. Superb development along almost perfect athletic lines, except for a slight increment of endomorphy in the thighs. From an athletic point of view, the best physique in the series although in this photograph he is a little overweight and "out of condition." No important dysplasias or weaknesses. Primary and secondary $g\pm$. Primary t 5, secondary t 3. Features well developed and symmetrical, but coarse and a little pudgy. Thick lips; broad, short nose; pimply complexion. General strength 5, hand strength 4. Coordination superb and suggestive of the great cats. A star football player and all-round athlete. A fighter of some renown both in and out of the ring (middleweight).

Temperament: Similar to that of a puppy. He is full of energy, playful, a great manifestor of affection; always good natured, ready for a frolic. He is hypersuggestible and is a follower rather than a leader. Easily influenced, he reflects the predominant attitudes of the immediate environment with acumen and vigor. He is gluttonous, a heavy eater. No indication of temperamental conflict. This is a somatotonic temperament, well buffered or blended with viscerotonia and perhaps a little pathologically free from cerebrotonia (cerebropenic). ψ 2–1–1.

Delinquency: Frequent early truancy. Three or four episodes of running away from foster homes at 15 and 16. At 16, identified temporarily with a gang which carried out extensive robberies. Arrested during that year for breaking and entering. No history of violence or destructiveness. Never a tough, but a sort of worshiper of the legendary Robin Hood character. Said to follow about after notoriously tough boys as a poodle dog might follow his master.

Origins and Family: Only child, village family. Father Old American and a powerfully built man who died of heart disease in his fifties when this boy was 15. He was improvident but in no social sense delinquent. Mother Scotch-Irish, short and muscular. She has been epileptic all her life and is described as tempestuous. Committed to a mental hospital when the boy was 14. Diagnosis: *epilepsy and paranoid condition.* Boy reared in the home until 14, thereafter in foster homes.

Mental History, Achievement: Left school in the seventh grade after the father's death. Mediocre record but always regarded by teachers as potentially better than the achievement indicated. IQ reports vary between 85 and 96, here called 90. Mental testers have commented that attention and concentration are poor.

His vocational plan is to "stay in the country." No special abilities. AMI that of a cherubic-looking youth with a round face and high color, a generous viscerotonic mouth, and wide-awake alertness. The whole personality is lively, jaunty, viscerotonically somatotonic. He is of the sort who when very young attract universal favorable attention.

Medical: Infancy history not known. No record of injury or of illness of any kind. PX reveals no significant pathology. Blood pressure moderately elevated.

Running Record: At the Inn he proved for the most part pleasantly tractable despite his tendency to attach himself like a romantic shadow to one or more of the actively delinquent youths. He would follow his mentor fervidly until the association was noticed by a staff member, but could then be whistled off rather easily. This youth is easily influenced and he is like putty under the predominating influence in his immediate environment. He seems to have a strong craving for identification with some tangible, visible cause, and his goal in life seems always that of pleasing some in-the-flesh master. During his period of association at the Inn he seemed gradually to transfer his loyalties from the comparatively more delinquent to the comparatively less delinquent personalities (staff). At camp, where close supervision was possible, he did excellently. On a farm where we were able to place him he did so well that the farmer indicated a desire to keep him permanently on the place. In general, when well supervised, he did good work. When unsupervised he tended to be lazy, shiftless, and to follow along into the nearest trouble.

On leaving the Inn he went to a farm and there he seemed to take to the soil. He pleased his employer and kept out of trouble. When inducted into military service he apparently continued in a pattern of good adaptation, stayed in until the end of the war. He got a job almost immediately following his discharge and during the intervening year has got along satisfactorily. He has gained about 40 pounds since our first contact with him, now is a very stocky and tolerably prosperous young man. He seems competent to earn a living and to keep out of trouble.

Summary: Chunky endomorphic mesomorph of good health and normal subaverage mentality. Easily influenced or hypersuggestible. Delinquency incidental to the latter characteristic.

ID 0–2–0 (2)
Insufficiencies:
IQ ....
Mop ....
Psychiatric:
1st order ....
2nd order 2
    C-penia (2–1–1)
C-phobic ....
G-phrenic ....
Residual D:
Primary crim. ....

Comment: Outlook presumably good. Free from any overt signs of delinquency for more than five years, and self-supportive during the whole of this period. Good military record. This is a good example of the sort of case sometimes charged up to "pure environmental delinquency." It is almost certain that in a good environment and under influences wholly good the boy would not have been delinquent. But such a statement is not very meaningful. Human behavior results from interaction between a responsive organism and a stimulating environment. If delinquent or unsatisfactory behavior is noted, the problem is to study and if possible work on both factors. If the breakdown of automobiles had always been attributed wholly to the roughness of the road there would not have been much improvement in automobiles, and under such circumstances I am not sure that roads would have reached their present state either. The problem is to attend to both sides of the picture. In the present case the boy is probably almost average. From the point of view of what average boys are he was but slightly and ephemerally delinquent. From the standpoint of what *first-rate* boys are he is about a 1918 Maxwell with a weak steering gear.

122.

COMPANY B, PLATOON 1, SECTION 2
Second-Order Psychopathy; with Minor Somatoroses:
Nos. 115–132

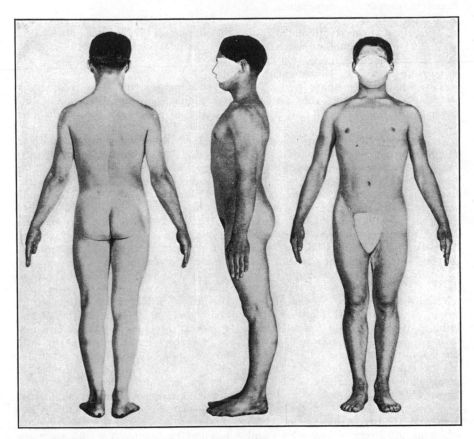

Description: Somatotype $3\frac{1}{2}$–$5\frac{1}{2}$–$1\frac{1}{2}$. A 17-year-old endomorphic meso-morph two inches below average stature. He is sturdy, well knit, will later be heavy. An excellent PPJ (see VHP, p. 199). To the untrained eye he now looks slender. At 30 he will be barrel-bodied and tubby. No dysplasias although the distal segments of the arms and legs are not quite as well developed as the rest of the physique. Primary and secondary $g\pm$. Primary t 3, secondary t 2. Features well developed but heavy and coarse; flaccid viscerotonic mouth. Large basketball-like head. Plethoric, ruddy color. General strength 4, hand strength 3. Coordination excellent. He moves with smooth grace but is too soft and too untempered (see p. 27) for fighting or for athletic competition.

Temperament: Somatotonia seems to predominate. He is restless, craves adventure and excitement. He is noisy and overbearing. Yet rich viscerotonia is also manifest. He is amiable, well oriented to people, an easy talker with good extraversion of affect. There are also signs of hyperattentionality and at times of cerebrotonic interference and self-conscious confusion. He seems to show an overloaded temperament, or to have what has sometimes been called the 4-4-4 problem at the temperamental level. ψ 2-1-1.

Delinquency: None, until suddenly at 17. No truancy and no court record. For two years before our contact with him he had been watched by police and had been known to be closely associated with a delinquent gang. One of the gang had recently committed a murder and this boy was questioned. Regarded by police as a youth who had been playing with delinquent fire but had probably not yet been seriously burned.

Origins and Family: Second of two, urban family of good standing. The father is Welsh-Irish and is a tall heavy man of good health history. He has been a successful artisan. The mother, of the same racial stock, has kept a good home and the family has had no agency contacts. Boy reared at home.

Mental History, Achievement: Finished the third year of high school and did fairly well, although failing in some subjects. He quit school as a senior after stormy disagreement both with school authorities and with his father over the question of participating in the physical education program, to which he objected. IQ reports fall between 95 and 104, here called 100. He is breezy, superficially alert, but does not seem to possess mental stamina.

No vocational plan and no special abilities. The AMI that of a tall, good-looking youth who, it seems to everybody, ought to be doing very well but isn't.

Medical: Normal birth and early development. No serious illnesses or injuries. PX reveals no significant pathology.

Running Record: It was soon evident both from this boy's behavior and from conferences with him that his disturbing problem was primarily sexual. He had had a late adolescence and sexuality had hit him like a tidal wave about two years later than is the case with the average boy. For some time he had been in the midst of what might be called a sexual somatorosis.[1] He had sought counsel with his father and others on the sexual problem, and pressure had been directed upon him to sublimate by means of athletics and "manly" physical activities of various kinds. This really did put him in a predicament. He is by nature as incompetent at conventional athletic games as the Queen of Bulgaria would be. Moreover he had the misfortune to attend a high school which boasted a successful and progressive director of physical education who did not know about gynandromorphy. The father had concurred in the view that the boy ought to be "urged strongly" toward physical proficiency. For two years the latter had been on the sexual prowl to an extent rarely understood or appreciated by people not familiar with this pattern of physical and temperamental endowment. It was the sex pursuit that had taken him into delinquent associations and the harvest (sexual experience) had been to his liking. He had been exploring sexuality as a four-year-old explores a Christmas tree.

---

[1] It should perhaps be noted that moderately gynandroid youths of high secondary *t* often show this characteristic of late adolescence and are often heavily endowed with sexual drive.

His response to a little insight into his own physical nature was good. His further response to the proposition that a temporarily excessive sexuality *might* be dissociated from delinquent identifications was also good. His response to our effort to get him to return to school was not good. However, he did raise his sights with respect to the quality of his sexual associations, abandoned his flirtation with delinquency, and returned to the good graces of his family. He is not, probably, the best moral influence imaginable for young girls; but he is now "respectable." He went into a defense industry, was thereby exempted from military service, seems to have got along very well during the intervening half-dozen years. He is now much heavier, and fairly complacent about life.

Summary: A very tall overenergized youth with moderate *g* and poor coordination. Average mentality; excellent health. Postadolescent flirtation with delinquency as a reverberation of sexual somatorosis.

ID 0–2–0 (2)
Insufficiencies:
  IQ ....
  Mop ....
Psychiatric:
  1st order ....

2nd order 2
Overloading, Hypersexuality
  (2–1–1)
  C-phobic ....
  G-phrenic ....
Residual D:
  Primary crim. ....

Comment: Outlook probably good so far as delinquency goes. He is now growing heavier and lazier, less dangerous in the poultry yard. In another decade he will probably be innocuous and may teach a Sunday School class. His story should be taken to heart by those whose lives or interests impinge in any way on the educational racket. It should never be forgotten that what is meat for one may be poison for another. If athletic and physical training programs, for example, are of value and importance to one kind of youth—as they doubtless are—it follows almost *ipse facto* that for other kinds of youths they may be harmful. The same is true of movements or emphases aimed at the development of any particular kind of ability. To insist that youths not gifted in music must learn to play the oboe would be a revolting idea. But it would be no harder on the youths than is the custom of exposing discoordinated gynandroid 4-4-4's to calisthenics and athletics.

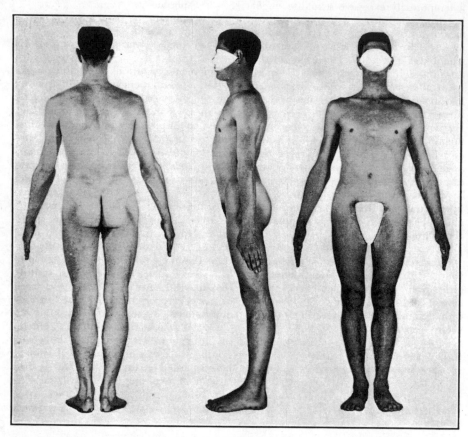

Description: Somatotype 4–4½–3½. A youth, age 19, of nearly midrange somatotype, seven inches above average stature. All segments of the body well developed, and no particular dysplasia. Trunk a little short for the long limbs. Moderately high waist. Primary $g\pm$—just a trace; secondary $g+1$. Long eyelashes, fine hair, features slightly feminoid, silky finish of the skin, gynandroid form of pubic hair. Primary t 3, secondary t 4. Features even, excellently molded, and sharply chiseled. He is a trifle too close to feminine beauty for conventional masculine standards. Hands and feet well structured. General strength 2, hand strength 3. Poor coordination. He handles himself awkwardly, is unhappy and out of place in the gymnasium, throws poorly, and adapts badly to games. He is gun-shy of boxing gloves. An endocrinologist friend of mine calls him "a case of subclinical hyperpituitary discoordination."

Temperament: The outstanding characteristic is cerebropenia. He seems to have no projicient impulse—no foresight and no inhibition. He is cocky, strutting, something of a bully; often starts fights or arguments which he cannot finish. After a half-dozen blows are struck he seems to become weak in the knees. He is in general somatotonic, but seems to believe himself tougher and sturdier than he actually is. The *persona* is that of major delinquency. He associates mainly with pool-hall toughs or near toughs, loves to stir up rows at dances and at similar gatherings. He reveals a good deal of underlying viscerotonia, becomes easily sentimental, is agglutinative and is well oriented to people. He loves crowds, celebrations, excitement. Perhaps the temperamental pattern is normal to that part of him which lies above the diaphragm, but taken as a whole, the boy has not yet learned how tough he isn't. ψ 2-1-1.

Delinquency: Early history of truancy and of destructive recalcitrancy in foster homes. Between 8 and 12, minor stealing, occasional running away, persistent mendacity. Between 12 and 18, in court difficulty five or six times for minor stealing and larceny, once for breaking and entering. One charge of breaking and entering at 20. This is not major delinquency but perhaps could be called "intermediate delinquency."

Origins and Family: A foundling in a large eastern city. Father unknown. The third illegitimate child of an Irish girl who, after producing one more, died a few years later in a state institution of "an unnamed infectious disease." This girl came from a family with a long delinquent and social agency record. Boy reared in a series of foster homes under agency management.

Mental History, Achievement: Finished two years of high school, quit during the third year after a series of disciplinary maladjustments and low grades. IQ reports range from 100 to 111, here called 105. The school history is interspersed with comments that the boy seems bright and ought to do better, that he is in some respects gifted, and the like. His personality was pleasing to many of his teachers.

No vocational plan. He has been a fair athlete and most of his ambition or fantasy seems to have been associated with the exciting fulfillments of high-grade mesomorphy. The AMI is based on a sort of natural straightforwardness. He is well composed, never seems to be embarrassed, and there is a manly, sturdy quality in his face. He has the mesomorphic trait of the steady, clear-eyed stare. Once described by one of my colleagues as "the most successful professional liar in the house."

Medical: Medical history essentially negative, except for enuresis persistent to age 14 and intermittent at least to age 20. PX reveals no significant pathology other than moderately carious teeth.

Running Record: His history at the Inn was on the whole unsatisfactory although we liked him and were usually glad to see him around. He never seemed to learn anything or to profit from experience. The concept of responsibility of any kind was apparently foreign to his mentality. He was good-naturedly careless on the work program, although when well supervised he did excellently. A number of outside jobs were started but he usually quit within a few days. He was easily influenced, followed after the more dominating delinquent personalities like a half-grown puppy. He seemed to be putty in the hands of a leader of any kind, but once turned in a new direction he never could maintain momentum under his own power. What he seemed basically to lack was cerebrotonia. On one occasion a good contact was made with him at a clinical interview and in the course of an hour he seemed to grasp the strengths and weaknesses of his physical constitution with almost conversional enthusiasm. However, a week later he started a fight at a dance hall in his regular old-time fashion.

We finally got him to complete a vocational course in one of the manual arts, and shortly afterward he was inducted into the service. After five years the story is this: He had a good time in the service and came out at the end of the war with a fairly good record. Then for six months he seemed to have no idea of what to do with himself and drifted. Finally he got a job, has now stuck to it for nearly a year. In some way the military experience appears to have done him good and to have raised his sights a little.

Summary: Chunky   mesomorph softer and weaker below the diaphragm than above it. Enuretic history and cerebropenic temperament. Normal mentality. Early delinquency and persistent irresponsibility.

ID 1–2–0 (3)
  Insufficiencies:
    IQ ....

Mop 1
Psychiatric:
  1st order ....
  2nd order 2
    C-penia. (2–1–1)
  C-phobic ....
  G-phrenic ....
Residual D:
  Primary crim. ....

Comment: The outlook has improved with maturation and it is probable that the military institution merits a good share of the credit. From the point of view of criminality, the boy may be cured. From the Promethean point of view, which is concerned with the better development of human potentialities, the outcome of the case is not much better than if the boy had become an alcoholic or a full-fledged criminal. His youth is gone and with it his chance for educational development. He has steadfastly refused to return to high school, has settled back to what will be at best a low level of conscious existence. At 26 he is far past his mental prime and was probably a better informed person at 16 than at any later period in his life. This makes Prometheus wince.

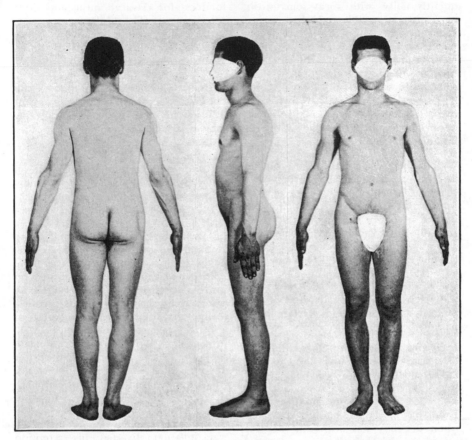

Description: Somatotype 3–5½–2. A chunky 20-year-old mesomorph of average stature. The face and neck and shoulders suggest extreme mesomorphy. Below the diaphragm, however, he changes over to a softer and more moderate mesomorph with comparatively weak legs. He possibly illustrates the hard-on-the-outside but softer-on-the-inside picture of which the psychoanalyst Franz Alexander has written. Primary $g\pm$; secondary g, no trace. Primary t 3; secondary t 3. Features evenly and strongly formed, a little too blocky or bunchy for the somatotype. Hands and feet of crude architecture. General strength 3, hand strength 3. Coordination good. He moves smoothly, is only fair at athletics, and is unable to fight successfully because of the relatively weak legs.

Temperament: *DAMP RAT* pattern, or arty-perverse and theatrical. He has inexhaustible energy, with somatotonia predominant. Willfulness seems to provide him with his *persona*. Frequently noisy, with vocal somatorosis, he is often in trouble and when crossed is inclined to go over into a sort of hysterical rage which may be accompanied by a deafening screech. He will slap smaller boys but that is the extent of his combativeness. One psychiatric clinic labels him psychoneurotic, with hysterical trends. He is affected, arty, has a superior air. Frequently accused, probably falsely, of homosexuality. ψ 2–2–2.

Delinquency: Truancy and willful or stubborn behavior during the early years of school. When corrected he would "screech like a wild Indian." No individual record of stealing, but at 15 and 16 involved with a gang which was responsible for extensive looting and for a number of burglaries. This boy was adjudged the most promising as well as one of the least guilty of the gang, and was referred to the Inn. History of epithetical and hairpulling warfare with parents between 13 and 16.

Origins and Family: Only child of a brief marriage, although both parents have numerous children by other marriages. There was an involved question as to just which of the mother's husbands was the father. Parents separated when this boy was born and he was reared by relatives, later joining the supposed father and stepmother, at 12. He promptly "rejected" these parents, and his real delinquency dates from the time when he joined them, against his will. "They are coarse, ordinary Negroes," he says.

Mental History, Achievement: Completed one year of high school with adequate grades, then refused to return to school. IQ reports fall within a narrow range at about 110. He is mentally alert, verbally superior, poor at mathematics.

Considered bright by teachers and called a gifted student of art and music, he "hates math."

No vocational plan except that of being "a cultivated person." Passionate fondness for classical music and great interest in art. The AMI that of a wide-eyed, polite, rather effeminate Negro boy who seems to have had an unusually bad case of family trouble.

Medical: Early medical history not known. No record of serious illnesses or injuries. PX reveals no significant pathology. Eyes protuberant but no other indication of hyperthyroidism.

Running Record: He did well on the work program and at camp was considered one of the half-dozen most satisfactory among a group of 60. Apparently grateful to escape a bad family situation, he was loyal to the staff at the Inn and remained well behaved and dependable throughout his stay there. He needed a certain amount of protection for he was offensive to some of our Irish mesomorphs because of his artiness ("airs," they called it); and because of a racial "aggressive defensiveness." He demanded a degree of democratic leaning over backwards, particularly at dances and at similar social functions. At dances he would cut in on the prettiest girls a little too often. A school program was planned for him, but the high pay for common labor during the war inflation diverted his attention from such childish matters. He got a job, kept it until he was inducted into military service, satisfied many of his cravings for fine clothes, jewelry, music records, and other items of cultural importance to him. After two years in the service he submitted an unfavorable report on the way things were run, but the service was at least neutral concerning *him* and his record could be called fair. Only recently released, he is now considering the question of returning to school, has not decided yet.

Summary: Midrange Negro physique of high secondary *t*. Good intelligence, good health. Moderate degree of hysterical somatorosis with some gynandrophrenic interference. A borderline *DAMP RAT*. Delinquency probably incidental or transitory.

ID 0–3–0 (3)
  Insufficiencies:
    IQ ....
    Mop ....
  Psychiatric:
    1st order ....
    2nd order 2
      Somatorotic (2–2–2)
    C-phobic ....
    G-phrenic 1
    DAMP RAT
  Residual D:
    Primary crim. ....

Comment: Outlook probably good. He has the IQ, the health, and perhaps he now has the motivation for at least a high school education. There has been no indication of active delinquency since our first contact with him, and there is little doubt that the familial or environmental situation played a major role in the "causation" of what delinquency there was. Yet this was not "pure" environmental delinquency, for a fairly conspicuous degree of second-order psychopathy is present. He is a hysterical psychopath, although of mild degree, and superimposed upon the hysterical trend is enough gynandrophrenia to render him uneasy in almost any environment. Insufficiently *DAMP RAT* for homosexuality, I think, he falls somewhere between that fraternity and the House of Masculinity. With a good education and a mellow outlook, such a position is tenable enough—or for that matter any other position; but until he attains these advantages he cannot be considered quite out of the woods.

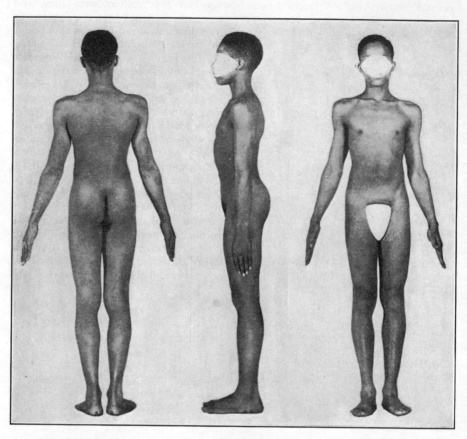

Description: Somatotype 4–4–4. A 16-year-old Negro youth of midrange somatotype and an inch above average stature. Immature physique. Mesomorphy perhaps slightly predominant. Ectomorphic (Nilotic) dysplasia in distal segments of arms and legs. Short trunk. A physique which will be heavy and soft in later life. Primary $g+1$, secondary $g+2$. Primary t 3, secondary t 4. Features feminoid and delicate for the stock, finely molded and regular. Hands, feet, skin, and teeth all show excellent texture. From a Negro point of view, he has aristocratic blood. Eyes remarkably large and luminous. He is what is sometimes called a Jamaica brown, in contrast with the heavily mesomorphic African West Coast black (see No. 113). General strength 2, hand strength 2. Coordination good in the graceful or gracile sense. Good dancer. Mincing, effeminate walk. Good at games in a minor way—plays softball well. Unable to fight.

Temperament: The pattern is that of well-sustained, seemingly inexhaustible somatotonia. He is primarily a young man of energy and of physical expression. Steadily aggressive but so successful and well poised in aggression that to casual observation he does not seem aggressive at all. He is direct, loves risk, is a natural leader, and never seems to strain in his somatotonic role. He is not pugnacious for he is rarely challenged. No indication of conflict or of poor integration between the second and third components. Temperamentally, as well as physically, he seems poised and well coordinated. Yet he has a "paranoid" obsession that society is "wrong"; that he must fight society; that to work would be immoral. From the standpoint of adaptation as a rollicking youth, this is undeniably a happy temperament; yet there is an undercurrent of both Dionysian and paranoid somatotonia which in the long run is maladaptive. ψ 2–2–1.

Delinquency: A persistent wanderer between 7 and 10. A frequent truant from school although well liked by teachers. He left home at 14, became a juvenile hobo, and wandered all over the country. Between 15 and 21, often in trouble with police for vagrancy and for minor stealing. At 19 he staged a country holdup with a rusty shotgun which later was found not to have been in working order for 50 years. He became a kind of beloved vagabond or irresponsible youth who found it possible to get along without working and considered life a game the object of which is to continue to get along without working. At 21 he boasted that he had never yet done a day's work for pay, and that rather than stoop so low he would rob a bank or even get married.

Origins and Family: Oldest of three, from a rural southern mountain country. Father a lean mountaineer who always enjoyed good health but was a ne'er-do-well. He deserted the family when the boy was 4. Mother, also of native stock, married at 14 and has enjoyed excellent health. She raised her family on a semi-migratory shack-renting pattern of life. Her husband is said to have been also her uncle.

Mental History, Achievement: Finished two years of high school with a poor scholastic record. He was quite an athlete in high school and was called a good baseball pitcher. Two IQ reports, 110 and 122, here called 115. He gives the impression of being mentally alert. He has humor and conversational poise; speaks with a modest reserve and on general, nonacademic subjects is informed well beyond his age. He is far from openminded about middle class "slavery" and American politics; says that if he had "the guts and brains" he would be a communist and would "clean out that sewer in Washington." After a long conference with him the writer felt some doubt as to whether or not to join up and march on Washington.

No vocational plan. He proposes to continue to be a vagabond. The AMI that of a tall, handsome, broad-shouldered youth with superb poise, a quiet southern drawl, and a shrewd knowledge of the weaknesses or soft points of social workers.

Medical: Early medical history not known. No known illnesses or injuries. Never sick a day in his life, he says, "except once, when the old sow bit a piece out of my leg. Next day the sow had a high fever." PX reveals no significant pathology. He even has excellent teeth and good foot structure.

Running Record: He spent a winter at the Inn, seemed to have a good time, aroused numerous female hopes, and played a merry game with social agencies. He was a great leg-puller of social workers; loved to get them excited about rehabilitating or saving him, but in the end he was usually satisfied with a very small advance. He was a gentle, not a ruthless grafter. For our part we registered him in two educational programs, got him a contract in professional athletics (with a small advance for signing), and interested a couple of businessmen in the project of "making a man of him." In the end he made a monkey of them. He was only kidding, just having a good time. We once or twice suspected that he might be a graduate student in sociology somewhere, out gathering material for a thesis. Apparently he was not.

He left for a CCC camp in a distant state but it developed that all he wanted of the CCC was transportation, for within a few days he moved on. Within a year the war broke out and he was inducted into military service. There he remained for a few months, deserted, was captured and sentenced to a term in the brig. During the period of desertion, however, he had enlisted on his side the good offices of a religious organization of conscientious objectors. They soon got him an honorable discharge as a conscientious objector. He disappeared for a few months, then enlisted again in another branch of the service, where he saw action at the front, reported that he was having a great time, and shortly thereafter was heroically killed.

Summary: Tall ectomorphic mesomorph of high *t*. Excellent health; college level mentality. Problem of wanderlust and restless vagrancy.

ID 0–2–1 (3)
Insufficiencies:
IQ ....
Mop ....
Psychiatric:
1st order ....
2nd order   2
*Restless wanderlust
(2–2–1)*
C-phobic ....
G-phrenic ....
Residual D:
Primary crim.   1
Irresponsibility

Comment: This story ought to have had a happy ending. Perhaps it did. If not, the margin of failure is possibly the difference between real life and romance.

When the boy left we regretted his going, for we felt in some poignant way inferior to him, and in his final departure from us we knew that the cause we represented had sustained an undeniable setback. He had looked at what we had to offer, had not even bothered to express scorn. To him we were the unfortunate and, I believe, the delinquent ones. We the stuffy weaklings caught in the sticky flypaper of everyday human moronity. This boy's internal life, and to some extent his external life, was that of a hero. In three parts of his make-up he walked the earth as a god who gazed serenely upon a swarming and inferior species, and made his notes. In the rest of his make-up he was perhaps a somatorotic delinquent, if that means anything.

126.

COMPANY B, PLATOON 1, SECTION 2
Second-Order Psychopathy; with Minor Somatoroses: Nos. 115–132

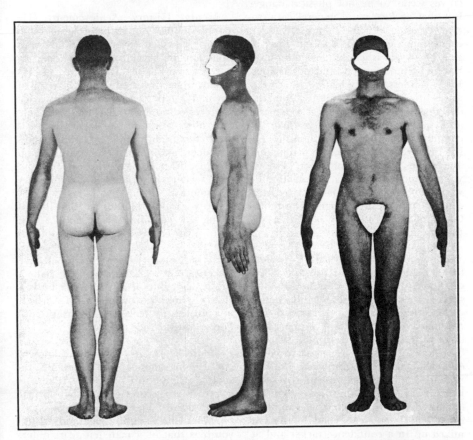

Description: Somatotype 2½–4½–4. A 21-year-old ectomorphic meso-morph five inches above average stature. He is heavier in bone than in muscle but all segments are about evenly developed. Primary $g+1$, second-ary $g\pm$. Primary t 3, secondary t 4. Features strong, well modeled, sharply chiseled. It is decidedly a handsome face. Hands and feet excellently formed. General strength 4, hand strength 4. Coordination that of an athlete, al-though he is too light and too gynandroid for first-rate athletic competition. A fairly good boxer but in no real sense a fighter.

Temperament: The predominant characteristic appears to be a somatotonic or somatorotic craving for the thrill of risk. He is devoted to various kinds of gambling, as a romantic lover to his mistress. His first love is that of danger, but it appears to be a kind of sublimated love. What he particularly craves seems to be not physical danger but that of *loss,* or of general catastrophe, together with the chance of sudden unearned gain. Which is to say, the passion of his life is gambling. Under alcohol he becomes violent and pugnacious. He is ruthless, overly mature in appearance, psychologically callous. But underlying these traits there is a remarkable physical relaxation, a love of comfort, gluttony, and sociophilia. He has intelligent orientation to people and an easy extraversion of affect. This is viscerotonic somatotonia, or somatotonic viscerotonia—as the somatotype indicates. There is little sign of cerebrotonic influence. Perhaps he has a pathological cerebropenia. ψ 2–1–1.

Delinquency: Much early and late truancy. Long record of juvenile delinquency, beginning at 7 or 8 with persistent stealing. Larceny and minor racketeering at 10. At 12, regarded as a confirmed delinquent and sentenced to one of the state correctional schools. This was followed by repeated runaway episodes, further larceny, and more racketeering. No delinquency of violence or of wanton destructiveness. He had lived by his wits and by gambling for a half-dozen years; had finally got mixed up in a confidence racket and at 21 had received a federal sentence.

Origins and Family: Fifth of six, small urban community. Father a powerful athlete of Portuguese-Irish extraction. A rough and ready character who never took a very active interest in his children. He expressed disappointment in this boy because of the latter's insufficient athletic prowess. The mother,

Irish, died at childbirth when this boy was 2. Latter then turned over to various relatives under intermittent social agency control. Three of the siblings died in early childhood. The remaining two turned out well in that they grew up healthy and have kept out of trouble.

Mental History, Achievement: He has the equivalent of eighth-grade education. Finished seven grades, then in and out of several continuational or correctional schools. Record of vigorous demurral against "education" in all of them. IQ reports range from 86 to 95, here called 90 and this agrees with general observation of the boy. He seems well removed from feeblemindedness but does not appear to be of quite high school caliber. He verbalizes poorly and has serious trouble with elementary arithmetic.

No vocational plan other than that of living by gambling. No special gifts. The AMI is based on the *persona* of bad luck or tough breaks. He tells his hard luck story with a certain massive sincerity, and indeed he has had a pretty bad time of it. Moreover he is a sturdy, durable young man in whom one intuitively feels that a certain confidence ought to be reposed.

Medical: Infancy history not known. No serious illnesses or injuries. PX reveals no significant pathology. There is a rather early preview of the normal middle-aged "obesity" of this somatotype, and the general appearance of the youth is that of a man ten years older.

Running Record: At the Inn he absorbed casework about as a captive seal absorbs fish. When favored, he showed momentary warmth or pleasure but never evidenced any overwhelming sense of indebtedness. His relations at the Inn seemed to constitute for him a pleasing and interesting game—one which he enjoyed playing out to the end of the string. He alcoholized himself with irregular frequency and when alcoholized was inclined to be truculent. During the intervening periods he was urbane and guardedly mendacious. He brushed aside efforts at educational or vocational rehabilitation as a honey-drunk bear will brush off bees. On the work program he showed judgment and insight in doing only what was necessary to meet the immediate exigency, from day to day. While he was with us all the money he was able to secure went into gambling rackets. Above everything he loved the race track. His *persona* seemed to become increasingly that of the sophisticated gambler, "in the know" and associated with a mysterious undercover element. He lived under many aliases and in his philosophy reflected a salty realism.

After more than a year at the Inn he moved on into more grown-up territory, apparently living by his wits and by gambling until the war came along and the military institution picked him up. He took to military life almost at once, expanding in both a physical and mental sense, and there he seemed to prosper. Gambling remained the one great interest; the inflation flood was on, and the money cream ran like water from faucets. After the war he reenlisted. Today he gives an impression both of greater relaxation and of greater security. "The military is a racket," he says, "but I like it."

Summary: A massive endomorph of great strength and energy. Good health and mentality within normal limits. Long history of delinquency and gambling, but none of destructiveness. An irresponsibility which perhaps approaches criminality.

ID 0–2–1 (3)
Insufficiencies:
  IQ ....
  Mop ....
Psychiatric:

1st order ....
2nd order 2
  Somatorotic love of risk
  (2–1–1)
C-phobic ....
G-phrenic ....
Residual D:
  Primary crim. 1

Comment: The outlook may now be good, and if so the credit belongs to the military institution. As matters now look the military has succeeded where all other efforts had failed. Such a statement should of course be tempered by one qualification: The youth has not risen to great intellectual heights in the Army, and he has probably devoted fully as great a proportion of his thought and attention to gambling as he ever did. But he has found an environment in which such interests are commensurate with good social standing so long as enough buoyant energy remains to meet routine requirements. He has plenty of energy and seems well adapted to his present pattern of life. He has of course not demonstrated in a noninstitutional environment that there has been any permanent change in his predilection to delinquency.

One point in this case is worth further speculation. Although the boy was a vigorous fellow with far above average strength and athletic ability, he was *in comparison with his father* a physical failure. Mesomorphically he was a disappointment to his father and to his own early ideal of himself. This may be an important fact in his history. A case might be made out that the social delinquency was intimately related to a true physical delinquency, or to a falling away from a desired state. It is certainly possible that many cases of delinquency in mesomorphs could be better understood in the light of this mechanism, which after all is perhaps no more than a particular instance of the universal human tragedy of the almost.

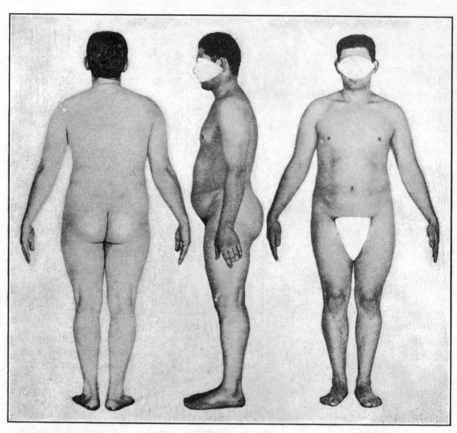

Description: Somatotype 5½–4½–1. A 22-year-old mesomorphic endomorph an inch under average stature. A massive and sturdy although (when photographed) slightly obese physique, with some underdevelopment of muscularity in the distal segments of the arms and legs. Primary $g\pm$, or just a trace. Secondary $g\pm$. He is not built for first-rate athletic competition, yet on the whole he is tough and durable. The physique has both tennis-ball buoyancy and golf-ball toughness without an extreme of either. Primary t 2, secondary t 2. The underlying architecture and basic lines of the body depart somewhat radically from classical ideals. Features are heavy, soggy, doughy. He has a surly face with no suggestion of clean chiseling. General strength 4, hand strength 3. Coordination good although he moves in a lumbering, bear-like manner. He is physically efficient in the way that a bear is efficient, and for the somatotype is a remarkably effective fighter. His physical courage is still a byword among his contemporaries. Never interested in athletics as such.

Temperament: Aggressive, overriding, somatotonically extraverted. Second component clearly predominant. He loves action, is fond of noise and confusion, identifies with boisterous carousing and with the *persona* of toughness. Yet he is viscerotonically relaxed, is fond of food and of loitering over food. He is amiable, sociophilic, agglutinative. Cerebrotonia seems to be the weakest component although he does show distressing aftereffect from alcohol and is fatigued by that drug. He seems to fight his booze—a cerebrotonic sign. There is a suggestion of overloading in the first two components and if he were to become psychotic he would be cycloid or Dionysian. ψ 3–2–1.

Delinquency: Much early truancy and frequent stealing before 10. Several times arrested for larceny between 13 and 16. Numerous charges of drunkenness, and three of larceny, between 16 and 18. Repeatedly in trouble with police for drunkenness at 18.

Origins and Family: Extramarital, father unknown. Mother Irish and an active, heavy woman who as a girl used a number of aliases, was many times arrested on morals charges, and was sent to women's reformatories. Boy turned over to agencies at birth and reared in foster homes.

Mental History, Achievement: Finished the eighth grade after much repetition and failure. IQ reports fall consistently between 90 and 105, here called 100. He gives the impression of normal mentality. He is alert and nobody's fool but is negatively conditioned to school in all its aspects.

No vocational plans or special gifts. His principal ambitions and identifications as a boy were in the direction of athletics. The AMI that of a big freckle-faced youth who is pleasantly extraverted and has a suggestion of Irish warmth.

Medical: Normal birth and early development. No serious illnesses although he has always been an upper respiratory delinquent. He has frequent prolonged colds that settle in the chest and leave him with a loud cough which seems to be everlasting. Alcoholic bouts are followed by severe hangovers and he often looks debauched. PX reveals severe dental caries and evidence of chronic sinusitis. He borders on the infectious syndrome.

Running Record: At the Inn he was a rollicking Irish boy who produced enough noise and confusion for three and was out for a good time. His idea of a good time was to spend money a little before he got it, to laugh at obligations, to get drunk when possible, to drive an automobile or truck as fast as it would go. After several fiascos at job placement we found that his passion for automobiles was so strong that he was prepared even to *work* at a truck driving job, and he undertook such a job. He smashed up two trucks, meanwhile making things lively for pedestrians and for other drivers about the city, but his employers stood by him and after three months he still had the job. He spent all his money on liquor and girls, was addicted to riotous celebrations involving a mixture of gasoline, alcohol, and sex. But he kept out of the hands of police for six months, and so we hailed him as a success.

After leaving the Inn he was drafted into military service. There he stated his preference for truck driving and was assigned to a transport unit. During his stay in the service there were numerous episodes of drunkenness, some AWOL incidents, and on one occasion when drunk he hit an officer. Yet he stayed in. His rollicking pattern is, no doubt rightly, well tolerated among military men. We received one report from him while he was overseas to the effect that he was having a "swell time" and was killing the enemy right and left—presumably with trucks. He stayed in the service for a year or more after the war and now, another year after discharge, looks as fat and prosperous as a sausage. His general behavior pattern is the same as before, except that he now has money and a little more alcohol. There has been no record of civilian delinquency against him since he left the Inn. He is still floundering, has no orientation to time, does not show signs of settling down. A military social agency reports him as "psychoneurotic."

Summary: Big, rollicking youth of midrange somatotype with a touch of *g*. Normal mentality; a first cousin to the infectious syndrome. Somatorotic and cerebropenic. Persistent alcoholism. Early delinquency.

ID 1–3–0 (4)
  Insufficiencies:
    IQ ....
    Mop 1
  Psychiatric:
    1st order ....
    2nd order 2
    Dionysian (3–2–1)
    C-phobic 1
    G-phrenic ....

  Residual D:
    Primary crim. ....

Comment: Outlook probably good as to delinquency unless moderate alcoholism and possibly chronic alcoholism in later life constitute delinquency. His life may become a race between obesity and alcoholism. A gluttonous 4–4–4, which he is, often grows so fat as to be unable to get around effectively and with the recession of locomotive acumen there is likely to be also a recession of alcoholism. The first component seems gently to sort of take over. The 4–4–4 is always interesting, wherever you meet him, and his possibilities are almost limitless. According to his temperament and to his mentality he may become obese or remain seemingly lean; once started in *any* direction, physically, mentally, or behaviorally, the 4–4–4 can go a long way if he wants to. This somatotype presents what seems to be the nearest human approach to Mr. G, who as everyone knows is a 7–7–7. It is a hard life to be even a 4–4–4, and if Mr. G with his 7–7–7 temperament, has made occasional mistakes in His human experiments perhaps they ought to be magnanimously forgiven.

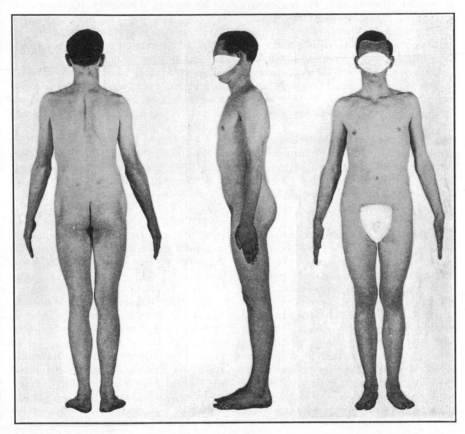

Description: Somatotype 4–4–4. An 18-year-old youth of midrange somatotype, four inches above average stature. Face endomorphic, neck solidly
mesomorphic, and the trunk is a little more heavily built than the limbs.
Arms and legs show ectomorphic dysplasia but no trace of asthenic flaccidity.
He is likely to become very heavy in later life. In middle age he will almost
surely pass 200 pounds. Primary $g+1$, secondary $g\pm$. Primary t 3, secondary
t 2. Features coarse, blunt, ill-shaped—he was called Pig Face by some of the
boys; viscerotonic mouth with suckling lips. General strength 3, hand
strength 3. Coordination fair. He moves awkwardly but gets around fast—
very noisy with feet and furniture. He is loosely put together. Not good at
athletics or at fighting.

Temperament: Somatotonia predominates. He is active, restless, but also hyperattentional, suspicious, and perhaps apprehensive. He is easily bored, cannot stand routine; seems never altogether at ease. He is also arty and has a strong trace of the *DAMP RAT* syndrome. Vocal somatorosis is a predominant characteristic, with uneven voice control and poor tonality. Cerebrotonic interference seems present in everything he does. There is little indication of viscerotonia. He has almost rhythmic periods of harsh hostility and irritability, suggesting a possible epileptoid factor. He overdresses, is meretricious, a little theatrical. This is an odd mixture of paranoid hardness and gynandrophrenic perverseness. He has been accused of homosexuality, probably unjustly. ψ 2–3–2.

Delinquency: Persistent truancy during the first three years of school. Incorrigibility and general perversity throughout grade school. Periodic violence and destructiveness all through childhood, with seemingly unprovoked outbursts of rage or fury. No history of stealing. He has been closely identified with delinquent associates, particularly with youngsters involved in some kind of sexual racket, but apparently he has been only a fringer in such business. He has been excessively bored with life and has always been a problem boy to teachers and vocational advisors.

Origins and Family: Youngest of three, urban family. Father a slender and well-regarded artisan of Scotch extraction who died of tuberculosis when the boy was 3. Described as a man of fine discrimination and of good stock. Mother Old American, short and stocky, died of the same disease three years later. Boy taken over by agencies and reared in a long series of foster homes. He was recalcitrant from the beginning but was always regarded as bright and "in some way promising."

Mental History, Achievement: Completed three years of high school and generally regarded as competent or bright, but frequently in trouble because of temper flare-ups and because of his moods of hostility. IQ reports fall between 108 and 121, here called 115. Well above average intelligence. He gives an impression of alertness but also of tension and instability.

No vocational plan. Gifted in music and he has toyed with the idea of being a musician. In some moods he would like to be an artist. In others he dreams of being a professional companion of rich old ladies. In all things he has been a dilettante. No interest in athletics. The AMI based on meticulously well-dressed gentlemanliness, and on a bright conversational alertness.

Medical: No history of illness or injury. PX reveals no pathology except advanced caries. Fingers are yellow with cigarette residue, and nails are badly bitten.

Running Record: His response to life at the Inn seemed to suggest a more or less thoroughbred dog who had been badly treated and never trained. He accepted friendliness but maintained a suspicious reserve. A highly discriminating youth with a somewhat arty *persona* he was regarded as close to the border of homosexuality, although probably not across that border. No one on the staff ever won his confidence. He never would apply himself to anything, could never save money. His principal interest was in music but it was an intermittent and superficial interest. He gave the impression of possessing a desire to sponge or exploit to the limit of tolerability, but he knew when to stop to keep out of trouble. He made several false starts and failures with jobs, finally refused the school program and drifted away from us. We had no disciplinary hold on him, since he was not in difficulty with authorities, and we seemed to have no way of reaching him.

After drifting for another year he was inducted into military service. He had a stormy time in the service with disciplinary difficulties and spent many months in the brig; but he stayed in and is now in retrospect rather pleased with the experience. A year after his discharge he is vocationally as undecided as ever but is happier, and has been playing with a number of more or less expansive and ambitious plans.

Summary: Ectomorphic mesomorphy with high *t* and an odd mixture of paranoid and *DAMP RAT* tendencies. Excellent health; mentality well above average. Early flirtation with delinquency, continued vocational confusion.

ID 0–4–0 (4)
Insufficiencies:
    IQ ....
    Mop ....
Psychiatric:
    1st order ....
    2nd order   2
        (2–3–2)

C-phobic ....
G-phrenic   2
    DAMP RAT
Residual D:
    Primary crim. ....

Comment: Outlook improving with maturation, although he is still not out of the woods. An unusual mixture of tendencies and apparently borderline in half a dozen respects. He is not far from homosexuality, not far from clinical psychoneurosis with a paranoid trend. More important for him, perhaps, he cannot be far from peptic ulcer and this may turn out to be his salvation, as it has been for many another of more or less similar temperament. The treatment or management which this ailment necessitates brings needed support to the first component and pours oil on the troubled waters of somatorotic tension. The ailment may constitute a natural remedy or natural safety valve for internal tension generated by the sort of personality which this youth presents. The latter, however, has not as yet reported any symptoms that suggest ulcer.

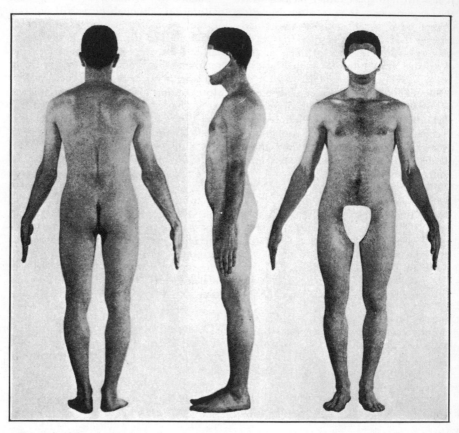

Description: Somatotype 2½–4½–3½. A 21-year-old ectomorphic meso-morph of average stature. Clean cut, rather jaunty general appearance, with an ectomorphic dysplasia in the arms. Arms brittle, suggestive of toothpicks in the distal segments. Primary $g\pm$, secondary $g+1$. Primary t 3, secondary t 4. Features well formed and almost too sharply chiseled. He is "good look-ing" in a somewhat brittle or Arrow-collar sense. The facial expression shows a certain "paranoid" hyperalertness. It is like the face of an underfed mas-tiff. Hands and feet fine. General strength 3, hand strength 3. Excellent co-ordination, although in a delicate, almost dainty sense. He is too brittle or too meticulously careful of himself for athletics, but is a very fine dancer.

Temperament: Exuberantly energetic and good natured, he shows what might be called a minor cycloid pattern. In the Dionysian phase he never rests, is a sort of professional clown and ubiquitous nuisance, although a well-liked one and a source of rich entertainment. In the quiet or depressed phase, which is of regular occurrence and is usually of short duration, he keeps out of sight; stays in bed if possible, is full of self-pity, cries easily. He comes out of this mood suddenly, changing in a moment from moroseness to the *persona* of a merry buffoon, and that is the role in which he earns his keep. He suggests the cycloid picture but lacks a sufficiently strong somatotonia for the development of manic behavior or (probably) for the development of a cycloid psychosis. There are no signs of orientational pathology. The psychopathy is clearly of the second order. ψ 3–2–1.

Delinquency: Early truancy and unusually persistent minor stealing. At 12, diagnosed *psychopathic personality with kleptomania*. Said to have "collected things" like a pack rat. He was a resourceful nuisance in foster homes, gleefully playing off one foster mother against another, and one agency against another. One or two later charges of larceny, and one of breaking and entering, at 15, just before we met him.

Origins and Family: Fifth of six, small urban community. Father French-Canadian. He had an early delinquent history, deserted the family when this boy was 2, later reported hospitalized as an alcoholic. Mother a French-Irish factory girl who "had never been strong" and died of tuberculosis at about the time the father disappeared. Boy reared in a series of foster homes under agency management. One sibling feeble-minded, one defective from congenital lues, two described as of weak constitution and one of these died during childhood.

Mental History, Achievement: Finished the fourth grade, then removed from public school and sent to special continuation schools, but no more measurable progress. IQ reports fall between 78 and 86, here called 83. He is bright and entertaining and is graciously verbose with a mendacity so thin and obvious that it seems intended to amuse rather than deceive.

He likes farms, expects to live close to the soil. No other vocational interest. The AMI (at 15) that of being an intriguing little fellow, as entertaining as a chipmunk, with his wide blue eyes and high energy, and his fantastic yarns centered around his adventures in foster homes. From long experience with social workers he has learned how to make 'em gasp with maternal indignation.

Medical: No early data. He has had numerous infections, trouble with ears, recurrent colds which settle on the chest, and he presents evidence of early rickets. Appendectomy and tonsillectomy. There is a heart murmur of long standing, and one clinic calls his heart enlarged. The X-ray looks to me, however, like that of a normally or perhaps dysplastically large mesomorphic heart. PX reveals only flat feet and defective, carious teeth.

Running Record: At the Inn he kept out of trouble with police and his buoyant sense of humor, even though a bit too earthy and practical, more than paid for his lodging and for what trifles he was able to steal. He failed good naturedly on all programs from work assignments to school. A clever mimic and an entertaining story teller, he had learned to relate his persecutions by foster parents in a really sidesplitting manner. At one foster home, on a freezing January night, they punished him for a trifling fault by taking off his clothes and burying him up to his chin in a vat of cow dung in the barnyard, where he soon froze solidly in. Still not satisfied, the fiendish foster mother shoveled snow and ice over his head, leaving only a small opening for him to breathe through. On another occasion a foster mother whipped him so hard that his chest caved in "and you can see that it has never grown right since." He was a great joy to the pederasts and undiscriminating homosexuals of the neighborhood, being always an available baggage to whom a dime or a package of cigarettes loomed large. This of course does not mean that he was a homosexual. He was an opportunist who liked dimes and had no inhibitions.

For two years after leaving us he did fairly well at farm jobs. He was then inducted into military service and after two years was discharged with no record of serious delinquency. Since then he has done farm work, has kept out of serious trouble despite a minor kleptoid tendency, has the same buoyantly optimistic manner as when we first knew him, and has a string of altogether wondrous stories of military life. He drinks a good deal now, and his attitude toward sexuality is decidedly Dionysian. When he visits the Inn everybody is sincerely glad to see him. The staff will usually drop whatever it is doing to gather around to hear the latest whopper. If later a little something turns up missing—no great matter.

Summary: Dysmorphic mesomorphy with good strength and poor coordination. Dull normal mentality; some degree of medical insufficiency. Second-order psychopathy with a cycloid trend. Just a faint trace of Dionysian irresponsibility.

ID 2–3–0 (5)
Insufficiencies:
  IQ 1
  Mop 1
Psychiatric:
  1st order ....
  2nd order 2
    Dionysian (3–2–1)
  C-phobic 1
  G-phrenic ....
Residual D:
  Primary crim. ....

Comment: Outlook probably good from his point of view and within his limitations. He certainly has made an "adaptation"; for five years now has got along under his own power and has kept out of trouble. His cessation of formal delinquency coincides chronologically with his contact with the Inn. If any other connection between the two events exists, we would be hard put to it to say what the connection is. The Inn makes no pretense of therapy, or of curing anybody of anything. The staff has felt that it does wonderfully well if it succeeds in *describing* a boy accurately or usefully. Sometimes, possibly, the description or its implications spill over a little to the boy himself so that a ray of understanding light breaks through. This may have happened in the present case, although not to any alarming degree.

COMPANY B, PLATOON 1, SECTION 2
Second-Order Psychopathy; with Minor Somatoroses:
Nos. 115–132

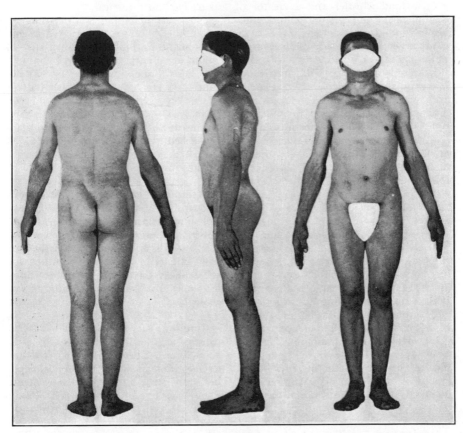

Description: Somatotype 3–5–3. A 15-year-old dysmorphic mesomorph of average stature. (The photograph used here was taken when he was 18.) All segments badly developed except the head and neck. The neck suggests that when the Potter started this one he may have had extreme mesomorphy in mind. Short, massive trunk with rachitic chest. Arms and legs long, heavy boned, but poorly molded and rather weakly muscled. Tremendous hands and feet. There is some ectomorphic dysplasia in the arms and legs but mesomorphy predominates strongly. Conspicuously large superficial veins show in the arms—a mesomorphic characteristic. Primary $g\pm$—there is just a trace of g in the lower trunk. Secondary $g\pm$. Primary t 1, secondary t 2. Features large but irregularly developed and asymmetrical. Broad, meaty face. The t is so low that he is attractive. General strength 3, hand strength 4. Coordination poor. Although he has abundant energy and strength there is nothing he can do in the way of athletic games and he cannot fight. Inept at anything requiring fine coordination.

Temperament: Somatorotic but in a sustained and even-tempered way. He is fresh or impudent to an extreme degree, a loud whistler and a creator of disturbances, but he is not tempestuous. No epileptoid characteristic. He is arrogantly assertive in a cocky, light-hearted pattern. Even at interview he will whistle through his teeth, will contrive to make a disturbance with rulers, pencils, and similar impromptu drumsticks. There seems to be always an undercurrent of unquenchable hostility along with hyperattentionality. The temperamental pattern probably reflects the somatotype accurately but at too high an energy level. He is just a trifle *DAMP RAT* or arty-perverse, although apparently never homosexual. ψ 2–2–1.

Delinquency: Early truancy and uncontrollability in school. A persistent runaway between 8 and 15. Minor stealing throughout childhood. Between 14 and 17, three times sent to state correctional school for stealing, running away, and automophilia. Known and several times arrested as a "looper" or temporary borrower of automobiles for joyriding purposes. He once stole and smashed up the automobile of a foster family, injured the occupants of the other car, and left the scene of the accident.

Origins and Family: Third of four illegitimate Negro children, small urban community. The father, who was never identified with the family, died later of syphilis. Mother often delinquent on morals charges and long treated for syphilis. She died of tuberculosis, when the boy was 7. Both maternal grandparents died young of tuberculosis. Boy reared with mother until her death, thereafter in foster homes under agency management.

Mental History, Achievement: Finished two years of high school with low grades. IQ reports fall between 80 and 90, here called 85. He gives the impression of a certain brightness and alertness but of impatient superficiality. He is restive and theatrical.

No vocational plan but quite an accomplished musician. He played several instruments in high school and talks of music in an arty, *DAMP RAT* manner. The AMI that of a well-rehearsed Freudian story. He has been caseworked for years, has learned to recite the insecurity-and-parental-mistreatment catechisms in a rapid offhand monotone interspersed by somatorotic gestures which for all the world suggest careless signs of the cross.

Medical: Early medical history not known. Many hospital referrals for minor ailments after 7 but no serious illnesses. Operations for hernia, tonsillectomy. He is myopic and partially deaf (congenital). Many times examined for tuberculosis but none found. He likes hospitals. PX reveals no significant pathology.

Running Record: Through several months at the Inn he made a fairly good record. There was no overt delinquency, he kept out of the hands of police, and carried out work assignments when closely supervised. He was a source of constant minor disturbance, was truculently race conscious, harangued other Negroes to "resist." The racial chip-on-the-shoulder once nearly precipitated a neighborhood war. He had acquired the habit of "ragging" an Italian tough or gangster of the neighborhood who according to the police was something of a big shot in local rackets. He would shout evil names at Giuseppe from the security of one of our third-story windows as the latter strolled below. On one occasion he grew unwary and complimented Giuseppe on the quality of his ancestry from the corner of the building. As he turned to dodge into the doorway he found himself in the eager embrace of one of the

Italian's henchmen. As Giuseppe proceeded to administer what he considered suitable appreciation of the compliments rendered, a number of our boys issued from the nearby front door and a neighborhood war began. Fortunately the Inn reinforcement included two or three powerful Irish mesomorphs and the Italian reinforcements were late in coming up. The rescue was accomplished with only light casualties on both sides.

After leaving us this boy drifted for about a year but kept out of police custody. He was then inducted into military service where he remained for the duration of the war. He got married and was hospitalized many times for various complaints. His duties were mainly confined to band work. After the war he reenlisted and has since sent in quite a favorable report on "what the Army does for you."

Summary: A slender ectomorph-mesomorph Negro with a strong trace of the *DAMP RAT* syndrome. Mentality better than borderline but poorly focused. History of hospitalitis with perhaps some physiological insufficiency. Somatorotic without an epileptoid tendency.

ID 2–3–0 (5)
Insufficiencies:
   IQ 1
   Mop 1
Psychiatric:
   1st order ....

2nd order 2
  Somatorotic (2–2–1)
C-phobic ....
G-phrenic 1
  DAMP RAT
Residual D:
  Primary crim. ....

Comment: The outlook may be favorable although he has not yet demonstrated an ability to live independently and keep out of trouble. Adjustment within the military institution seems to be satisfactory and ought to be a good omen. There are no very serious handicaps but it is worth noting that where the *DAMP RAT* syndrome is present, even to a mild degree as in the present case, the individual seems to *need* more intelligence than normally in order to make an adaptation. For a *DAMP RAT* an IQ of 85 may be borderline in about the same way that 70 is borderline for the average person or 60 for an extreme mesomorph. A 2–6–1 can usually do pretty well with an IQ of 65 but a *DAMP RAT* possibly needs 90 in order to enjoy the same chance of success or achievement. He has more ways of offending people and fewer natural defenses. For a somatorotic *DAMP RAT* Negro who cannot fight and has quite a long history of early delinquency, the chances of getting into trouble during the next few decades of American life may be worth considering. Yet this boy has not been in police custody since our first contact with him. On statistical grounds he could be presented as a success and a triumph.

131. *COMPANY B, PLATOON 1, SECTION 2*
Second-Order Psychopathy; with Minor Somatoroses: Nos. 115–132

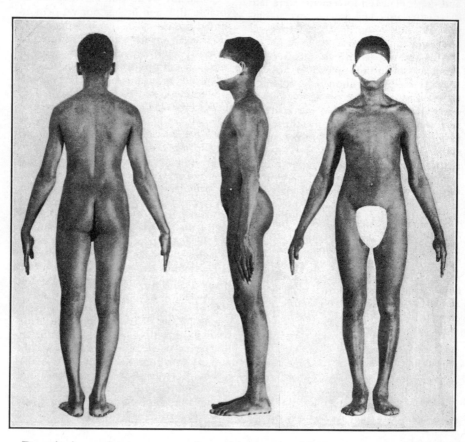

Description: Somatotype 2½–4–4. A 17-year-old Negro ectomorph-meso-morph two inches above average stature. A slender and sprightly body, pow-erfully built through the trunk, ectomorphically brittle in the distal seg-ments of the arms—Nilotic dysplasia. Primary and secondary g±. Primary *t* 4, secondary *t* 3. Features even, well formed, wholly Negro. General strength 3, hand strength 3. Coordination excellent. He handles himself with quick agility although the arms are too brittle for fighting or for the pre-dominantly popular athletic games.

Temperament: He is predominantly somatotonic, well energized, and buoyant, but the energy is poorly channeled and the picture is one of Dionysian somatorosis. He smokes two packages of cigarettes a day, is vocally strident, bids for the spotlight of attention but having got it can only make a noise or a confusion. No indication of cerebrotonic interference. No self-consciousness or hyperattentionality. There are frequent almost feminine outbursts of temper, but since he is helpless against other boys and can express only frustrated rage, the spasm soon passes. No suggestion of the epileptoid tantrum, with its rhythmicity and its prodromal signs. He merely flares up somatorotically, as dogs are inclined to do at one another. He is capriciously perverse and a little theatrical, faintly suggesting the *DAMP RAT* syndrome. ψ 3–1–1.

Delinquency: Persistent early truancy, minor stealing before 10, long association with street gangs as a fringer or follower. Half a dozen episodes of running away before 13 (but he never got far). Excessive addiction to cigarettes as early as 12. Often caught, at about that period, at such grave crimes as stealing rides in the subway. He was always one of the weak tailenders, the kind that *do* get caught at that sort of thing. Three charges of larceny, between 14 and 17.

Origins and Family: Only child, urban family. Father French-Irish, alcoholic, called irresponsible. He had quite a long agency history and was killed in an accident when the boy was 5. Mother Irish, in late years obese, twice sent to correctional schools as a girl for sexual delinquency. Later in trouble for keeping a disorderly house. Maternal grandfather an alcoholic. Boy reared intermittently with mother and other relatives, under agency management.

Mental History, Achievement: Finished the seventh grade after repeating three other grades. IQ reports fall narrowly between 79 and 87, here called 83. Optimistically, dull normal. Pessimistically, borderline. At first he seems brighter but with prolonged acquaintanceship the impression is revised downward. He blows with the wind, is easily talked into almost any acquiescence, but the new resolution is never kept for long. There seems to be no sustained focus of attention or of energy. Whatever "moral fiber" or "character" is, it is here woven of extraordinarily weak material.

No vocational plan or preparation. The AMI rests on an alert chipperness. Social workers write that he intends well, is a victim of bad associates, a casualty-of-the-broken-home; that he needs mothering and fathering. But social workers write this about everybody, and so far as it goes it is perfectly true—of nearly everybody.

Medical: Early history not known. No major illnesses or injuries. Long series of minor accidents. He is careless, accident-prone, as his father is said to have been. PX reveals poorly formed teeth and severe dental caries, moderately defective vision, flat feet.

Running Record: At the Inn he was known as Jitter. Cigaretty in the highest degree, hyperactive, often alcoholic, given to false starts and to ill-sustained gestures at reform, he was a kind of secondary nuisance. He seemed to want to be a *DAMP RAT* but the ruling spirits of that Order viewed him with austere disdain. He was never able to keep to a schedule under his own momentum. On various work programs the effort necessary to keep him at it always outweighed his achievement. On a work assignment he was like a terrier on a leash, always straining in a tangential direction. He was assigned to an industrial training program but there his frequent cigarette fires, alcoholism, girlish quarreling, and alleged intermittent illness led at last to abandonment of the project. We remember him for a certain tomboyish exuberance, however, and when he left here he was missed. Nuisance that he was, and dubious as the ultimate outlook may be, we are still glad to see him when he drops in.

Shortly after leaving, he was inducted into military service where he made a poor record and after somewhat more than a year was dropped. He drank heavily in the service, was irresponsible, and spent a large part of the time under hospital observation. A period of drifting in civilian life followed, and he was then placed in the Merchant Marine. There, after two years, he appears to be getting along. He has now grown quite fat and seems more composed.

Summary: Dysmorphic, poorly coordinated endomorphic mesomorph with a gynandrophrenic trend. Dull normal mentality; a trace of medical insufficiency. Somatorotic psychopathy. Alcoholism.

ID 2–4–0 (6)
Insufficiencies:
  IQ 1
  Mop 1
Psychiatric:
  1st order ....
  2nd order 2
   (3–1–1)
  C-phobic 1
  G-phrenic 1
Residual D:
  Primary crim. ....

Comment: Outlook still in doubt, although it probably has brightened within the past two years. His endomorphy is coming into full blossom now, and endomorphy acts on somatorosis like oil on troubled waters. There is no treatment for the somatorotic and Dionysian psychopathies like fattening. This boy has gained 40 pounds within three years. Add another 20 or 30 and he *won't be able* to make himself troublesome. We can then carry him as a complete success.

132.
COMPANY B, PLATOON 1, SECTION 2
Second-Order Psychopathy; with Minor Somatoroses: Nos. 115–132

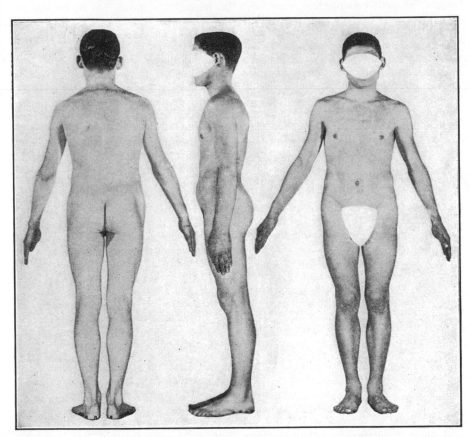

Description: Somatotype $3\frac{1}{2}$–5–$2\frac{1}{2}$. A 16-year-old endomorphic meso-morph of average stature. Extremely heavy skeleton but dysmorphic development of the various segments. Round, massive head with a short, thick neck. Short trunk, comparatively long arms and legs. Relatively poor muscular development throughout. The arms are almost asthenic but they show no ectomorphy. Such a physique tends to become heavy in middle life. Primary $g\pm$, secondary $g+1$. Primary t 1, secondary t 2. Features large and well developed but haphazardly formed and irregular—mongrel features. The whole physical pattern seems to express a mixture of stocks which did not blend well, and this may be one underlying cause of dysmorphy. General and hand strength 3. Coordination poor. He is clumsy. Limbs and trunk integrate badly. No athletic ability, unable to fight, unhappy in the gymnasium.

Temperament: A picture of magnificent relaxation and of unchallenged viscerotonia. He is lazy, manifests what might be called borderline viscerosis. His chief desire is to be comfortable; to be free to eat, relax, and spread out. He is then amiable and sociophilic. He shows no cerebrotonic interference, lacks aggression and drive. Yet he has a fairly good underlying somatotonia which is evidenced by agility on occasion and by a mountain-like stubborn resistance to being pushed in any direction. He wants to vegetate and proposes to do so. ψ 2–1–1.

Delinquency: None except secondary difficulties associated with stubbornness and failure to succeed in school. There has been smouldering warfare with the mother and with other siblings over the question of what he is to do. Familial alarm has been expressed over the quality of his associates. All of the older siblings are mesomorphic and have been aggressively successful.

Origins and Family: Youngest of five, urban family, both parents Jewish immigrants from Eastern Europe. The father is of average physique for this stock (a thickset endomorphic mesomorph) and has a good health history. He has been industriously successful in this country. Mother extraordinarily heavy but more mesomorphic than endomorphic and she has done well with her family. She has pushed the children hard. Boy reared in the home.

Mental History, Achievement: Finished three years of high school but then lost interest and refused to continue. IQ reports range from 93 to 105, here put at 100. He seems intelligent enough and has a good-humored outlook. He gives the impression of being mentally normal although lacking in the surplus physical and mental energy so often encountered in Jews.

No vocational plan and no particular interest in any direction other than being allowed to do as he likes. The AMI that of a mountainous youth who wears a friendly or humorous scowl on his broad face, is cooperative and good company but obviously has no intention of changing his mind on the question of school.

Medical: Normal birth and early development. Average birth weight. (Note: The very large babies are nearly always mesomorphs, not endomorphs.) Obese from the first year, walked at about 15 months, talked at 2 years. He seems to have had good general health although many times referred to clinics because of his size and weight. A "glandular" problem, the mother and boy have always been informed. There have been spasms of endocrine therapy, all of which seemed harmless although it was noted following one series of treatments that the pubic hair sprouted a little more than usual. Various diagnoses were made such as *hyperpituitary, hypopituitary, hyperthymus, hypothyroid,* etc. He weighed 34 pounds at the end of the first year, 140 pounds at 11, 300 pounds at 17. Never a very heavy eater, he does like sweets and insists on eating candy despite intermittently vigorous interdictions. PX reveals defective vision (congenital myopia) and excessively flat feet. Judging by the photograph and by the way he handles himself he is perhaps near his best or "correct" weight at 300 pounds, although with uncontrolled eating he no doubt could become heavy.

Running Record: After a series of conferences and consultations with this lad we became rather converted to his point of view that perhaps he had gone far enough in school and that college for a normal person may be a waste of time. His point was simply that higher education is not his racket and that there was already enough school achievement in his family. In the end he took the set and we brought no further pressure on him to go to college. In return for what he taught us we explained to him that endomorphy and viscerotonia may be normal on this pellet and not necessarily a result of endocrine pathology or of intrafamilial rejections. That relieved his mind no end. He agreed to finish high school although in his own way and at his own tempo.

After five years the interim report is this: He finished high school, held several jobs briefly in defense industry, and has saved money. Weight is about the same. He has long since forgotten about the "college foolishness." The family is still displeased with him, regarding him as a burden and a disappointment, but the warfare is less acute. His draft status was 4-F; overweight.

Summary: Extreme endomorphy with possibly a trace of viscerosis. Average mentality; good health.

ID 0–1–0 (1)
Insufficiencies:
   IQ ....
   Mop ....
Psychiatric:
   1st order ....
   2nd order 1
      Trace of viscerosis, stubbornly supported (2–1–1)

C-phobic ....
G-phrenic ....
Residual D:
   Primary crim. ....

Comment: Prognosis very good, although within his limitations and on his own terms. He has no intention of being untrue to his magnificent viscertonia and probably his position is defensible. To try to force the draft in order to make him burn brightly with somatotonic ambition would be comparable to attempting to make an athlete of an ectomorph—a common enough tragedy. This boy is delinquent in the literal sense that he is disappointing to somebody, but he is probably justified in his delinquency. The case is an important one in the series for it illustrates a corner in the distribution of temperamental psychopathy which is likely to be forgotten in any discussion of psychoneurosis. Viscerosis is of common occurrence but is seldom recognized as psychopathy. The viscerotics usually just relax and keep out of trouble. Yet they are in a literal sense as "delinquent" as somatorotics or cerebrotics. In this boy's case it is the somatotonic support of the viscerosis—not the latter in itself—that produces the 2 in the first psychiatric component.

133. COMPANY B, PLATOON 1, SECTION 3
Second-Order Psychopathy; Uncomplicated: Nos. 133–143

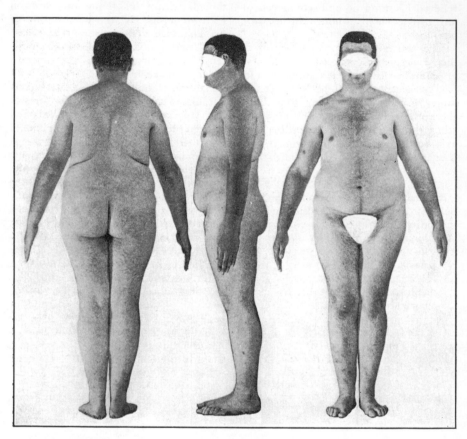

Description: Somatotype 7–2–1½. A 17-year-old extreme endomorph well over six feet in stature. A good example of the "short-fat type" for those who divide humanity into short-fats and long-thins. No particular dysplasias except a slight increment of ectomorphy in the arms and of mesomorphy in the face. Primary $g+2$, secondary $g\pm$. Primary t 2, secondary t 2. Features blunt and coarse but symmetrical. General strength 2, hand strength 2. Coordination good. He is surprisingly active and agile for the somatotype although far from athletic. He floats with a considerable portion of his anatomy above the surface—says he can sleep on the water "when it isn't too rough."

Temperament: Sustained, relaxed somatotonia. No strain, no trace of cerebrotonic conflict. He is happy-go-lucky, hearty, good humored, altogether unrestrained. A sort of rollicking, banjo-playing good fellow of infectious extraversion who never has to fight because never challenged. On the face of things a superbly adapted animal with great energy and with physical adequacy. At the Inn he was always up at six, was likely to have done a day's work by breakfast time (if in the mood), and by nine he would often have the staff in a good mood. His presence in the lobby destroyed the hope of cerebrotonic "peace," but also was sufficient to restrain untoward truculence. ψ 3–1–1.

Delinquency: History before 15 not known. Since then, frequently arrested for vagrancy, usually on the "idle and disorderly conduct" charge, or "common tramp" charge. Essentially a tramp or bum since leaving home at 15. Steadfast refusal to work or to accept regular gainful employment of any kind. A character well known to police and often regarded with suspicion, but with no known record of stealing or of violence. Occasional drunkenness. A frequenter of bars and dives.

Origins and Family: First of three, southern rural family of Scotch-Irish extraction. Both parents and one sibling died of tuberculosis when this boy was in his early teens. He spent a year or two with relatives, then became a tramp and had roamed the country at will for half a dozen years.

Mental History, Achievement: Left school in the eighth grade after a mediocre record. IQ reports fall between 80 and 85, here called 83, or about dull normal. He gives a first impression of better mentality, has a little of the Will Rogers personality, but there seems to be no mental purchase. His mind is like a fairly active compass needle that never quite comes to rest.

No vocational plan. He is an accomplished barroom entertainer, banjo player, singer of hill-billy songs, and moocher. The AMI is easily summarized in the short sentence, "He's got everything." The engaging smile, the southern accent, the towering and perfectly poised physique, the halo of mystery—these are too much for most men and he plays havoc with women of all ages.

Medical: Early medical history not known. He was repeatedly examined for tuberculosis both before and after our contact with him. No trace of that disease found. No known injuries or illnesses of any kind. PX reveals no significant pathology. He is a splendid specimen of mesomorphy, even to the details of good teeth and good eyesight.

Running Record: His relations with the Inn were almost wholly pleasant. Here at first as a casual vagrant seeking shelter, he returned many times, sometimes staying for several weeks. He always listened courteously to such efforts to convert him to middle class morality as we thought were polite, and he repaid these efforts with jolly entertainment, almost converting some of us to the barroom outlook. He became a well-known character in the lower South End dives, with his guitar and hill-billy songs, and his ten-gallon hat which he passed for nickels and dimes. Here he was never suspected of stealing, and while he was almost always just sufficiently intoxicated for joviality, we never saw him drunk. We always felt a pang of regret when he left, and everybody looked forward to his return. Among young women he left even more enduring monuments to the persuasiveness of his personality. During the seven years or so in which we have known him he has twice married young girls whom he had made pregnant, and after a period of living off the respective families has drifted away. Now known to be the father of at least three children. From a eugenic point of view this may be rejoicable.

When the war came along he was inducted into the service, but military discipline failed to impress him favorably. AWOL many times, he was finally given a discharge and he returned to his old haunts. He has gained 20 or 30 pounds, is perhaps a little more alcoholic, but is reported as otherwise unchanged. There has been no conversion and no dramatic deterioration. He is not regarded as a likely candidate for major crime. Perhaps his irresponsibility borders on criminality.

Summary: Superb mesomorphy of towering stature and excellent health. Dull normal or almost average mentality. No indications of first- or second-order psychopathy. Persistent vagrancy and irresponsibility. Never a thief.

ID 1–1–1 (3)
Insufficiencies:
    IQ 1
    Mop ....
Psychiatric:
    1st order ....
    2nd order 1
        C-penic irresponsibility
        (3–1–1)
    C-phobic ....

G-phrenic ....
Residual D:
    Primary crim. 1

Comment: Prognosis guarded. He seems to want to become a bum in the end. Psychiatric clinics to which he has been referred offer no more than the religious reiterations which happen to be the fashion of the moment. These tend to blame the ills of mankind on the failure of bewildered parents to achieve somebody or other's ideal of a monogamous family. Adam and Eve once encountered similar difficulties and they too have absorbed a modicum of blame. The difficulty is that such a failure is only a symptom, or a ramification of simpler and more fundamental failure. To explain personality difficulties in terms of the imperfect human family is like attributing failure to hit the moon to bad aiming of the gun. The family itself, as just now conceived, may be one of the worst of human delinquencies, and persistent promulgation of *that* delinquency might offer as rational an explanation of a youth's defections as would be contained in any specific analysis of his early and late relations with members of his particular family. This is suggested not as a hypothesis, but merely as something to think about.

134. COMPANY B, PLATOON 1, SECTION 3
Second-Order Psychopathy; Uncomplicated: Nos. 133–143

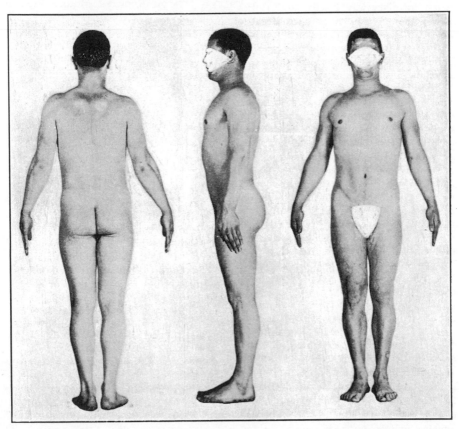

Description: Somatotype 3½–5½–2. A 21-year-old mesomorph five inches above average stature. A powerful, superbly developed physique. Stalwart mesomorphy smoothly buttressed with latent endomorphy. No apparent weaknesses or dysplasias. Primary and secondary $g\pm$. Primary t 4, secondary t 4. Features strong, well molded, cleanly chiseled, although the face is a trifle too large and has a trace of puffiness. General and hand strength 4. Excellent coordination. He looks and handles himself like a movie hero. Probably too slow and easy-going for first-rate athletic competition. Rarely pugnacious or truculent, but he is reported to be an efficient fighter when provoked. We never saw him provoked.

Temperament: Predominantly cerebrotonic. He is normally quiet, watchful, tight-lipped. He is self-conscious and hyperattentional, with a restrained voice that is difficult to follow. But he is not always true to this pattern. There are periods of somatorotic disturbance, when he gives way briefly, and rather unconvincingly, to a sort of reckless abandon. In these periods he apparently forgets that he is an ectomorph and behaves for the moment like a buccaneering mesomorph. (Probably all healthy ectomorphs *dream* of doing that sort of thing. This one lives out the dream from time to time.) When the somatorotic mood is on his nostrils expand, the face takes on a haughty expression, as if he were a medieval prince, the voice becomes austere, ringing, and full. His mesomorphic first region takes over and for the moment he is living on the grand scale, with paranoid austerity the predominant *motif*. During such moments he usually does something that later will require patient and remorseful undoing. He has a good voice for singing but, being cerebrotonic, of course cannot sing in public. When the somatorotic mood is on, though, he can pour it out for a moment or two as if such a thing as cerebrotonia never existed. Another thing he does in the somatorotic mood is recklessly throw away friendships and loyalties—for he is then a scornful and overriding prince. In consequence he has been called changeable and untrustworthy. The expansive moods are of irregular occurrence, but there may be as many as half a dozen such moods in the course of a month. ψ 1–3–1.

Delinquency: Good early school history with no record of truancy—rare in this series. Arrested for stealing at 12. Several repetitions of stealing between 12 and 15. Larceny at 15 and sent to correctional school. Half a dozen further episodes of stealing between 15 and 20. Four times returned to correctional institutions. He says he steals when the "big mood" is on.

Origins and Family: First of two extramarital children. Father described as the black sheep from a good family, Old American. Called "a cutup who was hell on women." Mother French-English and described as a pretty girl. She came from a rural family in which there is no record of delinquency other than the illegitimacy indicated. Parents later lived together until the boy was 3, then separated. Boy sent to a foster home under agency management. He remained in one home until 16, when both foster parents died. He then appears to have embarked on a spree of delinquency.

Mental History, Achievement: Completed two years of high school with fair grades. IQ reports range narrowly between 100 and 112, here called 105.

Vocational ambition that of becoming a professional singer, and despite the obvious cerebrotonia he had been encouraged in such a plan by adult acquaintances. The AMI that of a tall, pale, aristocratic-looking youth who, except in the somatorotic mood, suggests drawing rooms and afternoon tea rather than jails.

Medical: Early history not known. No record of any illnesses or injuries. Apparently he has enjoyed excellent health. PX reveals no significant pathology. He has well-formed hands and feet, good teeth and good vision—rare in this series.

Running Record: At the Inn he at first was quietly defiant, liked to leave the impression of being a kind of "lone highwayman." His somatorotic episodes were quite clearly demarcated and usually occurred on warm evenings. In the more reasonable mood his main interest was in singing. We tried to encourage this as an amateur hobby; to discourage it as a professional aim. It was thought worth while to send him to a famous school for voice training, and his reaction to the inevitable disappointment in this experience (inevitable, probably, in every case of predominant third component) was a sharp one. For a short time after this he went on a kind of binge of prowling and drinking—probably did some stealing, although he was not caught. The Inn tolerated the reaction, persuaded other agencies to do likewise. We empathised the tragedy poignantly enough—there may be no greater human tragedy than that of being *almost* a singer. For a time the boy was regarded as deteriorating. With the peculiar attraction for homosexuals that a high *t* component carries, he was suspected of indulging in the racket of prostitution in that field, although he showed no *DAMP RAT* characteristics and therefore the problem of homosexuality did not worry us. (It did, however, worry a psychiatrist to whom he was referred.)

After about a year of contact with the Inn he seemed to have burned off his predilection to delinquent behavior and showed some curiosity about himself. He then entered into a series of discussions or conferences which led to an expression of what appeared to be a degree of insight into himself. Shortly thereafter he joined the maritime service, where until the end of the war he made a good record. During the half-dozen years since he left the Inn he has committed no delinquent acts so far as is known. He seems not yet to have found a satisfactory vocational pattern, but from the point of view of criminality he can be considered as being entirely reformed.

Summary: Tall ectomorph with high *t,* good coordination, and a mesomorphically dysplastic first region. Mentality better than average. Good health. Second-order somatorotic psychopathy with an episodal pattern. A kleptoid difficulty which seems to have cleared up abruptly.

ID 0–3–0 (3)
  Insufficiencies:
    IQ . . . .
    Mop . . . .
  Psychiatric:
    1st order . . . .
    2nd order   3
      Episodically somatorotic
      (1–3–1)
    C-phobic . . . .
    G-phrenic . . . .
  Residual D:
    Primary crim. . . . .

Comment: Outlook probably good. Considered very good so far as active delinquency goes. Possibly good from the point of view of the general development and usefulness of the boy, although that hope may be as fatuous as it is faint. He has reneged with enthusiasm on the idea of returning to school. The case might be presented as a good example of environmental delinquency, for it is highly probable that the familial mess played a role in the motivation of the delinquency; but there is more in the picture than that, and we need to bring up into daylight the dark continent which is the pattern of the man himself. We could say, I think, that such a background would have made many a man delinquent. Possibly it would have driven most men to some kind of crime, although I would not go so far as to affirm that. Certainly there are some who would never have responded by stealing and by breaking into enough houses to be sent four times to correctional institutions.

This youth is of peculiar interest because of being both a well-developed and a pronounced ectomorph, in fact the only one in the series. The fully blossomed ectomorphic constitution is encountered on the Harvard and other college campuses in droves but at the Inn it was a great rarity (see p. 729). Note that this boy, although an extreme ectomorph, is free from the asthenic characteristic and (therefore?) shows no trace of the third psychiatric component.

135.

COMPANY B, PLATOON 1, SECTION 3
Second-Order Psychopathy; Uncomplicated:
Nos. 133–143

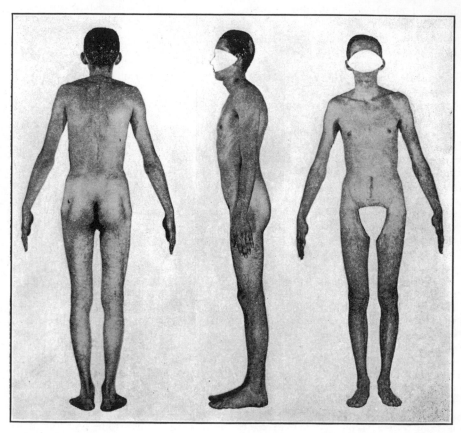

Description: Somatotype 1½–2½–6½. A 20-year-old well-developed ecto-morph five inches above average stature. A physique uniformly ectomorphic except in the first region where there is a dramatic increment of mesomor-phy. He has the neck of a more mesomorphic physique. Arms *not* asthenic. Primary and secondary *g*±. Primary *t* 3, secondary *t* 4. Features fine, regular, strongly developed—a handsome face. General strength 2, hand strength 4 (165 lbs. grip strength in each hand). Good example of peripherotonic strength (see p. 29). Coordination excellent. He moves gracefully, throws well, good at minor games. Not good at fighting.

Temperament: Predominantly somatotonic with frequent minor outbursts of violent or somatorotic impatience. He has excessive physical energy poorly controlled—has been called "temperamental." He often becomes truculent and is frequently challenged and forced to back down, perhaps after furious verbal combat. Little evidence of inhibition, and little natural restraint manifest in any field. There seems to be a constitutional cerebropenia. When well fed he shows a rich underlying viscerotonia, has good orientation to people, and easy communication of feeling; is greedy, dependent, eager for affection and approval. The temperament probably reflects the physical endowment accurately, with overloading in energy. ψ 3–1–1.

Delinquency: Early incorrigibility in foster homes, truancy, violent outbursts of temper with destructiveness. A ruthlessly persistent early sexual aggressiveness, beginning at about age 12 and resulting five years later in the diagnosis "moral delinquent" at a local psychiatric clinic. At 19, a failure in school and a waster or drifter, with delinquent associates. No record of stealing, however, and regarded as only on the verge of serious delinquency.

Origins and Family: Fourth of eight, urban family. Father Old American, of average stature and medium build. He was an artisan for many years but has been an intermittent drunkard and deserted the family at the time of the death of the mother when our boy was 6. The paternal relatives are a healthy lot, apparently of solid middle class stock. Mother of Old American and Scandinavian extraction, and a large, muscular woman who through a period of eight years after marriage gave birth to one child a year, seemed to remain "strong as an ox," then suddenly died, apparently of apoplexy, in the middle thirties. The maternal grandmother, of about the same physique, followed the same course. She produced eight children within nine years, then suddenly died in her mid-thirties. Most of the maternal relatives are very large people. One cousin confined in a state mental hospital. Boy reared in the home until 6, then in a long series of foster homes under agency control.

Mental History, Achievement: Finished high school, entered a local college, failed out during the first year. IQ reports range from 120 to 132, here called 125. He gives the impression of sharp, incisive mentality which has been poorly disciplined. Reactions are fast and accurate, general information and vocabulary excellent, but he is not in the habit of thinking problems through. Shows poor insight and poor judgment on occasions.

No vocational plan. Drifting and confused for two years. A good ball player but not quite good enough for professional competition. He plays one or two musical instruments, likes jazz, does well on mechanical aptitude tests. The AMI that of an obviously intelligent but self-centered and undisciplined youth who is violently impatient and seems to have ants in his trousers.

Medical: Normal birth and development history. No serious illnesses or injuries. PX reveals no significant pathology.

Running Record: Through several years of intermittent association at the Inn he remained somatorotic, especially with respect to sexuality, and was occasionally alcoholic. He made numerous false starts at programs and was often a disappointment but he showed no signs of deterioration, was involved in no major delinquency, and within the limits of what seemed to be an essential irresponsibility he got along. Because of the comparatively high IQ he was taken in hand by one of our staff who maintained a close contact with him for several years. The boy strained the patience of a patient man, although in the end he seems to have responded. He was twice returned to college on the school program with the result that he eventually finished one year, doing well in mathematics and mechanics. He was then placed in a defense job but spent the $80 a week as fast as he got it.

Finally he was inducted into military service. There he got along and seemed to have a good time, meanwhile starting a family. Following the war he was settled down to a job which for two years now he has held successfully.

Summary: Endomorphic mesomorphy with some athletic ability, excellent health, and better than college average mentality. Somatorotic, irresponsible, on the fringe of delinquency. Good military adjustment.

ID 0–3–0 (3)
> Insufficiencies:
> > IQ ....
> > Mop ....
> Psychiatric:
> > 1st order ....
> > 2nd order 3
> > > *Somatorotic (3–1–1)*
> > C-phobic ....
> > G-phrenic ....
> Residual D:
> > Primary crim. ....

Comment: Outlook probably good so far as delinquency is concerned, although this youth has disappointed the original hope of the Inn. He was considered potentially good college material and an attempt was made to cajole or inveigle him into applying himself to educational objectives. Instead, he is now applying himself vigorously and with success to reproductive objectives. The problem here seems to have been restlessness arising from somatorosis. On one side he comes from very large, and in this case apoplectic stock.

A strikingly large proportion of the somatorotic delinquents of the series have this same kind of organic background. Apparently the mean weight, particularly of the mothers of these boys, is far above the mean for the general population. Many of the delinquent mesomorphs come from tremendous mothers. A direct relationship between mesomorphy of forebears and delinquency is unlikely, but there may be a relationship between the former factor and somatorosis, especially in cases where the offspring inherited the energy of the parent but without developing quite the corresponding grossness and vigor of body. This may be an instance of a "syndrome" which could be called *disappointed mesomorphic expectancy*.

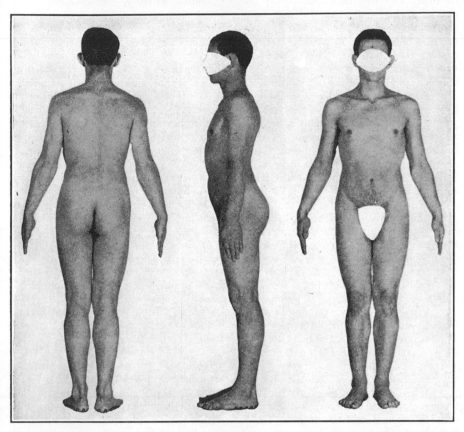

Description: Somatotype 4–4½–2. A 21-year-old endomorphic mesomorph of average stature. A dysmorphic and moderately gynandroid physique with a very heavy skeleton. Muscular development in the first region
and in the arms and chest has fallen a little behind the bony structure. At
one stage the Potter seems to have had extreme mesomorphy in mind. Primary g+1, secondary g±. Primary t 2, secondary t 2. Features prominent
and rather badly molded. Hands and feet coarse. General strength 4, hand
strength 3. Coordination excellent. He moves with the smooth muscular balance of the cat family and is a fairly good natural athlete although he has
too much gynandromorphy for effective fighting.

Temperament: Unrestrained, assertive, loud. Vocally truculent and psychologically callous to an extreme degree. Viscerotonically and somatotonically extraverted; well oriented to people, relaxed, fond of comfort and of food. The first two components are overwhelmingly dominant, but also there are signs of cerebrotonic interference. The voice is harshly strained despite its loudness—it has a strident quality whenever the boy seems to encounter the least trace of opposition. The eyes are hypermotile and there is a sharp watchfulness, like that of the predators. The pattern seems to be one of temperamental overloading, with most of the emphasis on the first two components. He gives the impression of a slightly manic tendency and of a paranoid trend. ψ 5–2–1.

Delinquency: Early history of violent temper tantrums and of destructiveness. Early school truancy. Destructiveness and stealing in school between 8 and 13. One teacher commented that he had too much energy. Frequent runaway between 12 and 17, and during these years many episodes of stealing. A participant in vigorous intrafamilial warfare from about the age of 9. Carried on guerilla warfare with parents for eight or nine years. Sent to correctional schools for stealing, at 14, but promptly ran away. At 16, stole a large sum in another city and was sent to a state mental hospital for a period of observation. Diagnosed *not psychotic.*

Origins and Family: Second of two, urban family, both parents Jewish from Poland. Father short and very heavy, described as "energetic, irritable and tyrannical." Has very high blood pressure. He has done fairly well with his small business, has been in and out of hospitals for many years with such diagnoses as *psychoneurosis* and *neurasthenia.* Mother also short and very

heavy, described as "energetic, aggressive, overbearing." Boy reared at home and he too seems to have been energetic and overbearing in an overenergized family where nobody knew how to hit.

Mental History, Achievement: Finished two years of high school despite himself. IQ reports range from 102 to 115, here called 110. He gives the impression of possessing adequate, practical mentality. He is alert, watchful, and when he wants to be is adaptively reactive. No trace of psychotic disorientation. No intellectual interests.

No vocational indentification and no plan other than that of successful prosecution of the warfare with the parents. The AMI that of a tremendously energized, overgrown Jewish boy who has good native intelligence and is obviously harmless from a physical point of view.

Medical: Normal birth and good developmental history. Walked and talked at 1 year. Weighed "about 40 pounds" at 13 months—a pediatric triumph. No record of serious illnesses or injuries. Defective vision. PX reveals no further pathology except flat feet and moderately elevated blood pressure.

Running Record: At the Inn he resolutely declined to participate in the work program, associated with the most delinquent group, ran up bills with local tradesmen, was suspected of stealing. Meanwhile he spent much energy and time proselyting the staff and boys to an orthodox Freudian interpretation of the origins, causes, and previous course of his war with his family. In the main he seemed to be right, too. The Freudians got their basic philosophy of life from the study of just such families.

Following a conference of psychiatrists, it was decided to let the boy be sent to one of the state correctional schools where he could be closely supervised and could be protected from all contact with his parents. He thus escaped finally from the home nest. After a year of detention he announced that he had had a good time—that he approved of the school. Exempt from military service because of his record, he then entered upon a job in a war industry; for three years now appears to have got along satisfactorily on his own. Meanwhile he has burgeoned out into a "very handsome 200-pounder."

Summary: A big gynandroid endomorph of great energy and no fighting ability. Normal mentality; good health; second-order psychopathy suggestive of both a manic and a paranoid tendency. Delinquency secondary to intrafamilial warfare.

ID 0–3–0 (3)
  Insufficiencies:
    IQ ....
    Mop ....
  Psychiatric:
    1st order ....
    2nd order   3
      (5–2–1)
    C-phobic ....
    G-phrenic ....
  Residual D:
    Primary crim. ....

Comment: Outlook good, at least from a police point of view. There was a period of singularly persistent criminality in his history, but the permanent or enduring pathological characteristic seems to be temperamental, not criminological. He is somatorotic, manic to a degree, paranoid to a degree. Loaded with energy and therefore with aggressiveness, but helpless at physical combat, he can no more conform to a conventional Anglo-Saxon or Irish stereotype of masculine comportment than a dolphin can frolic with collies. He makes war with his lungs and with fierce gestures; only as a last resort with the slapping palm. That is hard for an Irishman to understand.

With the advent of success and prosperity in his family, during the past decade, quite an effort was made to force a new outlook on this physically exuberant youth who is but one generation removed from Polish peasantry. He was cajoled into dancing classes, into listening with hypnotic ecstasy to "noises made on musical instruments." He didn't care for these things, and he "told the old bitch to go to hell." In his home there was never any discipline; no dependable order of punishment; only loud castigation and bribery. The one method for getting the boy to do something was to offer bribe compounded on bribe. The method for stopping him was to outyell him. Parents and child seem to have been more or less on an equal footing from the time when the latter could talk. The boy's delinquency, he himself readily explains (having been told so by half a dozen psychiatrists and by fifty ordinary people), was a way of striking at the parents. The general pattern is frequently enough encountered also in non-Jewish families where heavy bodied, vigorously energized but noncombative somatotypes prevail. Such characteristics are not "racial" unless the underlying organic structure is racial.

COMPANY B, PLATOON 1, SECTION 3
Second-Order Psychopathy; Uncomplicated:
Nos. 133–143

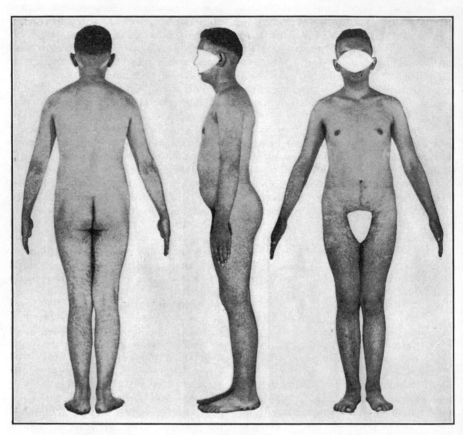

Description: Somatotype 5–3½–2½. A 17-year-old mesomorphic endomorph four inches above average stature. A very large, overgrown youth
with well-balanced segmental development and no particular dysplasias.
This is a physique which may become tremendously heavy in later life. Primary $g+1$, secondary $g+1$. Primary t 3, secondary t 2. Gross, prominent features of blobby shape. Coarse skin. Hands small, weak, and poorly formed;
feet extremely flat and weak. Distal segments of arms and legs poorly muscled although heavy boned. Hair approaches the consistency of steel wool.
Heavy muscling in the trunk and thighs. General strength 3, hand strength
2. Coordination fairly good. He moves smoothly and with agility. Inept at
all games and at fighting. His hitting power is perhaps no greater than that
of the average woman of his weight. Good slapping power.

Temperament: Superabundant energy is the predominant characteristic. He is heavily endowed with both viscerotonia and somatotonia but shows no overt indications of any interference from the third component. He seems rarely to get anything done because some *other* activity always interferes. He is adventurous, dominating, personally overwhelming. He is also relaxed, comfort-loving and amiable—all to a high degree. There is no cycloid tendency. He steadily maintains a high level of energy expenditure and appears to have the physical structure to stand up under the terrific strain which his heavy somatotonic endowment puts upon it—as a tennis ball stands up under the play. If pathology is present in this temperament it must be a question of pathological cerebropenia. ψ 4–1–1.

Delinquency: History of excessive truancy before 10. At 12 he was a frequent runaway and was often a juvenile bum or vagrant. Between 12 and 15, picked up several times by police in distant states as a runaway and juvenile vagrant. Many episodes of minor stealing during the adolescent period; one charge of forgery at 15. He spent two years in state correctional schools between 14 and 17. At 16, sent to military school but he deserted after a brief stay. Several times in trouble for alcoholism and vagrancy between 17 and 21, and called destructive or violent when drunk.

Origins and Family: Extramarital, father unknown. Mother a strongly built French-Canadian woman who immediately turned the boy over to an agency. Boy adopted shortly after birth, but both foster parents died when he was about 10. He was then taken over by agencies and reared in foster homes.

Mental History, Achievement: Finished one year of high school with low grades. Started military school, also courses in welding, in electrical work, in nursing, and in embalming; always quit after a few weeks. He starts many things but soon gives up, always good naturedly. He has been like a bird dog who, after being put on the trail of game, is soon observed pointing field mice. IQ reports range narrowly in the region of 100. He appears to be of just about average mentality. Social intelligence is excellent. He is well oriented to people, possesses a keen sense of the best inital approach to different kinds of personalities in order to get what he wants.

No vocational plan or ambition except that of having a good time. The AMI rests on good nature, geniality. He is round-faced and round-bodied, jovial, Dionysian. Everybody likes him, especially before he begins to borrow.

Medical: Infancy history not known. No record of serious illnesses or injuries. Never hospitalized except for intermittent venereal infections. PX reveals no significant pathology except carious teeth.

Running Record: At the Inn he appeared to have a rollicking good time and in general he paid his way by being an amiable and entertaining character. He absorbed "social service" readily, maintained friendly relations with nearly everybody, and succeeded in getting along with an astonishingly slight compromise with his essential distaste for work. His identification seemed not to be with delinquency in an active or positive sense, but only in the negative and literal sense. He had experienced no inner reform or conversion. He was satisfied with his irresponsible pattern of life and proposed to continue in it. He had a firm hold on one hind udder and proposed to hang on. During his stay at the Inn he showed ability as a politician both in his relations with other boys and in those with the staff. He adroitly handled at least four different social agencies, playing one off against another, and thus living reasonably well without the humiliation of meniality in any guise. He gave us the general impression of being too good a politician ever to have to work very hard, and his native intelligence seemed more than adequate for a political career. However, he had little resistance to alcohol and his sights were low. Whenever things appeared to be going well with him he was fairly certain to turn up drunk within a day or two. He was lazy, indolent, refused to project his consciousness more than a few hours into the future. Perhaps he was a moral moron.

After continuing for another year in the general pattern described, he was involved in court difficulties following a series of alcoholic episodes and left this vicinity, later communicating from another eastern state. There he was exempted from military training because of the previous record, and for another five years appears to have got along without further serious difficulty. He does not work very hard, is not thrifty, has accumulated much avoirdupois, together with a wife and children, and he may be said to be doing well. He is also said to be somewhat immoderately alcoholic.

Summary: A massive endormorph-mesomorph with Dionysian cerebropenia. Good health and normal mentality. Rollicking or irresponsibly exploitative way of life with incidental delinquency and mild alcoholism.

ID o–4–o (4)
  Insufficiencies:
    IQ ....
    Mop ....
  Psychiatric:
    1st order ....
    2nd order 3
      Dionysian C-penia (4–1–1)
    C-phobic 1
    G-phrenic ....
  Residual D:
    Primary crim. ....

Comment: Outlook probably good from the standpoint of delinquency; poor from that of civic responsibility and of the Methodist virtues. In a few years the endomorphy will have blossomed like a magnolia and then the tempo of his life may slow down to a complacent amble. It is a reasonably safe bet that the alcoholism will then diminish spontaneously. I think that alcohol rarely becomes a serious problem in the presence of an extreme natural cerebropenia.

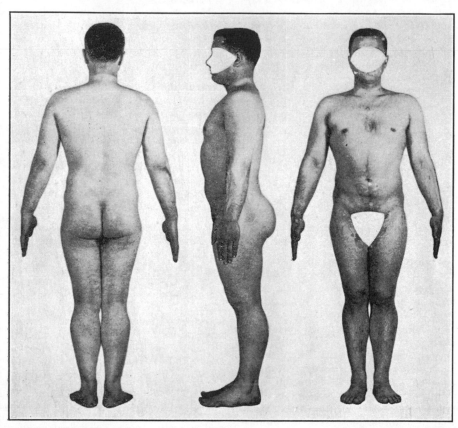

Description: Somatotype 5–5–1. A 21-year-old endomorph-mesomorph an inch under average stature. The neck is slender for the somatotype and the waist is high. Long, heavily muscled trunk with endomorphic legs. A well-proportioned, well-molded balloon-tire physique in its general lines. Primary $g+1$, secondary $g\pm$. Primary t 3, secondary t 3. Features strongly developed and regular but pudgy. Broad, round moon face. General strength 3, hand strength 2. Coordination very good—he gets around with agility. Too soft for successful fighting or for serious athletic competition. This might be called a tennis-ball physique because of the great bounce and buoyancy, in contrast with the tougher and harder golf-ball physiques of the mesomorphs with lower endomorphy.

Temperament: A case of astonishing somatorosis. Despite his ineffectuality and awkwardness he is tirelessly hyperactive and into things like a colony of ants. He has a *persona* of stubborn defiance and lives up to it with remarkable energy. Social workers, thinking him frail, try to pet him whereupon he buzzes like an infuriated wasp. He is irresponsible, wants to play, is not interested in tomorrow or even in this afternoon. He shows a peculiarly jagged somatotonic assertiveness rather than the cerebrotonic restraint that might be expected from a quick look at the photograph. Despite the big and crude bones the somatotype photograph appears to insist that he is an ectomorph. If this is so, the expressed temperamental pattern seems to reverse the morphological dominance. But I think it would be well to watch this boy for a couple of decades before insisting that such a reversal has in fact taken place. ψ 1–3–1.

Delinquency: Remarkably persistent early truancy and frequent running away before the age of 10. At 11 he ran away and was picked up in a distant western city, repeating the experience four or five times within the succeeding three years. At 14, arrested for "improper advances" toward little girls. At 14 and 15, a few episodes of minor stealing, but only of the most petty sort. Frequently in trouble for vagrancy. After 15, no active delinquency except that of running away and of uninhibited sexual curiosity.

Origins and Family: Second of three, urban family. Father English and a slender, frail man who has always been a clerk and has a reputable history. Mother an energetic woman of French-Canadian extraction who is said to have been a juvenile delinquent before marriage. She deserted after the birth of the third child, then became "alcoholic, immoral, irresponsible." Children reared by relatives. Both the other siblings have been involved in delinquency.

Mental History, Achievement: Finished the eight grade with a poor record. IQ reports vary from 78 to 114, here put at 95. He gives an impression of alertness but of mental inadequacy, or silly superficiality.

No vocational plan, no special interests or abilities. The AMI that of a pathetic, unwashed, poorly coordinated youth who rather increases his appeal by his "manly" defiance.

Medical: No serious illnesses or injuries. History of enuresis which stopped at 12. A hyperactive, nervous child. Psychiatric referral when he was 8 elicited the diagnosis *nervous child*. PX reveals no significant pathology except carious, badly formed teeth. He has remarkable strength for the physique and defines a good antithesis to the asthenic characteristic.

Running Record: His performance at the Inn was at least interesting to watch. He identified himself with a delinquent pattern, set up a *persona* of toughness and endeavored with singular persistence to live up to it. He boasted of imaginary holdups, claimed heroic proficiency at the art of rape, often attempted to drink and suffered abysmally in consequence. Alcohol always produced emesis. He engaged to his utmost in somatorotic vocal disputation about the lobby, shirked work assignments, tried hard to be a pest, but he was so amusing a pest that no hand and scarcely a voice was raised against him.

During his stay he experienced a sort of religious conversion, announced the intention of becoming a missionary, seemed to emerge from his negativism for a time and to give up the Robin Hood struggle for recognition as a delinquent. He even attempted to return to school on an educational program, although this effort soon petered out. When he left, the mood for reform still prevailed. We carried him on the records for a time as "a success."

However, the good intentions lasted only for a few months and then he was a vagrant again. Within the past six years he has wandered back and forth across the country many times, resting up for a few months after each voyage. Exempt from military service, he has held a number of jobs for short periods, was married some time ago and is now a father. He has gained about 25 pounds, now presents a more substantial and more mesomorphic appearance than he did when photographed. He is apparently having a good time of life. At last report he was "looking for a job" and was trying to borrow money from a social agency to "prevent the loss of his automobile." Except for the vagrancy there has been no delinquency of record since our first contact with him.

Summary: Mesomorphic ectomorph with comparatively heavy skeletal structure and low primary *t*. Normal subaverage mentality. Enuretic and somatorotic history but good general health. Persistent vagrancy.

ID 1–3–0 (4)
  Insufficiencies:
    IQ ....
    Mop 1
  Psychiatric:
    1st order ....
    2nd order 3
      Somatorotic, with possible reversal of a morphological dominance (1–3–1)
    C-phobic ....
    G-phrenic ....

Residual D:
  Primary crim. ....

Comment: Outlook possibly good. He may live long and have a lot of fun. First-order psychopathy can be ruled out, since there has been no history of attentional divagation. Insufficiency of IQ is not involved. Health in the strictly clinical sense can be called good except for enuresis, and this disorder may derive from cerebropenia rather than from any more specific physiological cause. The boy is "constitutionally inadequate" in some fundamental sense, and there may be no role in life where the inadequacy would not make itself felt. Even with an IQ of 150 he might be unable to make an ordinary adaptation.

He seems to be constitutionally somatorotic. That might account for the vagrancy, to some extent, but not for the slovenly ineffectuality, the lifelong history of failure, the inadequate physical development and bad coordination. He has some degree of deepseated physiological insufficiency which appears to be more fundamental than an endocrine dyscrasia, more general than a central nervous system defect. Some day we may be able to describe such a picture in terms of its underlying chemistry, but probably not until psychology—the description of the behaving organism as a whole—has taken long strides toward developing the same kind of operational frame of reference that has made chemistry useful. We still need a periodic table for temperament.

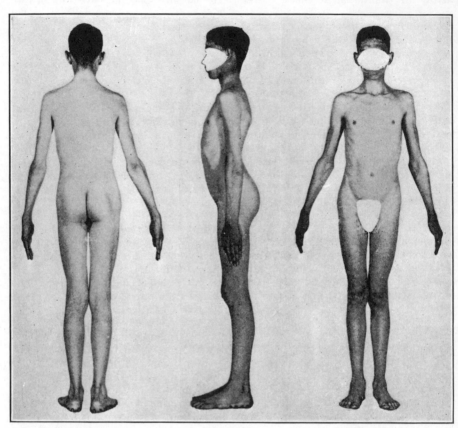

Description: Somatotype 1½–2½–6. A 16-year-old mesomorphic or dys-morphic ectomorph two inches above average stature. Immature physique for 16. Superficially he looks helpless but the bones and joints are heavy enough for mesomorphy. Note the heavy elbows and knees. Apparently a case of arrested mesomorphy. No trace of asthenic flaccidity. Muscle development scanty throughout the physique, yet energy is high and well sustained. Primary $g\pm$, secondary g, no trace. He is hard like a little hickory nut. Primary t 1, secondary t 2. Features far too heavy and coarse for the physique as a whole. Nose and ears crudely molded. Hands and feet large and strong. General strength 4, hand strength 4. Coordination poor. He walks as if he were on stilts, throws badly, not at all happy in the gymnasium.

Temperament: The picture is that of high energy without normal inhibition. He is somatorotic in the higest degree, with a harsh stridency of vocalization which surpasseth ordinary imagination. He is hard, harsh, often called paranoid. Somatotonia has the upper hand virtually all the time. Under alcohol he becomes at first even more wildly somatorotic, later depressed and unhappy. He is a disturbing factor in any situation. One of the staff says "that boy's voice cuts like a rusty buzz saw." He is vital, but chaotiç and undisciplined. ψ 2–4–1.

Delinquency: Uncontrollable as an infant; incorrigible as a small boy. Early truancy, mendacity, stealing, and school difficulties before 10. Noisy, tempestuous, and assertive from infancy, yet never able to fight, and there is no record of any delinquency of violence. Minor stealing between 10 and 16. Throughout the half-dozen years before our contact with him he was delinquent in the sense of demanding an enormous amount of attention and care, but free from court delinquency. He had been a disturbing element in every environment. A flagrant disobeyer of rules, he had been smart enough to keep out of serious trouble.

Origins and Family: Third of nine, urban family, both parents immigrant from Italy. Father short, thick and vigorous; at times regarded as a sort of professional exploiter of social agencies. He showed astuteness and vigor during the Volsteadian era. Mother short, hard and wiry, with an early history of minor delinquency and carried by one agency as "feebleminded." Many of the maternal relatives are delinquent. The record of the immediate family as a whole shows between forty and fifty agency contacts since the birth of this boy, who was reared in the home. On one hospital record there is the comment "This family is over-hospitalized . . . often as many as four or five of them here at one time." One agency has more than three hundred pages of records on three of the siblings.

Mental History, Achievement: Graduated from high school after a stormy history of truancy, running away, and minor delinquency, but with fairly good grades. He then drifted for four or five years. IQ reports range from 102 to 116, here called 110. Of his essential intelligence there was never any question. He gives the impression of astute mental alertness, is watchful and sharp, seems to know what he wants. His language is replete with Freudian terminology and he is a veteran of hundreds of hours of psychiatric consultation, having been followed closely by one clinic for half a dozen years.

Vocational plan. To be a musician. He has some talent in this direction, had already been on several programs of training before our contact with him. The AMI is based on his really outstanding history with social agencies, medical clinics, psychiatrists, and rehabilitation programs. He is sufficiently intelligent and sufficiently vigorous to impress people favorably.

Medical: Normal birth and early development. History of more than forty hospital contacts arising from children's diseases, pneumonia, sensory defects, abscesses and infections, many minor accidents, half a dozen operations, and psychiatric referrals. Numerous psychiatric diagnoses arranged around the recurrent terms *anxiety neurosis* and *psychoneurosis*. PX reveals scoliosis, flat feet, dental caries.

Running Record: At the Inn he was difficult to handle—a noisy and disorganizing influence, tempestuous and destructive. Yet he was unquestionably bright and from the beginning it was clear that within the limits of his own outlook he had a certain integrity of purpose. He was put on the college program, a special piano was provided for him, and arrangements were made to continue his training in music. In the course of six months he virtually destroyed the piano. At one count 68 cigarette burns were found on it, the front was torn off (so that it would make more noise), many keys were broken. In the words of one of the staff he seemed to use the piano "more as a dummy for bayonet practice than as a musical instrument." For him music appeared to offer primarily a medium of expression for his violent somatorosis. He was too impatient to learn to play anything all the way through, and it became clear during the course of two years that music was offering him not a vocational future but a channel for the untrammeled expression of aggression. Meanwhile in his college work he got along, despite outbursts of temper and violent critical reactions. He managed continually to give the impression of being on the verge of cracking up, yet some of us had the feeling that he had matters pretty well in hand and that in his way he was having a good time.

Exempt from military service on medical grounds, he finished college in due time, gave up the idea of music as a profession, quickly married, and went to work at a white-collar job. For four years now he seems to have done very well and is regarded as a success.

Summary: Timberline mesomorphy with excessive energy and poor coordination. Somatorotic temperament. Mentality well above average; vigorous general health despite minor ailments. Early delinquency of a minor and probably irrelevant nature.

ID 1–3–0 (4)
Insufficiencies:
  IQ ....
  Mop 1
Psychiatric:
  1st order ....
  2nd order 3
  (2–4–1)
  C-phobic ....
  G-phrenic ....
Residual D:
  Primary crim. ....

Comment: Outlook apparently good, and there may never have been anything more seriously wrong with him than what one of my colleagues used to call "a normal Italian somatorosis." Certainly music did not offer him an optimal vocation, and once he arrived at a decision to abandon that ambition, the somatorotic pressure seemed to subside appreciably. Prior to our contact with him he had for nearly a decade been in very close association with psychiatrists and psychoanalysts. Once when asked his occupation he replied, "talking with psychiatrists." It is possible that the psychiatrists "saved him," and that to them belongs the credit for the comparatively good outcome of the case. Yet the real improvement in his behavior seems to have been associated with his escape from psychiatrists and with the awakening and implementation of a desire to get through college. Whether the happy awakening took place because of or despite the psychiatry we are not now able to say. Perhaps in another decade the boy himself will be able to answer that. In any event here is a case of troubled Italian somatorosis of the first water on which psychiatry, time, maturation, the Inn, or Mr. G has poured quieting oil.

140. COMPANY B, PLATOON 1, SECTION 3
Second-Order Psychopathy; Uncomplicated: Nos. 133–143

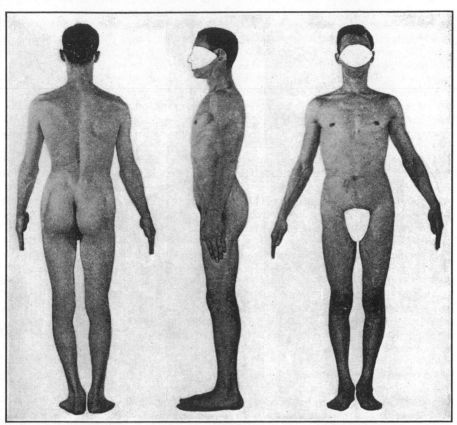

Description: Somatotype 1½–5–3½. A 22-year-old Italian mesomorph of average stature, with secondary ectomorphy. An example of the "timberline" (see p. 23) characteristic often seen in Italian mesomorphs. Heavy bones but the distal segments of the legs are brittle and there is a suggestion of sharp angularity throughout. The physique as a whole is so tense and strained that the boy seems nearly spastic. Primary g±—a strong trace; secondary g, no trace. Waist slightly high with a gynic flare at the hips. He presents a good antithesis to secondary g with his rock-quarry body surface and prominent superficial blood vessels. Primary t 3, secondary t 2. Features illformed and asymmetrical. Expression lowering-paranoid or threatening. Hands and feet large and crude. General strength 4, hand strength 3. Coordination rather poor. Of enormous bodily energy but unable to express it smoothly. Movements jerky or harsh. Not good at athletics or at fighting.

Temperament: Somatorotic, or harshly and jaggedly somatotonic. It is a violent, stormy temperament showing little trace of "free" viscerotonia; no signs of comfortable relaxation. He is strident, wrathful, strained. Long history of gastrointestinal oversensitivity. Tolerates alcohol badly—it makes him ugly and violent rather than smoothly extraverted. A clinician's first question would be, Where is the ulcer? This is one example, or one kind, of the peptic ulcer temperament. ψ 4–2–1.

Delinquency: Early truancy and incorrigibility in school. Described as violent tempered and destructive at 8. Long association with delinquent boys and considered a gang leader at 16. Arrested for armed robbery at 17. Between 17 and 20, numerous brushes with police but never alcoholic and regarded as a canny, elusive youngster.

Origins and Family: Second of four, small urban community. Father French-Canadian. Described as an athletic 200-pounder who led a violent life and died in the mid-thirties of a cardiac ailment. Mother a muscular 200-pound Irish woman who has long been a semi-invalid because of high blood pressure and complications. The family life said to have been one of chronic warfare with occasional light casualties on both sides. Boy reared in the home.

Mental History, Achievement: Finished the eighth grade. Was considered bright by some teachers but lacked the disciplinary adaptation to go to high school and was "too deep in rackets." IQ reports range from 100 to 110, here put at 105. Clearly of average mentality or better.

No vocational plan and no special abilities except that of first-rate athletic strength. The AMI that of a threatening looking youth with the elastic tread of the great cats and the universal passport of extreme mesomorphy.

Medical: Very large baby. Walked and talked at about 12 months. No serious illnesses or injuries. Between 17 and 20, referred to medical clinics by various agencies because of complaints of nervous tension, digestive upsets, stomach pains. No peptic ulcer yet diagnosed. PX reveals no significant pathology. Moderately high blood pressure.

Running Record: At the Inn he was a tough egg—quarrelsome, ruthless, and a terrific fighter. He would sometimes start a quarrel and end it by a knockout blow before the other boy was quite aware of what was going on. He had a hair-trigger temper and in his angry mood was a prodigious destroyer of property. On occasion he threatened members of the staff with annihilation. Other boys reported that he carried a gun but we never saw the gun. Because of his relatively good intelligence we attempted a series of conferences with him and seemed to strike a chord of interest in the business of photographing and describing physical constitutions. He was astonished to discover that in bodily power and agility he fell in the upper 2 per cent of the population. This appeared to result in some degree of quieting down or of relaxation. At any rate his ferocity toward smaller and mesopenic boys decreased. As he grew aware of his true power he seemed to use it a little more discriminatively. When he left he announced an intention of "getting in on the big money in the labor racket."

Exempt from military service because of the delinquent history, he appears to have had a good time through the war boom and he kept out of police hands. He was employed in a succession of defense plants, at one time earned $110 a week. He is married now, seems to have settled down to a steady job, and is no longer considered an active delinquent by police. He once stated that the Inn made a "right guy" of him by showing him his picture.

Summary: Extreme mesomorphy with first-rate fighting and athletic ability. Harsh, somatorotic temperament with an attitude of ferocity. Average or better than average mentality; good general health with premonitory signs pointing toward peptic ulcer. The criminality seems to have been aborted.

ID 1–3–0 (4)
  Insufficiencies:
    IQ ....
    Mop 1
  Psychiatric:
    1st order ....
    2nd order 3
      Somatorotic ferocity (4–2–1)
    C-phobic ....
    G-phrenic ....
  Residual D:
    Primary crim. ....

Comment: Present indications are favorable but with such a personality the prognosis should be guarded, at least until he crosses age 30 and 175 pounds. He has something in common with an ambulant barrel of gunpowder. For a long time there will remain the latent possibility of violent explosion with mortal consequences. He *ought* to develop a clinical case of peptic ulcer and therein will lie his best insurance, for the treatment of ulcer is to exert every medical resource toward marshalling the full enveloping power of the first component. Every effort is made to protect the ulcer patient from irritating influences and usually to fatten him to the limit of his normal capacity. Since peptic ulcer occurs almost exclusively in somatorotic personalities we may perhaps be justified in looking upon ulcer as an important natural deterrent of delinquency. For this youth the favorableness of the prognosis may depend inversely on the degree of resistance to ulceration in his gastric and duodenal mucosae.

141. *COMPANY B, PLATOON 1, SECTION 3*
Second-Order Psychopathy; Uncomplicated: Nos. 133–143

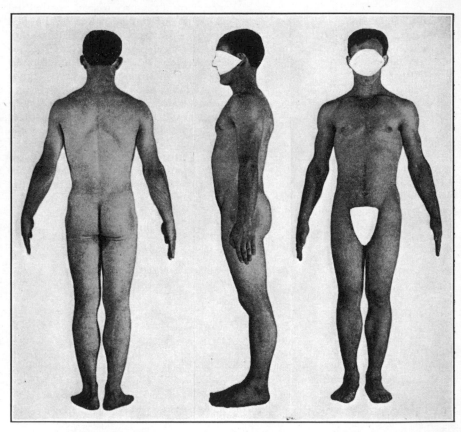

Description: Somatotype 2–7–1. A 20-year-old extreme mesomorph of average stature. Traces of ectomorphy in the face, otherwise no dysplasia. This is a fighter's physique with heavy muscular development throughout. Primary and secondary *g*, no trace. Primary *t* 4, secondary *t* 3. Features rugged and well developed but slightly angular, and the face has a hard, ferocious look. General strength 5, hand strength 4. Coordination excellent. He is a first-rate athlete and fighter, although he probably could not withstand severe punishment in the face—that would be his weakness.

Temperament: A violently impatient and somatorotic personality. He seems always on the verge of turmoil; has a hair-trigger temper, views the world from the vantage point of an Airedale who had been weaned at the wrong moment. No epileptoid or cycloid characteristics. There seems to be no leaven in him, no trace of humor or of sweet compassion. Yet he has high physical energy. All his mannerisms are threatening and he is a hard and effective fighter, striking without preliminary bluster. But there is little *systematic* hostility—not much paranoia. His whole pattern of performance seems to shout down angrily the primary *g*. He has often been called paranoid and one psychiatrist labelled him *paranoid, prepsychotic. ψ* 4–2–1.

Delinquency: Destructiveness and uncontrollability in school and at home, as early as 7. Sent to state correctional school at 12 as a stubborn child. At 14, he assaulted and badly beat a teacher. Sent to correctional school at 15 for "immoral relations"; to another at 18 for robbery. At 19 and 20 he became something of a vagabond and developed a technique of preying on homosexuals, decoying and robbing them, then "giving them a damn good beating." Charge of assault and battery at 20. Dishonorable discharge from CCC for malicious destructiveness and assault and battery. Long history of violence but little or none of furtive theft.

Origins and Family: First of four, suburban family, both parents Scandinavian. Father alcoholic but not otherwise delinquent. Mother very heavy and muscular, described as reliable and honest although somewhat ineffectual. Boy reared in the home until sent to correctional schools.

Mental History, Achievement: Finished high school with low grades. On several school teams and considered an excellent high school athlete. IQ reports fall between 110 and 120, here called 115. He gives the impression of possessing competent or perhaps college average mentality.

No vocational plan other than an ambition to be a champion prize fighter. He had done fairly well in some amateur tournaments. The AMI based on a *persona* of hard realism, or perhaps of objectivity. He has little to say, never smiles, likes things "straight from the shoulder," wants a spade called a soiled shovel. Despite the constant threat of personal violence his manner and address suggest a certain competence and efficiency.

Medical: Early history not available. No record of serious illness or injury. He appears to have enjoyed the best of health. PX reveals no significant pathology. A vigorously healthy youth from biologically good stock.

Running Record: Through several intermittent stays at the Inn he remained tempestuous and rather haughty, like a Viking caught inland. We felt that he was constitutionally sound and psychiatrically salvageable; therefore we made a number of efforts to start him in college on a school program. From these he finally demurred altogether, but he did in the end participate in a series of discussions of his own constitutional endowment, and he became greatly interested in why he was *not quite* of championship material as a fighter. In his later weeks in the House he seemed to relax a little and to reveal more viscerotonia than was at first manifest. But we did not win his confidence entirely. He was like a snapping turtle who finally would protrude the precious neck about a half inch. With his ugly temper he was a great destroyer of property and a wrencher-off of things. He appeared to be expressing an unsatiated or paranoid spite against people in general, but he also appeared to have something to offer. We bore him with such fortitude as we could muster. After starting several programs, and impatiently tossing each aside within a fortnight or less, he decided to migrate to another state and start afresh. For the succeeding year we do not know his adventures in detail, but know that he kept out of trouble. In communications he credited the Inn with "straightening him out."

With the advent of war he was inducted into the service where he remained for the duration. He had a stormy time; was several times punished for insubordination, but in a strictly military sense his record was acceptable. No weakling, he was presumably a good soldier under stress when it mattered. He accumulated a wife, some children later, and following discharge from the service he appears to have settled down to a routinely reputable way of life. He has held a job successfully now for two years.

Summary: Healthy mesomorph of almost extreme degree with good athletic and fighting ability, although with a gynandroid interference. "Ulcer type" somatorosis; persistent early destructiveness and criminality. He seems to have straightened out in the military service.

ID 0–4–0 (4)
Insufficiencies:
  IQ ....
  Mop ....
Psychiatric:
  1st order ....
  2nd order 4
   Ulcer type somatorosis
   (4–2–1)
  C-phobic ....
  G-phrenic ....
Residual D:
  Primary crim. ....

Comment: Outlook now probably good so far as active delinquency is a consideration. The ferocious and toothy Airedale is now older, fatter, and is exposed to less immeditae irritation. It should not be supposed, however, that the Airedale has been magically transformed into a viscerotonic Pekinese or a delicate-minded Irish setter. That kind of transformation does not happen in one lifetime, or perhaps in fifty generations. This youth has "made an adaptation." Just how much would be necessary to provoke the old violence and the old criminality to come again to the surface is speculative, and the hope is that it will remain speculative. It might be a good idea, too, to pray for a *good* ulcer.

COMPANY B, PLATOON 1, SECTION 3
Second-Order Psychopathy; Uncomplicated:
Nos. 133–143

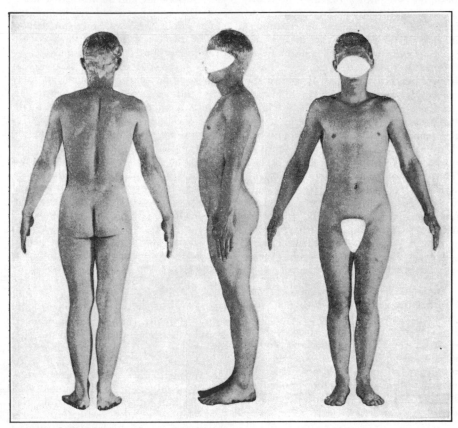

Description: Somatotype 3–5½–1½. A 21-year-old mesomorph an inch above average stature. All segments well developed with strong muscling throughout. He approaches extreme mesomorphy. A lithe, panther-like physique. No noticeable dysplasias, although the waist is a little too high or gynandroid for first-rate athletic performance. Primary *g*+1; secondary *g*, no trace. Primary *t* 3, secondary *t* 2. Features ill shapen and pudgy; low forehead. He has a Scandinavian scowl. General strength 4, hand strength 4. Coordination good in the sense that he handles himself effectively and is a good fighter and athlete. Yet his bodily movements are jerky. He has poor poise and is harsh and threatening in manner.

Temperament: A pattern of sustained somatotonia with wanderlust. He is restless beyond ordinary reasonableness. Suggests a piece of machinery that whirs continually without meshing. He must always be going somewhere or planning something big and new. Although he is physically relaxed and fairly well poised there is no restfulness in him. To hitchhike to Chicago and back over the weekend is a normal routine. He has a sexual somatorosis, waves from which lap continuously against the banks of our respectable middle class pretense of nonsexuality. He is also a Promethean dreamer who seems to get the fabric of his dreams confused with that of real life. Yet within the limits of his desires he seems almost competent. There is no indication of conflict, no sign of cerebrotonic interference—only a sort of generalized and sustained somatorosis. He is not paranoid toward individuals; not paranoid in the concrete, but he is paranoid-Promethean toward society in the abstract. ψ 2–3–2.

Delinquency: A runaway as early as 8 and a frequent truant during the succeeding four years. Often a vagrant from 12 to 16. Between 16 and 18 almost continuously vagrant and known as a juvenile hobo. Numerous minor or incidental contacts with police, always in association with vagrancy and minor stealing. No delinquency of violence or destructiveness.

Origins and Family: Second of four, small-town Old American family. Father a large energetic man of excellent health and with an athletic history. Also known as a man of intellectual interests. Mother a tall, heavy woman of "ineffectual mentality." She too has enjoyed excellent health, and the family as a whole are "middle-class respectable." Boy lived at home until he left at 16 and became a hobo. All of the other siblings turned out well.

Mental History, Achievement: Finished one year of high school with a good record. Two IQ reports fall at 117 and 125; here called 120, or about average college intelligence. He gives the impression of good native mentality, with superficial and sophisticated interests. For an 18-year-old he knows too much about the way American democracy works, too little about the way children are supposed to think it works.

No vocational plan. He is quite an accomplished musician but will play only "hot jazz." He loves rhythm, action, and noise. The AMI that of a tall, broad-shouldered, handsome youth with a breezy and self-confident manner.

Medical: Early medical history not known. No record of serious illnesses or injuries. PX reveals no significant pathology. Apparently of excellent general health.

Running Record: Through a period of nearly two years he made irregular visits at the Inn, where he was courteous, amiable, always pleasant. Every member of the staff was glad to see him when he turned up. He would usually bring presents, minor remembrances; would distribute cigars, small articles, liquor, or cigarettes with remarkable shrewdness. During this period he traveled tremendously, knew a great number of people, kept in close touch with agencies and individuals who could give him what he wanted, and had at least a dozen women in this city more or less astir. He always seemed to have money although its source was a mystery. We knew only that he neither worked nor received the money from home. Here he toyed several times with programs of various sorts, once or twice aroused hope in us. On one occasion we registered him for high school on the school program. He attended for half a day. Several times we secured jobs for him, but he never actually started work on any of them. In the end we felt that he had come nearer to converting us middle class morons to his philosophy than vice versa.

After his last visit to the Inn he "hit the road" as usual, and shortly thereafter the war broke out. He immediately enlisted, deserted after a few months, was a vagabond for a time, reenlisted and again deserted; reappeared after a year and enlisted for a third time in a third branch of the service. This time he went overseas and came back within a year with some medals and ribbons, but he soon deserted for the third time. After the final desertion he was a nomad for three or four years, was finally apprehended for a serious robbery and is now under federal detention.

Summary: Tall ectomorphic mesomorph of high *t*. Excellent health; college level mentality. Problem of wanderlust and restless vagrancy, with a trace of criminality and irresponsibility. A little Dionysian; a little paranoid, with a touch of oneirophrenia or dream addiction.

ID 0–4–1 (5)
Insufficiencies:
  IQ ....
  Mop ....
Psychiatric:
  1st order ....
  2nd order 4
  Restless wanderlust (2–3–2)
  C-phobic ....
  G-phrenic ....
Residual D:
  Primary crim. 1

Comment: Outlook doubtful but far from hopeless, even from the point of view of respectability. He shares with many of the better-endowed youths of the series an essential and seemingly irreconcilable hatred of what has been called the middle class moral outlook. When we last saw him he intended to remain a professional parasite and vagrant. But he is resourceful and intelligent. His superb health and freedom from degenerative tendencies like alcoholism indicate that it will be a long time before he breaks down. He is perhaps more likely to jump from vagabondage to the economic aristocracy, through marriage or some other happenchance, than to join the oppressed and toiling middle classes.

This case might be "explained" in terms of the syndrome of *disappointed mesomorphic expectancy* (see p. 524). Although mesomorphic, the youth is distinctly less so than his father, and is less powerfully athletic than his father. He was in this sense a disappointment to the latter, and very likely was also a disappointment to his own one-time expectations or hopes. If you like to sit and construct explanations of personality around one datum, the case offers good hunting. His delinquency might be called an expression of a "masculine protest," and that case would be nicely strengthened by the fact that just enough gynandromorphy is present to cut him off hopelessly from first-rate athletic achievement. But such explanations are too easy by far, and I think the job is to inhibit indulgence in them until description has been carried well beyond its present boundaries.

143. COMPANY B, PLATOON 1, SECTION 3
Second-Order Psychopathy; Uncomplicated:
Nos. 133–143

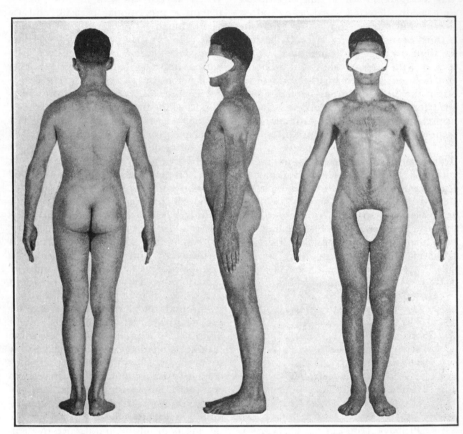

Description: Somatotype 3–4½–4. An 18-year-old moderate mesomorph four inches above average stature. Heavier in bone than in muscle and all segments imperfectly—although about equally—developed. The Potter seems to have started to make a more pronounced mesomorph but somehow wavered. No dysplasias. Primary $g+1$, secondary $g\pm$. Primary t 3, secondary t 4. Features strong, well developed, finely molded and chiseled. A handsome face. Fine hands and feet. General strength 3, hand strength 3. Coordination excellent. A fair athlete, a fine dancer, good at all minor games. Not much of a fighter. Too gynandroid for competitive athletics.

Temperament: He is somatotonic, with frequent emotional tantrums. Stridently noisy and aggressive, he seems too full of energy. When crossed he is inclined to fly off the handle, to become loudly profane, and to attack violently if some weapon is at hand. He does not attack with his fists, is not a hitter. This boy is one whose hatreds are sustained. Known to carry a knife and said to have used it on various occasions, he is feared even by some of the tougher mesomorphs. He easily becomes furious; on one occasion attacked a staff member with a screw driver. He grows harder or more paranoid under alcohol. He seems to dream of himself as a sort of Robin Hood avenger. ψ 2–4–2.

Delinquency: Much early truancy. Arrested several times at 12 and 13 for stealing. Frequent runaway from foster homes during this period. Broke into automobiles at 15 and 16, finally sent to a correctional institution at 17 for this habit. Larceny at 18.

Origins and Family: Extramarital. Father said to have been an Irish taxicab driver. Mother a stocky Lithuanian-Polish girl who had a record of alcoholism, promiscuity, and "stubborn child" charges in her teens, was later a show girl. The boy spent his first eight years with the mother, who became a chronic alcoholic, developed very high blood pressure, and died at about 30 after producing two other illegitimate children. It is reported that she and her siblings produced "no less than ten illegitimates." Boy turned over to foster homes at 8.

Mental History, Achievement: Finished the seventh grade after several failures of promotion. IQ reports fall between 85 and 95, here called 90. He gives the impression of being alert, but suspiciously so or paranoid. There is little indication of mental stamina and none of intellectual potentiality.

No vocational plans or special gifts. The AMI that of a healthy looking, alert boy with a puzzling expression. He seems to smile with his viscerotonic mouth but there remains a hard, menacing look in his paranoid eyes. One social worker referred to him as "that baby-faced boy who looks like a killer."

Medical: Early history not known. No serious illnesses or injuries. Reported as enuretic at least to 14. PX reveals no significant pathology except dental caries and astigmatism.

Running Record: He stayed at the Inn intermittently during two years, disappearing several times on mysterious errands which probably were merely tramping trips. Once he left for the CCC but soon deserted and returned. Once removed by police for breaking into automobiles. His two principal interests or rackets were breaking into automobiles and robbing homosexuals. He would lead the latter on, then rob or blackmail them. He was accused of homosexual prostitution, was said to have been supported by "aunties"—elderly homosexuals with money. He was an extremely difficult boy to handle and only one or two members of the staff could do anything with him. There was always something elusive or mysterious about him. We had the feeling that he was potentially more competent or useful than his history indicated, yet he was one of the few whom we regarded as dangerous. The Inn owns a collection of knives which from time to time were extracted from him. On one occasion he did stab another boy, but inflicted only minor scratches. Police twice suspected and questioned him with respect to shootings, once when an unsolved murder was involved, but the crime was never charged against him. He called himself Billy the Kid. Perhaps the fact that he liked that appellation rather improved the prognosis. Dogs who like to be thought biters

rarely are. Yet he was a real trouble-
maker and caused perhaps as much disturbance as any other one boy, bringing
in our friends the police on a number
of occasions. We seemed to accomplish
little with him, although he retained a
warm respect for one of our staff and
apparently confided fully in the latter.
There were many hours of consultation
or counseling. Possibly some beginnings
of remotivation were accomplished.

Shortly after leaving the Inn he appears to have had one final delinquent
fling and was involved in a holdup. Almost immediately following this he enlisted in military service, liked it, stayed
in for four years, with intermittent difficulties, and after the war entered another branch of the service. There has
been no further record of formal delinquency. He has not yet faced the test of
getting along without institutional support and the outcome of the story is still
to be seen. It may be good or very bad.

Summary: Slender midrange youth
with a trace of primary *g* and too much
energy. Mentality normal subaverage;
history of enuresis. Somatorotic, with
epileptoid and paranoid tendencies.
Persistent early delinquency.

ID 1–3–1 (5)
Insufficiencies:

IQ ....
Mop 1
Psychiatric:
  1st order ....
  2nd order 2
    Paranoid-epileptoid (2–4–2)
  C-phobic ....
  G-phrenic 1
Residual D:
  Primary crim. 1

Comment: Outlook still uncertain.
This is a decidedly interesting personality, with his epileptoid tendency toward
violence and his gynandroid interference with the normal masculine expression of violence. He is only slightly gynandroid, possibly could be called a
borderline gynandrophrene. If he were
just a little *more* gynandroid he would
be harmless, but as he is he is tough
enough to be dangerous, at least during
the acute episodes of fury. However, he
has wisely "stayed in," and in the service he bids fair to ride out the rough
waters of the most dangerous period of
life. During the decade to come it is
probable that endomorphic blossom, fatigue, and other advance benefits of
middle age will render him comparatively safe. But this is a dangerous pattern of personality and one often involved in crimes of violence—with
weapons.

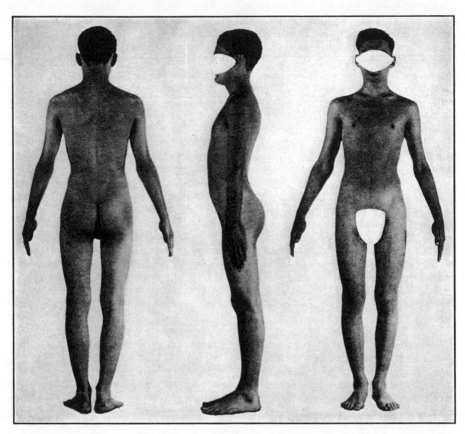

Description: Somatotype 3–4–4½. An 18-year-old youth of nearly mid-range somatotype three inches above average stature. A well-proportioned slender physique with balanced development of all segments. No dysplasia. Primary $g\pm$—a trace; secondary $g\pm$. High waist. He has the high cheek bones and broad upper face of the blond East Baltic stock. Round, fat face with a conspicuously viscerotonic mouth. Primary t 4, secondary t 3. Features large and a trifle gross, but the face has good general proportions. He will be fat jowled in middle age. Hands and feet well formed. General strength 4, hand strength 4. Coordination excellent. He moves with the sure grace of an athlete but his arms are too weak for fighting and he is too lightly built for contact athletics. Too gynandroid to be a good runner.

Temperament: He might be described as a normal submanic. Hyperactive, bumptious, and overflowing with energy like a terrier, he lightly suggests the textbook picture of hypomanic behavior, although without any overt incoherence or flight of ideas. With him it appears to be a normal pattern in about the sense that the wild and destructive hyperactivity of a young terrier is normal. He appears to have no inhibitory component and he boils over with action and energy without interruption. There seems to be no cycloid pattern in it—no periods of exhaustion and depression. Health is *high*. Mesomorphy and somatotonia are at the extreme. In him there is an underlying ruthlessness that bodes ill for bunnies. This physical organism looks as if it could stand the pressure of a submanic way of life for at least as long as it is young. With a less solidly constructed or with a slightly gynandroid organism of this pattern the question of future manic-depressive psychopathy might well be raised, but this youth gives no very strong indication of such a future. ψ 5–2–1.

Delinquency: Excessive truancy from the first year of school. At 12, sent to a state correctional school because of truancy. Persistent minor stealing between 8 and 13; three episodes of larceny. Spent nearly the whole of the three years between 13 and 16 at correctional schools: larceny and "stubborn child" complaints. Often a runaway between 14 and 17; returned by agencies from other states. Arrested for drunkenness and brawling at 17.

Origins and Family: First of six, urban family. Father Portuguese, of about the same physique as the boy. Irregularly employed, has heart disease, and described as "a tempestuous drunkard and stabber." Paternal grandfather died of chronic alcoholism. Mother, Portuguese-Italian, died of tuberculosis when the boy was 12; described as "a finer person than the father." Boy reared in the home until 6, then in a variety of foster homes. At 6 he was adjudged uncontrollable at home. All of the siblings called "difficult children." Only one other known to have a court record.

Mental History, Achievement: Finished a year of high school. IQ reports fall between 91 and 108, here put at 100. He gives an impression of bright alertness, but only within the range of his highly practical and direct interests. Has always shown prodigious energy and has been a great favorite with social workers.

No vocational plan other than continued exploitation of his effective AMI, which is that of being such a dynamically vital youth that you can scarcely resist joining in the dance with him. He has the knack of telling tall stories, real whoppers which far surpass the romantic fiction of the pulp magazines, and it is largely by means of these stories that he makes his way. I confess now and then postponing more important business in order to hear out his thrillers. They were based uniformly on the theme of his sexual conquests.

Medical: Large 9-pound baby; walked at 10 months, talked at 12 months. No record of serious illnesses or injuries. Several minor accidents incidental to a somatotonic life. He has always been careless, and as resilient and tough as a golf ball. He is a prodigious eater. PX reveals no significant pathology.

Running Record: His stay at the Inn was intermittent for about a year. Because of the normal mentality and perhaps also because of the irresistible AMI, we tried him on all four levels of program: House work program, outside jobs, vocational training, and school program. He was equally irresponsible and equally objective or uninvolved with respect to all of them. Jobs he would quit as soon as a few dollars were brought to hand. School and training programs were started only, so it seemed, to realize an initial or immediate benefit. He seemed to override life like a toy balloon. With alcohol he floated higher and even more buoyantly. On one occasion a staff member was assigned to "stay with him" until he did at least one work assignment. The boy then put on a regular one-ring circus with an attack of acute appendicitis. Referred to a local clinic he came back next day as buoyant as ever. Diagnosis: *acute psychogenic illness, hysteria.* He gave the general impression of having a good time with life and of making a game of ball of it. On only rare occasions did any person or event give him serious pause. Two or three of our more belligerent mesomorphs attempted to push him around, but none ever tried it more than once. When he fought he was a whirlwind—a puncher and a butter. He could catapult himself into the midriff of a youth seemingly twice his size, and could double up the latter like a jackknife. His one real interest, or obsession, was sexuality. Other agencies credited the Inn with exerting a beneficial effect on this youngster. It was reported that he became less alcoholic while here, that he quit stealing, and that his sexuality was brought under better control, despite his romantic boasts to the contrary. (His goal, he said, was to sire an average of twelve children a year.) So far as we knew he actually sired only one during the time of our contact with him, and this one was eventually made legal by his being married to the girl for a while.

For another year or so he floated like a cork on the turbulent tides of life, and then came the war. After being dropped from one branch of service as intractable, he entered another and stayed in for two years before being given a medical discharge. He is now again on the drift, as formerly; is much heavier and more alcoholic. Some of the bright buoyancy seems to be gone. One social worker speaks of him as "now an ugly customer."

Summary: Extreme mesomorphy with tremendous strength and dangerous fighting ability, despite short stature. Good health; normal mentality; moderate alcoholism. An irresponsibility and exploitativeness so pronounced that in adult life they probably partake of criminality.

ID 0–3–2 (5)
Insufficiencies:
  IQ . . . .•
  Mop . . . .
Psychiatric:
  1st order . . . .•
  2nd order   2
    S-orotic. C-penic (5–2–1)
  C-phobic   1
  G-phrenic . . . .
Residual D:
  Primary crim.   2

Comment: Outlook possibly good from the boy's point of view. He is in fairly good position with respect to various social agencies, and may never have to work. But he is coming into his middle twenties now, and to him that is middle age. He hates and fears the thought of growing older, as most mesomorphs do.

Dr. Alfred Adler, who was of just about the same somatotype and stature as this boy, used to explain somatotonic aggression as a compensation for short stature. He seemed to feel that the aggression was induced by a kind of physical inferiority—by the shortness. But shortness in nonmesomorphs is not associated with aggression. Rather the opposite. The important thing in personality study is to be sure that one starts by looking at, and by accurately describing the organism. The first job is to get the most fundamental things in fundamental position. Otherwise you get into verbal flypaper. In the case of the boy in question Adler's approach to personality study would seem to fill the bill admirably. The boy is short, and he is extremely aggressive. From the two facts a whole series of conjectures and generalizations might follow. But they would be nonsense if the essential fact —the extreme mesomorphy—were to be omitted from the picture.

145.　COMPANY B, PLATOON 1, SECTION 4
Second-Order Psychopathy; Multiple Complications: Nos. 144–164

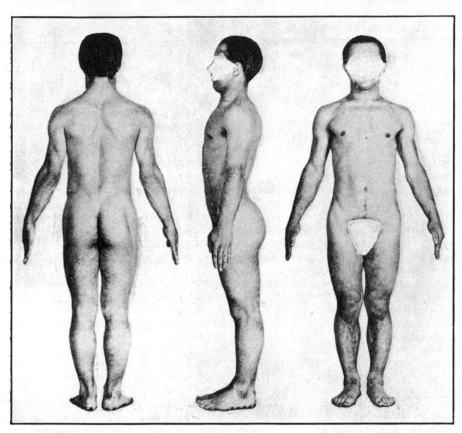

Description: Somatotype 2–7–1. A 17-year-old extreme mesomorph four inches under average stature. Remarkably heavy bones and heavy muscular development in all segments of the body. Long trunk, short neck and legs. Average stature for his Portuguese breed and he is taller than either parent. All of his immediate ancestors short and blocky. No weaknesses or dysplasias. Primary and secondary $g\pm$. Primary t 3 although he is too pudgy and squat for classical standards. Secondary t 2. Features strongly developed but bunchy and coarse, as is the entire bodily texture. General strength 5, hand strength 3. Coordination excellent. He functions as a well-integrated unit; is as physically sure of himself and as cockily alert as a circus tumbler.

Temperament: A somatotonic temperament with signs of cerebrotonic restraint pathologically absent. He is somatotonic like a monkey. You never feel like relaxing when he is around. He is aggressive and has a distinct tinge of the feminine but he is in no sense a *DAMP RAT*. Noisy and irresponsible with alcohol, but also sociophilic and as a rule amiable. He is easily communicative of feeling—cries easily. Perhaps his outstanding characteristic is monkey-like alertness. ψ 2-2-2.

Delinquency: Early truancy and unmanageability in school. Troublesome in foster homes. At 12 referred to a psychiatric clinic and called "an acute problem—stubborn, vindictive. mendacious, vulgar." Between 12 and 15, minor stealing, running away, and defiance of authorities. Arrested for vagrancy at 15. At 16 a barroom hanger-on repeatedly involved in sexual delinquency such as pimping and the like. Episodes of drunkenness at 16. Sent to state correctional school three times, at 15 and 16, on these minor charges—really for persistent toying with the fringes of delinquency.

Origins and Family: Fifth of eight, urban family. The father, Irish and called slender, died of tuberculosis when this boy was a small child. He is said to have been of borderline intelligence; was a juvenile delinquent. The mother, Irish-English and of average physique, was married at an early age and shortly after the death of her husband was institutionalized as epileptic and feebleminded. The children were turned over to agencies. Boy reared in a long series of foster homes.

Mental History, Achievement: Finished the eighth grade after vigorous school maladjustment. IQ reports fall between 80 and 90, here called 85. He gives a first impression of better native mentality, seems bright and responsive but devoid of mental stamina. His conversation reveals paucity of general vocabulary although it is rich in both anatomical and physiological Anglo-Saxon.

No vocational plans. Gifted in music but not identified with the *DAMP RAT* syndrome. The AMI is based on monkey-like mischievousness. He has a bright gleam in his eye which is too much for you and he has learned fragments of pious *ejecta* concerning family misanthropies and associated adventures.

Medical: Early history not known. Numerous referrals to medical clinics for minor complaints although no serious illnesses. At least four minor operations; frequent hospitalization for acute upper respiratory infections and the like. Several psychiatric referrals, no diagnosis. Called "sexually very troublesome" at 7. Reached puberty at 10, and then *decidedly* troublesome. PX reveals no significant pathology except severe dental caries.

Running Record: Many contacts at the Inn through a period of two years. An early plan for getting him on the school program soon failed decisively. He was placed in numerous minor jobs most of which terminated abruptly. After a few days he would seem to ignore a job just as a monkey seems to forget about one of his playthings. His mentality and energy were focussed on sexuality. He seemed incapable of developing interests or conversation outside the general theme of the sexual pursuit. From the first he was alcoholic and a bar-fly, haunting local saloons whenever released from direct supervision. He was a popular character in these places, picking up money and other favors by crooning and playing the harmonica. In one of the nearby saloons he built up quite a following. Often some of his following would accompany him to the Inn and would have to be brushed off like mosquitoes.

As to the work program, he never objected to work but we encountered the utmost difficulty in drawing his attention to it. On the whole he had the better of the interchange and we were unable to preach him a telling sermon. He never was sold on middle class humdrummery at all. Finally he was inducted into military service and for a few months we awaited news with bated breath.

He stayed in until the end of the war, with minor court martials and other difficulties arising from alcoholism and from his peculiar susceptibility to the AWOL bug. After the war, at 20, he seemed maturer and more secure, although showing unmistakable signs of alcoholism. After a brief look around in civilian life he reenlisted—jumped back in like a ground hog who had seen quite a long shadow.

Summary: Moderate mesomorphy with high energy, slightly asthenic extremities, and a trace of *g*. Monkey-like somatorosis, expressed especially in the third panel (see p. 826). Early pubescence. Mentality dull normal; health fair. Alcoholism from about 15 and progressive, with minor associated delinquency.

ID 2–4–0 (6)
Insufficiencies:
  IQ 1
  Mop 1
Psychiatric:
  1st order ....
  2nd order 2
   Monkey somatorosis (2–2–2)
  C-phobic 1
  G-phrenic 1
Residual D:
  Primary crim. ....

Comment: Prognosis guarded. The alcoholism appears to be firmly established, although it has not interfered fatally with his ability to get along under protection of the military institution. He is sufficiently bright and personable to win a sort of mascot place for himself in an average military unit. So long as he stays there he may perhaps live what for him constitutes an optimally good life. But if he comes out, problems will follow like flocks of migrating blackbirds. He has really a little of almost everything but psychosis the matter with him, and with the IQ at 85, time—in the garments of wisdom, fatigue, and endomorphic blossom—may fail to cope with so much rough water.

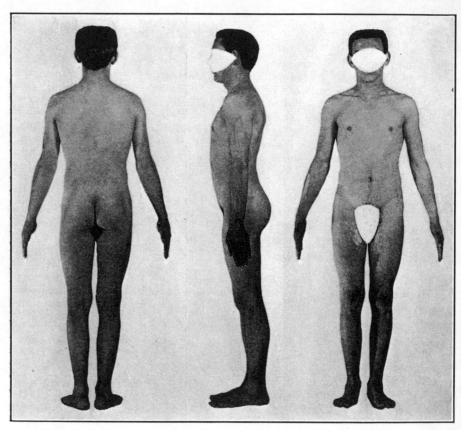

Description: Somatotype 3–4½–3. A 16-year-old moderately mesomorphic youth an inch above average stature. First region more mesomorphic than the rest of the body. The distal segments of both arms and legs are weak and badly formed although heavy boned. Waist moderately high. Primary $g\pm$—just a good trace; secondary $g\pm$. Primary t 3, secondary t 3. Features nondescript but well balanced and he is regarded as a "pretty good looking" boy. High color, alert face. Hands and feet well formed. General strength 3, hand strength 3. Coordination excellent. He moves with poise and self-possession. Enjoys local fame as a jitterbug dancer. Not athletic, not a fighter.

Temperament: A vigorous and emotionally extraverted youth. With so much structural weakness he could not quite be a leader, but he was part of the "political nucleus," or one of the inside gang at the Inn and seemed in a sense to be a dominating factor. At the inner councils of this singularly powerful and troublesome agglutination he was known as The Sage. He was aggressive, bossy, vicious when crossed. When he hit he hit for the face, suddenly and as hard as he could. He seemed to love both inflicting and receiving physical injury, was called by psychiatric consultants sado-masochistic. Without provocation he would sometimes attack other boys, apparently from sheer desire to hurt and to be hurt. Almost helpless at fighting, he would usually sustain injuries, then would come happily to the clinic to have them dressed. He liked the smarting of alcohol and of antiseptics on fresh cuts and abrasions. But his chief delight seemed to come from relating the "far greater damage" he had just inflicted on the enemy. He was unquestionably courageous and fearless of pain. The original intent of the Potter seems to have got over into his temperamental pattern. Yet by mesomorphic standards he is hopelessly gynandroid and physically inept. Affectively extraverted to a remarkable degree, he had periodic emotional spasms or outbursts which one psychiatrist called *convulsive fugues.* At another clinic he was called *hysterical.* The temperamental picture seemed to involve a degree of both viscerotonic and somatotonic extraversion extending well beyond what the physique would support. ψ 4–3–2.

Delinquency: Truancy during the early years of school. A persistent runaway at 10. Incorrigibility and uncontrollability in foster homes at 12. Minor stealing between 12 and 16. Diagnosed *unstable, temperamental, with amoral trends* at 17. Numerous referrals to psychiatric clinics between 17 and 19.

Breaking and entering, handbag-snatching, and larceny at 17. Larceny, robbery, and automobile stealing at 18. To state correctional school at 18. Between 18 and 20, numerous charges of drunkenness and many episodes of larceny. Involved frequently in street brawls and gang fights. A case of persistently tough identification.

Origins and Family: Fifth of fifteen, urban Irish family. Father a powerfully built man. A heavy drinker and said to be quite a fighter when drunk. His contact with his family has been irregular and stormy. He is a lover of boxing, follows prize fighting closely; attempted during the boy's early childhood to teach the latter to box and fight. Mother described as a large energetic woman and quite a fighter in her own right. Because of the large family and low contributing power of the father, most of the children were taken over by agencies and reared in foster homes. Our boy was at home until 10, thereafter in a long series of foster homes. Of the fifteen children only one has died, only three are institutionalized and but four, so far as we know, have been involved in delinquency of record.

Mental History, Achievement: Finished one year of high school. Always a truant and a school delinquent. IQ reports vary from 83 to 99, here called 90. He gives the impression of being more intelligent than mental tests indicate— an impression shared by some of his early teachers.

No vocational plans or special gifts. The AMI really that of unbridled emotionalism, or extraversion of feeling with easy weeping and hysterical repentance. Periods of emotional bathos are of almost rhythmic occurrence. During the interim the boy may have little to say but maintains an ominously knowing facial expression in which there is the challenge of mystery. He generates the atmosphere of being a big shot, or a dark criminal. One big 4–5–2 social worker could scarcely contain herself when the boy was around. She said "He excites me."

Medical: Early history not known. Enuretic to 15: Temper tantrums from early childhood. As a child and later he has been a groaner and a noise-maker during sleep. Between 14 and 20, frequent episodes of somnambulism and periodic "convulsive fugues" which usually occurred when he was alcoholized. At 17, called *epileptoid* at one clinic; at another called *hysterical*. No history of serious illnesses or injuries. PX reveals only dental caries and defective vision.

Running Record: He was at the beginning placed on the school program to finish high school. It soon developed, however, that he had no such intention. He used the school program for a time as a sort of racket, attending school for a few days now and then, just to keep us hopeful. Later several efforts were made at job placement, but similarly without good result. Occasionally, when caught in just the right mood, he would do an excellent job at something. But such an occasion was nearly always prodromal to an alcoholic spree. While he was at the Inn most of his energy and attention seemed to be devoted to planning or carrying out delinquent activities. Finally he got entangled in episodes of larceny that extended beyond our jurisdiction, and he was returned to one of the correctional schools.

He shortly ran away from the correctional school and disappeared for a time. It was learned later that he had gone to another city and had enlisted. After three years in the service he was given a psychiatric or medical discharge. Meanwhile he accumulated a wife and family. For two years since separation from the service he has worked fairly

regularly and seems to be getting along. He drinks moderately and is said to be "difficult" but is referred to locally as a success.

Summary: Gynandroid midrange somatotype with weak extremities. Emotional extraversion and epileptoid temperament. Mentality normal subaverage; enuretic and somnambulistic history. Persistent alcoholism and early delinquency. Identification with toughness.

ID 2–4–0 (6)
Insufficiencies:
  IQ ....
  Mop 2
Psychiatric:
  1st order ....
  2nd order 2
  Epileptoid—Dionysian
  (4–3–2)
  C-phobic 1
  G-phrenic 1
Residual D:
  Primary crim. ....

Comment: Outlook still highly uncertain. Since his contact with the Inn his only delinquency of record transpired within the succeeding two months, but if he has really changed his philosophy of life it is probable that the military institution earned the credit. It was clear enough at the Inn that he needed stronger medicine than we could give him. He has gained nearly 40 pounds since we first saw him, and with each pound the prognosis with respect to active delinquency has doubtless improved. Yet he remains a dangerous person. He is only slightly gynandroid, is tough enough to be a killer, and he is emotionally unstable enough, under unusual provocation, to stop at nothing. His course of life for the next two decades should be of great psychological interest.

COMPANY B, PLATOON 1, SECTION 4
Second-Order Psychopathy; Multiple Complications: Nos. 144–164

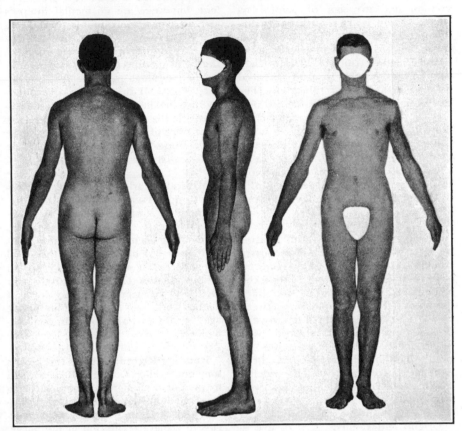

Description: Somatotype 4–4–3½. A 20-year-old youth of midrange somatotype an inch above average stature. Trunk and neck comparatively massive. The arms and legs show a trace of asthenic failure. The Potter seems to have started to make a powerful physique but his attention must have wandered when he got to the extremities. Primary $g+1$; secondary g, no trace. Primary t 3, secondary t 3. This is a comparatively well-groomed, clean-looking youth. General strength 3, hand strength 3. Coordination excellent. He moves with catlike agility but he is soft. The g deprives him of real toughness or athletic ability. Despite this he is good at minor games, even plays baseball fairly well. He is of course unable to fight effectively against fighters but he compensates with excessive pugnacity and thus at least avoids the bottom of the peck order.

Temperament: The general picture is that of outwardly adaptive and decorous behavior. He moves quietly, like a gentleman, with neither somatorotic aggression nor any sign of painful restraint. There is no conspicuous manifestation of *any* of the primary components, but there is a certain dearth of positive characteristics, or a lack of character in his behavior. He is of a neutral gray, seems to escape implications. The temperamental problem, if there is one, may be that of cerebropenia or lack of normal inhibition. Although his impulses are not strong he has too weak a hold on the reins of his impulses. There seems to be an absence of directive control. In many ways he suggests feminine dependence. He is a day dreamer. ψ 2–2–2.

Delinquency: Truancy and stealing in foster homes as early as 8. Repeated trouble with the police for stealing between 8 and 12. At 13, sent to state correctional school for stealing and on a "stubborn child" complaint. Between 13 and 17, many episodes of larceny and breaking and entering; returned twice to correctional schools during this period. All of his delinquency has been stealing. There has been no tendency toward violence, no identification with toughness.

Origins and Family: First of five illegitimate children. Father unknown. Mother, called feebleminded, came from a large and delinquent French-Canadian family. She ran away from a foster home at an early age and was a millworker at 15, a year before this boy was born. Later she had various court difficulties on morals charges and gave birth to at least four more illegitimate children. All these like the first were turned over to agencies and reared in foster homes.

Mental History, Achievement: Finished the eighth grade after several repetitions. IQ reports fall mostly between 80 and 90, here called 85. He gives a first impression of average mentality, for his appearance and address are excellent, but there are no mental interests and no evidence of durable mental fabric. He responds superficially well but does not appear ever to have initiated the habit of thinking.

No vocational plans or special abilities. The AMI that of an extraordinarily nice looking boy who dresses meticulously and is well mannered. There is a faint trace of whimsy about him and he has a kind of ebullient good humor. He is decidedly likeable.

Medical: Early history and development not known. Hospitalized frequently in early childhood for children's diseases, colds, and the like. There have been a number of infections and abscesses, together with the usual appendectomy and tonsillectomy, but no serious illnesses. He has excessively poor teeth and an estimated $2,000 worth of dental work was done on him before age 17. PX reveals no additional pathology.

Running Record: At the Inn he was sometimes called Cinderella. He seemed to present a Cinderella complex, or to see himself subconsciously as an aristocrat and to resort to fantasy and shortcuts to achieve realization of the image. This is characteristic of people of high *t* component who are lacking either in mentality or in courage. By physical heredity he is, in part at least, a refined and high-grade being—one of nature's luxuries; but he is caught in a situation where he must struggle with coarser and tougher organisms at a contest in which they have the advantage. His solution of the problem was to become a sneak thief, accepting meanwhile such minor opportunisms as presented themselves. (For example, he was attractive to homosexuals and he made a practice of picking up what change he could by a kind of assignation—*homosexualitas op-portunitatis.*) He showed a moderate although steady alcoholism, and with the alcohol there was euphoria together with some increment in aggression. A strong effort was made to develop in him an insight into himself, and to lead him to accept the obvious way out for high *t* component people—educational development or, in the case of the really weakminded, interest in "things cultural." But this effort bore no fruit. He was a weak-willed youth, easily influenced by his immediate associates and seemingly incapable of the sustained effort necessary for standing on his own feet. He tended to agglutinate with the furtively delinquent element and to follow along particularly with one of our more persistent practitioners of larceny. We encouraged him to enter military service on the theory that since he tended to reflect the dominant attitudes of his immediate environment, he might respond well in a military setting.

He probably was a victim of bad luck. He enlisted before war was declared, at a time when military morale and discipline were perhaps at an all-time low. The military did not hold him. He soon deserted, was presently involved in larceny, also in breaking and entering, and was jailed. He got a dishonorable discharge from the service. Six years of drifting and of delinquency have followed, and he has spent about half of this time under detention. He is now more alcoholic and somewhat confused. Several times during the war he tried to reenlist but was always rejected.

Summary: A Cinderella youth of midrange somatotype. Mentality dull normal; immunology slightly defective. Weak fabric. Alcoholism and persistent appropriativeness. Bad luck or bad timing with the military institution.

ID 2–4–1 (7)
  Insufficiencies:
    IQ 1
    Mop 1
  Psychiatric:
    1st order ....
    2nd order 2
      C-penia (2–2–2)
    C-phobic 1
    G-phrenic 1
  Residual D:
    Primary crim. 1

Comment: Outlook now considered doubtful or poor. He is regarded by authorities as a chronic criminal, and when his ID is reviewed he seems to have a little of nearly everything wrong with him. Yet he impressed everyone, seven or eight years ago, as being a lad of promise, and I have twenty of my graduate students' words for it that he has an honest face. This boy is what used to be called a weak character. He is simply weak, in various ways, and no amount of polysyllabic circumnavigation of Robin Hood's barn can alter the matter. Yet he may also have had a particularly bad piece of luck in getting into the service just when he did. Had he got in a year later he would very likely have been on pension for the rest of his life, and with no essential alteration in his outlook. Followers of Dr. Alfred Adler will see in this youth a case of "masculine protest."

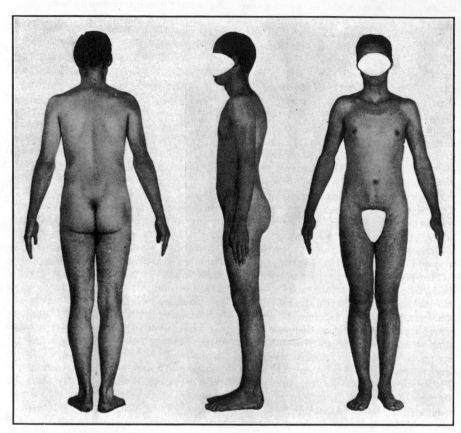

Description: Somatotype 4–4–4. A 17-year-old youth of midrange somatotype, an inch above average stature. No particular dysplasia although the arms show a trace of asthenic failure. Excellent segmental harmony. Primary $g\pm$—a trace; secondary g, no trace. Primary t 4, secondary t 4. He has an attractive face with smiling eyes, and cleanly chiseled regular features. The eyes are steady and wide apart. A fine looking youth. His picture was picked as showing the "most honest face" among a series of twenty pictures shown to one of the writer's graduate classes in psychology at Harvard. Hands and feet finely molded, rather small and weak. General strength 2, hand strength 2. Coordination excellent. He is good at bowling and at other minor games, and is a good dancer but cannot fight.

Temperament: He is somatorotic, harsh, has often been called paranoid. Extremely strident speech. It is a picture not of paranoia but of *harsh* somatotonia. He releases great energy, requires little sleep, is courageous, and has a true love of danger; succeeds to a large degree in dominating his environment. Many of the younger boys are frightened by him, while the older ones consider him good entertainment. He is a *raconteur* of such prowess that he was known at the Inn as the Arabian Knight. When well fed he is sociophilic, but there are few if any signs of cerebrotonic inhibition. ψ 4–2–1.

Delinquency: Excessive truancy and frequent running away before 10. Between 12 and 16 he was an intermittent vagrant, wandering all over the country. Numerous episodes of minor stealing and three larceny charges during that period. Between 16 and 20 he was a real wanderer, crossing the ocean at least twice and traveling about in European countries. First sent to state correctional school for vagrancy and larceny at 13; returned eleven times between 13 and 18. He tells fantastic stories of his jaunts and adventures, and these stories are his principal stock in trade. He recites them almost as an epic poem. At one psychiatric clinic labeled "pathological liar," but this seems a little unfair and decidedly unimaginative. He is really a kind of dramatic artist. Between 18 and 22, intermittent vagrancy, and one charge of forgery.

Origins and Family: Second of three, urban family. Father a Russian-Jewish immigrant who married the mother after the first child was born, maintained the family for about a decade, then disappeared when our boy was 8. Said to have been short and muscular, nonalcoholic, and "successful." The mother, Irish and pretty, was in difficulty because of morals charges both before and after marriage. She deserted the children when the father disappeared. Children then reared in foster homes under agency management.

Mental History, Achievement: Finished the eighth grade with low marks and a poor record. IQ reports range from 75 to 83, here called 80. He gives an impression of mental alertness with poorly focussed mentality. With his great energy the flow of language is profuse, but not always apt.

Vocational plan: To be an explorer or traveler. At 22 he is already a widely traveled young man. The AMI is based on his story-telling ability, backed by a good deal of real knowledge of the world.

Medical: Birth and development history not known. No serious illnesses but long history of intermittent enuresis, extending at least to age 20. Hernia repair at 17. PX reveals carious teeth and excessive sweating of the hands and feet.

Running Record: For a year this youth was one of the colorful characters at the Inn. Despite the gynandroid trace he was no "sissy" or weakling, and his romantic imagination and Arabian Nights yarns provided a highlight in the sometimes drab life in the House. He was an exploiter who lived largely by his wits and did not always bother about his assignments or promises. There were periods of surly hostility and paranoid resentment. But on the whole he was one of the least unsatisfactory "Inn-keepers" and nostalgic memories of him still linger in the place. During his stay at the House there was no delinquency of record. Twice he started the school program but in each instance he proved too much for it after a few days and he dropped it. He would not adapt to scholastic work, although he had a persistent proclivity for writing fiction and poetry. On several job placements he did poorly, always proving "too independent." On the work program at the House he sometimes did excellently, especially when given a free hand.

The war came along and he was an early volunteer. He got overseas, was in several campaigns, and remained in the service until the end of hostilities, although not advancing beyond the lowest rating. There were minor disciplinary difficulties. After the war he returned to his old haunts for a while but was very unhappy and restless; within six months he reenlisted, reporting that he was "better off in than out." A year later, however, he was out again and reported breath-taking prosperity from a mining adventure in the West. His endomorphy is blossoming.

Summary: Short, overenergized mesomorph too centrotonic and a little too gynandroid for athletics. Mentality dull normal; medical history fair but intermittent enuresis and hernia trouble. Second-order Dionysian psychopathy. A somatorotic wanderer.

ID 2–3–0 (5)
    Insufficiencies:
        IQ 1
        Mop 1
    Psychiatric:
        1st order ....
        2nd order 3
            (4–2–1)

C-phobic ....
G-phrenic ....
Residual D:
    Primary crim. ....

Comment: Outlook considered uncertain by local authorities, and the boy is regarded as "highly unreliable." Yet he has kept out of trouble for five years and made a creditable military record. The steady and pleasant advance of endomorphic blossom is all in his favor. It will possibly have taken the sharp edge off his somatorosis. One of his problems is that his IQ is not quite sufficient to keep up with his somatotonia and in consequence the tail seems to wag the dog. Perhaps the central problem is cerebropenia rather than "IQ," and it may be that many alleged IQ problems are really problems of cerebropenia, which by definition is lack of power to inhibit visceral and somatic processes while achieving the function of attentional focus. IQ and cerebrotonia are emphatically not synonymous concepts. Previous studies (see *Varieties of Temperament,* p. 406) have shown that the positive correlation between the two is less than .20. However, the presence and effective management of the third component in the equation is doubtless necessary to intelligent behavior. Cerebrotonia is not IQ, but either cerebropenia or cerebrosis can impair the IQ.

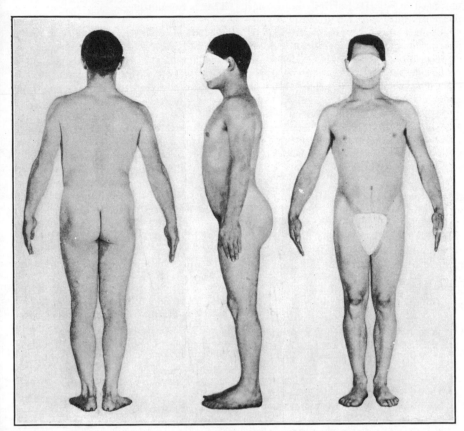

Description: Somatotype 3½–5½–1½. A 22-year-old chunky mesomorph, four inches under average stature. A powerful, almost extremely mesomorphic physique with great concentration of strength through the trunk and first region. Arms and legs less powerfully developed, particularly in the distal segments. Primary $g\pm$—just a good trace; secondary g, no trace. Not quite a fighter's physique. A fighter requires freedom from g and good arms and good legs. This is centrotonic mesomorphy—central concentration of the strength (see p. 29). Primary t 4, secondary t 3. Features strong and harsh looking, but symmetrical and fairly well molded. Hands and feet distinctly too small. He has a paranoid Irish eye in a massive Jewish face. General strength 4, hand strength 2. Coordination fairly good, and energy tremendous, but he is not an athlete and is a slapper and pusher rather than a hitter.

Temperament: He is somatorotic. Energy seems to be excessive and seems to boil over irregularly, like a badly managed stew. He hurries about ineffectually, fails to get below the surface of undertakings. Suggests a water bug darting about on the surface of a pond. Superficially aggressive and assertive, he undertakes much and completes nothing. The somatotonia seems thin, although a Dionysian component is intermittently present. More conspicuous is a steady and an essentially hard or ruthless hostility, directed both toward individuals and toward society. ψ 2–3–1.

Delinquency: Early incorrigibility, destructiveness, lying, stealing, and firesetting in foster homes. Truancy and troublesomeness during the first years of school. Involved repeatedly and persistently in heterosexual adventures, beginning at age 7. Transferred from one grade school at 12 because of this problem. Removed from high school at 16 as a "sexually corruptive influence," after impregnating two girls. Accused of rape. Careless and destructive of property. Breezily irresponsible in all relationships. No charges of stealing after 14.

Origins and Family: Illegitimate, father presumably Italian. Mother a muscular Italian immigrant who died of "a blood disease" in her early thirties after producing five children. Boy reared in foster homes under agency management.

Mental History, Achievement: Finished two years of high school despite deportmental difficulties. IQ reports fall uniformly near 100. He gives an impression of mental alertness but of poor mental focus. Suggests a barnyard cockerel.

No vocational plan. He "never gave it a thought." His mind has been centered on sexuality, with other considerations pushed back out of the attentional focus. The AMI depends on a kind of

vibrant energy and bright-eyed alertness. He is intent, and his black eyes bore keenly into the face of a listener. This is no moron.

Medical: No early data. No hospital referrals and he seems to have enjoyed excellent health. PX reveals advanced dental caries with many teeth already gone, and a systolic heart murmur. Fast, hyperactive deep reflexes.

Running Record: At the Inn he was as uncontrollable as a March hare. Hastily lapping up what material benefits were forthcoming, he was up and away about his business, which appeared to be mostly sexual. He handled work assignments irresponsibly and did the same with outside job placements, but the Inn liked the "IQ 100" and twice started him on a high school program. Each time he quit within a fortnight. In the House he was rowdyish, vulgar, sexy, and several times got drunk. Once he was caught by police at a homosexual orgy, but we did not regard him as therefore a homosexual. He was obsessed with sex *in general*. We attributed his flirtation with homosexuality to what we called *homosexualitas curiositas*. The motivation appeared to be that of mischievous adventure and exploratory curiosity.

For a year after leaving the Inn he lived a wild life, was several times arrested on sexual charges. Once held over for grand jury investigation but not sentenced. With the outbreak of war he was inducted into military service, and the uniform seemed to give him what he needed. Shortly after induction he reported to one of our staff, "This is it. The uniform does it. Now I'm set." He may have been right. At any rate he stayed in until the end of the war, got married. After a year or so of postwar hesitation he accepted a job and held it for a few months. During the year prior to the present writing he is reported as "mainly at loose ends."

Summary: A slender well-energized mesomorphic Italian of normal mentality. Just a suggestion of medical insufficiency; somatorotic satyriasis with associated delinquency.

ID 1–3–1 (5)
Insufficiencies:
    IQ ....
    Mop 1
Psychiatric:
    1st order ....
    2nd order 3
    Somatorotic (2–3–1)
    C-phobic ....
    G-phrenic ....
Residual D:
    Primary crim. 1

Comment: This story is not finished but the outlook may perhaps be called good. It is possible that the somatorosis has quieted down with maturation and that the manifestations of sexual delinquency can be classed under the general heading of "wild oats." There would then remain the question of an essential or general irresponsibility and a minor question of physiological insufficiency as shown by a heart murmur and early decaying teeth. The latter are signs merely of physical *imperfection,* and neither would necessarily interfere with the normal adaptation of a personality or even with longevity.

His history raises the bugaboo question of homosexuality. It has long been known that boys normally pass through a phase of exploratory curiosity and of nonspecifically directed sexual expression. In the natural course of events some of this interplay results, perhaps by trial and error, in boys themselves becoming the recipients of one another's sexual attentions. Occasionally goats, sheep, calves, ducks, and the like are similarly favored if they happen to be in the environment. This is the "homosexual" phase. I think it is not a homosexual phase at all, but in reality a literally *hetero*sexual phase, in the sense that *anything* will do; just *what* doesn't so much matter. The suffix *hetero-* here would mean simply that the impulse is turned outward or otherward, anywhere. At the time when we knew the present youth he was still on a sort of sexual spree which had already lasted for more than a decade. Homosexuality was to be explored, along with every other possible aspect of the general question. Yet he was never a homosexual in any meaningful sense of that term, but might be more accurately described as a *literal* heterosexual.

150.

COMPANY B, PLATOON 1, SECTION 4
Second-Order Psychopathy; Multiple Complications:
Nos. 144–164

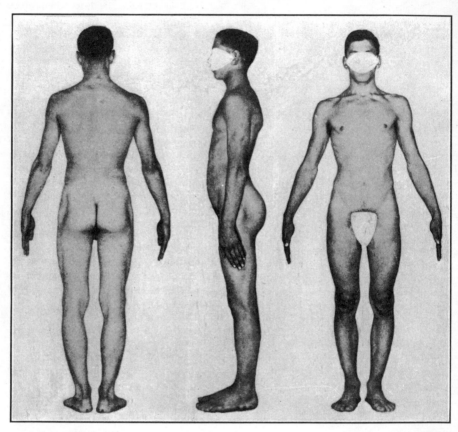

Description: Somatotype 2–5–3½. A 17-year-old moderate mesomorph of average stature. A lean, well-proportioned youth with heavy skeletal development throughout. No conspicuous dysplasias although the waist is a little high. Primary *g*±; secondary *g*, no trace. An essentially hard, masculine physique. Primary and secondary *t* 3. Features bold, a little too heavy for the general architecture as a whole, but regular. Aquiline Italian face. General and hand strength 3. Coordination fair. He handles himself with despatch but movements are jerky. Only fair at athletic games and at fighting.

Temperament: Somatorotic in both a Dionysian and a hostile sense. He is quarrelsome, arrogant; is forever starting quarrels he cannot finish and is a noisy crybaby. He is at the same time both somatorotically aggressive and viscerotically dependent. In consequence he is nearly always in a noisy quarrel of some kind with "his best friend." Great emotional and coprolalial heroics ensue. Psychopathy is pronounced but of the second order. There is no question of attentional or orientational trouble— no indication of a psychotic component. He always knows what he is doing and is well oriented to the whole situation. There is an unmistakably gynandroid interference but no suggestion of the *DAMP RAT* syndrome. He is not artyperverse but quarrelsome like a mother hen. ψ 5–2–1.

Delinquency: Excessive truancy from the first years of school. Persistent running away between 8 and 14. Sent back three times from distant states, at 13 and 14. To correctional school at 14. Quarreling, and later open physical combat with the mother, beginning at about 13. Charges of larceny, receiving stolen goods, automobile stealing, alcoholism between 14 and 17. To correctional school at 16 and 17.

Origins and Family: Only child, urban family. Both parents Portugese immigrants. Father described as a vigorous, healthy, improvident alcoholic who "gave up the battle" and retired from the drama when the boy was 8. Mother large and excessively muscular, described as a "hypomanic go-getter who can fight like a man." Her second husband committed suicide. The third is now a chronic alcoholic. One social worker says "there's a reason." Between the mother and the boy, after the latter got big enough to fight, spirited warfare has been routine. Boy lived at home until age 16, except for a year at correctional school.

Mental History, Achievement: Finished the eighth grade after a very unsatisfactory school history. IQ reports range between 90 and 100, here called 95. Poor verbal ability. Good social intelligence, and he knows how to use it to extract what he wants from the immediate environment.

No vocational plan. He enjoys a magnificent hatred of teachers, of whatever variety. The AMI rests on good exploitation of a generous viscerotonic endowment. Rapport with people is excellent. He tells Dickens-like yarns in the Freudian vernacular, is quick to follow up an opening, and has a practised eye for sociophilia or softheartedness in others. Plays several musical instruments, has good rhythm and harmony. Has rehearsed the story of maternal rejection, with the help of psychiatrists and social workers, to the point where it yields him a fairly good living *via* agency symbiosis.

Medical: Normal birth, big baby. Talked and walked at about 12 months. Excellent health history. No serious illnesses or injuries. Overly fond of sweets and something of a glutton. PX reveals no significant pathology.

Running Record: At the Inn his sociophilia soon made him well acquainted with everybody, but by the third day the hostile somatorosis had caused many to regret the acquaintanceship. It seemed impossible to please him or to fit him into any kind of program, either of work or of training. He soon established himself as a vigorous malcontent, quarrelsome, disregardful of rules, flauntingly alcoholic, irresponsible in the highest degree. After about three months the Inn gave up on him as far beyond the reach of its methods and equipment. He was exempted from military service on psychiatric grounds —*psychopathic personality.*

During the ensuing half-dozen years he has remained intermittently in contact with the home nest, seems to have carried on the warfare with the mother unabatedly but has been handicapped in this enterprise by having to spend about 50 per cent of the time in correctional institutions. All of the later charges against him have had to do with stealing, although he seems to be increasingly alcoholic. Weighing now close to 200, he looks bloated. One of his earlier acquaintances says he has become a "fat souse."

Summary: Heavy mesomorph-endomorph of excellent health. Normal or about average mentality. Temperament Dionysian, quarrelsome, and gynandrophrenic. Some alcoholism and persistent stealing.

ID 0–5–1 (6)
Insufficiencies:
  IQ ....
  Mop ....
Psychiatric:
  1st order ....
  2nd order 3
    (5–2–1)
  C-phobic 1
  G-phrenic 1
Residual D:
  Primary crim. 1

Comment: The outlook is thought to be poor by most of those who know this youth. He seems to be going downhill, has become more identified with delinquency, is considered almost a drunkard. But there are still some considerations in his favor. First, he has almost an average IQ. That means that if the motivational problem should ever be solved—if the boy should ever *want* to snap out of it—he very likely can. Second, there has been the mother problem. Here really *is* a mother problem, and this fool of a youth has not even yet severed relations with the home roost. That card is not yet played, and when it is played a dramatic change might take place. This is one kind of case that sometimes is reached helpfully by psychoanalysis, or even by a reading of Freudian scripture. The boy is close to that hysterically extravert type of personality that Freud originally studied with shrewd insight. Third, he has excellent health, and a copper-lined digestive tract. Perhaps he can resist alcoholic deterioration for a long time. Fourth, his positive delinquency has been confined mainly to furtive stealing—no destructiveness or open declaration of criminality. Finally, there is no indication of first-order psychopathy. I do not therefore suggest his nomination for the presidency of the Epworth League, but this is a case in which the prognosis should be considered still unsettled.

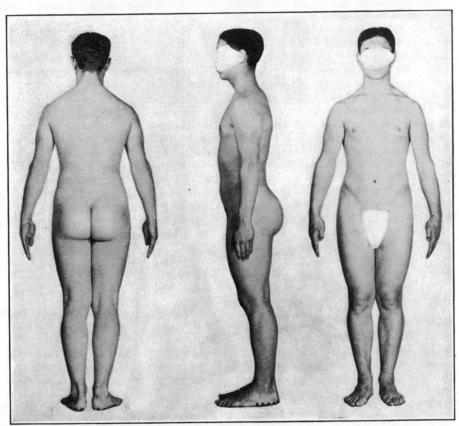

Description: Somatotype 5–5–1½. A 17-year-old heavily built mesomorph-endomorph an inch above average stature. He is both heavily mesomorphic and endomorphically pneumatic. Such a physique might become
enormously heavy ("gross") in later life. Small head. No particular dysplasia
except a decrement of mesomorphy and increment of endomorphy in the
face. Primary and secondary $g+1$. Primary t 3, secondary t 2. Features flabby
and crude. Mouth flaccid with heavy, suckling lips. General strength 4, hand
strength 3. He is about equally strong all over and can fight a little, although
he cannot fight the hard mesomorphs. Good coordination but he is slow.
Excellent swimmer. Not good at any other type of athletics. Too slow for
baseball, basketball, or first-rate fighting.

Temperament: He is temperamentally confused. There are signs of cerebrotonic predominance, but also strong indications of viscerotonia and intermittent spasms of attempted somatotonic aggression. He is usually quiet both as to bodily movement and as to speech. When he moves nothing gets knocked over. Chairs don't scrape, doors and covers never slam, boards rarely creak. He steps restrainedly with no noise from the heels. He is hyperattentional. The eyes are as watchful as those of a mouse in a strange grain bin. There is a childlike intentness about him. All this is normal cerebrotonia. Yet he often gives the suggestion of being grossly relaxed. When he sits he sprawls on the middle of his back, seems to have no backbone. Arms and hands overly relaxed. There is also a strong somatotonic component but this is jaggedly or unevenly expressed. He has periods of energetic vigor. There are brief outbursts of extraversion, many false starts at big undertakings. After dark, on warm nights, he loves to go out on long prowls, like a night animal. A stubborn persistence in stealing may also be an indication of poorly integrated somatotonia. There are no tantrums, no indications of epileptoid psychopathy. He is a dreamer, and may live a primarily oneirophrenic life. He has a facet of romantic wistfulness. The temperamental picture seems to be that of overloading, with the first and third components a little predominant. ψ 2–2–3.

Delinquency: Called unpredictable and uncontrollable by his father at 3. Stealing and running away from foster homes between 6 and 10. Persistent stealing at 12, and kept at state correctional school almost continuously between 12 and 15, although with frequent episodes of running away. Sent to a private school at 15 and soon expelled for complications of minor delinquency. Expelled from public school at 16 for repeated stealing. He then ran away and at 16 and 17 wandered all over the country. Several times returned by agencies from other states. Returned to correctional school at 17, after charges of breaking and entering and larceny. No trace of violence in his history and no open defiance. A good-natured, smiling youth with an apparent compulsion for stealing.

Origins and Family: Youngest of six, urban family. Father Scotch-Irish. He has "fits" which were never diagnosed but sound like petit mal epilepsy. Paternal grandfather, aunt, and uncle were epileptic. Mother Scotch-Irish and a large, loosely built woman who died a few weeks after this boy's birth. She had had high blood pressure and associated complications "for years." Maternal grandmother epileptic. Boy lived for ten years with relatives, then found uncontrollable and turned over to foster homes under agency management. One sibling confined in a school for the feebleminded, another said to have "seizures."

Mental History, Achievement: Finished two years of high school after difficulties noted. IQ reports run from 83 to 96, here put at 90. He gives just about that impression. Although far from feebleminded he is equally far from being bright.

No vocational plan, no special abilities. The AMI that of an apologetically overgrown and pleasant-looking youngster of poor posture who presents a history of mischief which, from looking at him, you wouldn't quite believe.

Medical: No early data. No record of serious specific illnesses although throughout childhood he was frequently referred to medical clinics because of dizziness, weakness, spots before the eyes, shortness of breath, and the like. During the early teens there were several fainting spells. Many efforts have been made to change him into a mesomorph through exercises, physical education, endocrine therapy. Although he is surrounded by epilepsy on both sides of his heredity there have been no epileptoid indications unless the periodic compulsion to steal is epileptoid. His history is that of insufficiency and weakness. PX reveals no significant pathology. He has low blood pressure.

Running Record: He was unobtrusive, at times easily fatigued, outwardly well behaved. Within the limits of an essential physical incompetence he did work assignments faithfully and well. He showed no agglutinative tendency at all, was never on the inside with any group, seemed to belong nowhere. He had a characteristic tendency to attach himself closely for a time to some one person, weak like himself, and the two would presently be caught at furtive theft. He did well for a time at three or four dead-end jobs like dishwashing and hospital orderly work, but was unable to control the tendency to steal. From here he went into military service.

The physical and disciplinary requirement of the service proved too much for him. He wandered away, was brought back by military police four times within a period of six months. Finally he successfully deserted and disappeared. Four years later federal authorities picked him up in a rural community where he had been working and had kept out of trouble. At the present writing he is still under detention.

Summary: Dysplastic, nearly midrange physique without athletic ability. Mentality in the lower normal range; general insufficiency; some evidence of temperamental overloading; epileptic heredity. Persistent furtive stealing.

ID 1–4–1 (6)
  Insufficiencies:
    IQ ....
    Mop 1
  Psychiatric:
    1st order .... (?)
    2nd order 3
    Overloading, possibly "compulsive" (2–2–3)
    C-phobic ....
    G-phrenic 1
  Residual D:
    Primary crim. 1

Comment: Outlook doubtful rather than poor. It is difficult to reconcile his persistent delinquency with his essential weakness. People with this kind of physique, and normal mentality, usually behave whether they want to or not. I suppose it is impossible to be a successful criminal for long with a physical personality as vulnerable and lacking in natural defenses as this boy's unless a high-grade and alert mentality is present to compensate for the weakness. His behavior suggests a lack of orientation to reality which seems to border on first-order psychopathy. Perhaps he has a psychotic component. But it is probably more likely that the combination of physical inadequacy and temperamental overloading has simply been too much for him. If that is the case the outlook may be relatively good, for the boy's generous endomorphic endowment will now be blossoming and a good endomorphic bloom is nature's elixir for temperamental confusion. With the possibility that a psychotic component may be present this will be one of the most interesting cases in the series to watch.

152. COMPANY B, PLATOON 1, SECTION 4
Second-Order Psychopathy; Multiple Complications: Nos. 144–164

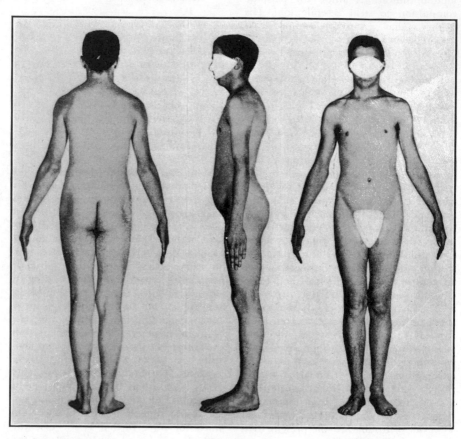

Description: Somatotype 4–3½–4½. An 18-year-old endomorphic ecto-morph five inches above average stature. There is a dramatic mesomorphic dysplasia in the first region and the somatotype as a whole is almost mid-range. Ectomorphic arms which present a distinctly asthenic appearance. Legs ectomorphic. Lower trunk massive. In later life he will be heavy. Primary $g+1$, secondary $g\pm$. Primary t 2, secondary t 2. Features show traces of delicacy but they are lumpy and ill-molded. Face large, pasty. General strength 2, hand strength 2. Coordination good in the sense that he moves smoothly but it is feminoid coordination. From the point of view of athletics and physical combat he is almost as helpless as a seal out of water. The arms are weak flippers, scarcely adequate for slapping.

Temperament: He boils over with somatorotic energy; is given to impulsive and overwhelming but unsustained enthusiasms; starts many undertakings but finishes none. Not epileptoid, in the tantrum sense, and not quite cycloid. Aggressive as a fox terrier, he keeps his immediate environment in turmoil but has periods of exhaustion. No indication of cerebrotonic restraint. The pattern is somatorotic, not Dionysian. ψ 3–2–1.

Delinquency: Called uncontrollable at 2. Persistent truancy and incorrigibility during the early school years. Stubbornness, defiance, destructiveness between 8 and 12. Several "stubborn child" complaints at 12 and 13. Minor stealing at all ages. Between 14 and 17, four times sent to state correctional schools.

Origins and Family: Fifth of eight, urban family, both parents Polish immigrants. Father tall and muscular. He has about twenty court convictions for disorderly conduct, drunkenness, neglect of family. Said to have kidney disease. Mother heavy and muscular, considered of borderline IQ, and described at social agencies as a "grasping and unreasonable person." Boy reared in the home with almost constant agency help. Of the other siblings, three are reported delinquent. None finished high school. This boy is the one runt in a family of oversized mesomorphs—a perfect setting for Adlerian overcompensation.

Mental History, Achievement: Finished the eighth grade after many failures and numerous episodes of defiance. IQ reports range narrowly between 90 and 100, here put at 95. He seems bright but there are no sustained mental interests and he was regarded as mentally defective by some of his school teachers.

No vocational plans or special achievements. The AMI is based on vivacious monkey business or game-cock strutting. At 15 he smoked fat black cigars, boasted of gangster achievements obviously lifted from daily comics, pretended to a toughness which Al Capone might envy. He is in some sense refreshing, makes people laugh and forget his persistent delinquency.

Medical: At 1, called "wizened and hyperactive." No other early data. No record of serious illnesses although many times referred to clinics by social agencies because of "undernourishment." For years he complained vigorously of aches and pains of many sorts. Enuretic at 14. There were more than twenty clinic referrals but no pathology was discovered. PX reveals no significant pathology except carious, poorly formed teeth and a defective eardrum.

Running Record: Despite two years of intermittent effort we failed to break through to this boy's motivational inner fortress. Because of his nearly average IQ the Inn tried hard to keep him on the school program. He was started in four different high schools, always showing great enthusiasm and drive for a week or ten days but in no instance lasting a month. Within the second week he would become careless, would truant, then would grow defiant and would disappear for a few days. After four repetitions of this performance the staff decided that the boy didn't want to go to high school. On work programs in the House and on outside jobs the same pattern held. He would do well for a few days but would then bring all manner of somatic complaints to bear—finally would bolt. Meanwhile by his somatorotic clowning he kept nearly everyone pleased and hopeful of him. He was incontinently fond of following the horse races. For about a month the plan of making a jockey of him was uppermost. This plan was abandoned only when it developed that work other than riding would be involved. In the House he was destructive and was a source of disquietude because of ready availability for toilet familiarities and unmentionable exercises. In no true sense a homosexual, he was always delighted to pick up a quarter or dime by any kind of monkey business (*homosexualitas don't-give-a-damitas*). His *persona* was that of being a satellite, hanger-on, or court jester to any available big shot. He spent most of his time hunting the big shot but never seemed to find him.

Exempt from military service, he has for another half decade followed the same general pattern. Indigence and parasitism with occasional minor stealing. With the coming of the war inflation he was placed in several defense jobs, one at $80 a week, but he never kept such a job for more than a few weeks. The big money overwhelmed him. Later he did hold a job for several months, but during the year prior to this writing has again been drifting and seeking social agency help. He now seems more furtive and dishevelled. At the agency where he is best known he is beginning to be considered a derelict.

Summary: Dysmorphic scrub-oak mesomorphy with comparatively weak chest and arms. Nearly average mentality. Obscure physical insufficiency. Somatorotic psychopathy. A touch of primary criminality.

ID 2–3–1 (6)
Insufficiencies:

IQ ....
Mop 2
Psychiatric:
  1st order ....
  2nd order 3
    Somatorotic (3–2–1)
  C-phobic ....
  G-phrenic ....
Residual D:
  Primary crim. 1

Comment: Prognosis guarded. Well into his twenties now, the elfin characteristic which won him a home half a dozen years ago is all gone. He now has a dull eye and his prematurely seamed face looks like the face of a middle-aged bum. He is a little heavier but no taller. Something went wrong at some point with his physiological development and growth. A review of his medical history would indicate that the mishap took place at least before age 1. Overenergized as he is, he was the weakling in a family of tremendous mesomorphic vigor. His life suggests a match which started to flare but failed to ignite properly. He has some kind of legitimate physiological grievance despite the failure of many clinics to discover specific pathology. A first-order insufficiency—a physiopathy—is present, although we do not know its nature. We see only its stunting effect, and psychopathy which may be etiologically associated.

153.

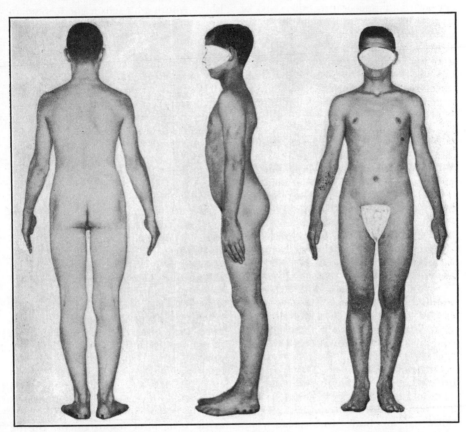

Description: Somatotype 3–5–$2\frac{1}{2}$. A 17-year-old dysmorphic mesomorph three inches under average stature. All segments of the body stunted or arrested, except the legs. Heavy bone structure throughout. Suggestion of gnarled mesomorphy. Chest and arms the weakest segments. Primary $g\pm$; secondary g, no trace. High waist because of stunting of the chest—not, in this case, because of gynandromorphy. Primary t 2, secondary t 2. He is microcephalic with coarse and irregular features. General strength 4, hand strength 3. Coordination only fair. Although highly energized and courageous he is not good at any kind of athletics, is not an effectual fighter. He likes and seems to feel an affinity for the gymnasium.

Temperament: A sort of brazen imp, but with traces of cerebrotonic straining in the role. Apprehensive, tense, he suffers intermittently from acute fatigue. One of our workers comments, "That boy is as twitchy as a frog's leg." When supported by one or two other boys of greater strength and mesomorphy he becomes malicious. He tends to be destructive and pollutive, like a rat in a granary. He often starts fights but never finishes one. The picture is that of unrelaxed or visceropenic somatorosis in the face of interfering cerebrotonia. ψ 1–3–2.

Delinquency: Much early stealing and persistent truancy. He had the habit of breaking into automobiles at 7. At 8, called a chronic thief and "excessively mendacious." At 9, arrested for firesetting; at 11, for pouring sand into gasoline tanks, a trick at that time fashionable. At 12, credited with wrecking a steam roller—several boys tampered with it and started it down a hill. He did not begin to steal automobiles until 13. With another boy he killed a pedestrian in a stolen automobile at 15. After further episodes of car stealing, sent to state correctional school at 15. Several complaints of "unnatural acts" at 16.

Origins and Family: Third of five, urban family. Father a tall, slender French-Canadian taxi-driver described as "only mildly alcoholic." Mother called a well-built Irishwoman. She died of pneumonia when our boy was 4. Before marriage she had had illegitimate children and had been involved in minor delinquency. Children reared in foster homes under agency management. Of the four other siblings two have died, one is serving sentence for major delinquency.

Mental History, Achievement: Finished the eighth grade after a stormy school history. IQ reports fall between 75 and 93, here put at 83. Because of

hyperactivity and a cerebrotonic or birdlike alertness he gives a first impression of better mental endowment, but further contact vitiates the impression.

No vocational plan or special ability. The AMI that of a pale, "undernourished" youth who tells a good Freudian story and gives every indication of neglect.

Medical: No early data. Many referrals to medical clinics, at least twenty in all, but no serious illness. He had the usual tonsillectomy and appendectomy, children's diseases, minor injuries, nosebleeds, skin infections, and has been an object of concern because "underweight." Twice examined at hospitals for epilepsy. The electroencephalogram shows a typical "epileptoid graph" but no other indications of epilepsy found. Frequently diagnosed *psychopathic personality,* and one psychiatrist added "will need institutional care." PX reveals advanced dental caries.

Running Record: During the early weeks of his contact at the Inn he was as wild as a hawk. We found him destructively incorrigible and could do little with him. One psychiatric clinic recommended institutional care. Later, through acquaintances made at the Inn, he found a heterosexual outlet apparently for the first time. Contemporary with this achievement, although not necessarily because of it, there was a dramatic behavioral improvement. During the last month of his stay with us he quieted down remarkably and held a job.

After leaving the House, however, the somatorosis reappeared in full force. He was soon involved in delinquent episodes arising from automophilia, was again sent to state correctional schools. After one arrest he was inducted into military service, and there he has remained to the present writing, through a period of more than three years. He reports favorably on military life, says he spends a good deal of time in the hospital "mostly because of getting hurt," but gets everything he wants and has a good time. The "outcome" of this case will not be apparent until the boy is released from the service and has faced a year or two of civilian life, but the interim report puts a bright feather in the military cap.

Summary: Midrange or slightly ectomorphic somatotype with comparatively heavy skeletal structure. Somatorotic energy. IQ almost borderline. Some obscure physiological insufficiency, but health passable in general. Second-order psychopathy. Persistent automophilia.

ID 2–3–1 (6)
    Insufficiencies:
        IQ 1
        Mop 1
    Psychiatric:
        1st order ....
        2nd order 3
            Somatorotic (1–3–2)

C-phobic ....
G-phrenic ....
Residual D:
    Primary crim. 1

Comment: The outlook may be good from the point of view of avoidance of further legal delinquency. He will not reflect intellectual credit on his generation, but may become a passable citizen. The somatorosis will doubtless recede with age and with increase in bodily weight. He has no psychotic indications and no early indication of alcoholism. There is evidence of an obscure physiological insufficiency, and if a cautious medical examiner for a life insurance firm were to review the total picture he might recommend hesitancy in selling life insurance to this kind of risk. The youth is just about "borderline" physically, mentally, and behaviorally. He is virtually certain to be incapacitated, in one way or another, during a large part of his life, and the prognosis for longevity would not appear to be good.

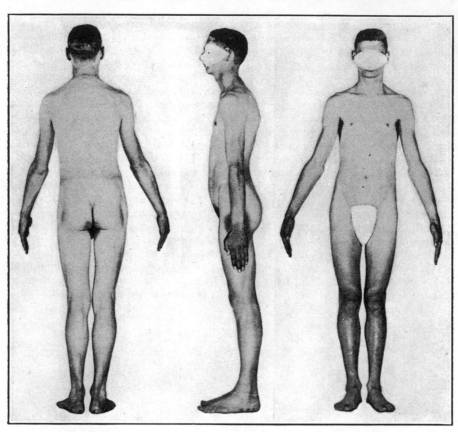

Description: Somatotype 2½–4–5. A 16-year-old mesomorphic ectomorph two inches above average stature. All segments of the body poorly muscled but heavy boned. Ectomorphic arms and legs. Chest asthenic. Neck and face mesomorphic. Very small head. Superficially the physique looks delicate and fragile but ectomorphy is only slightly predominant. Good example of arrested mesomorphy. In later life the body will fill out to moderate fullness. Primary g±; secondary g, no trace. Primary t 2, secondary t 2. Features irregular, ill-formed, too large for the face. There is a hard, untamed, or rodent-like expression. Hands and feet large and strong for the somatotype. General strength 3, hand strength 3. Coordination poor. He moves jerkily and awkwardly although incessantly. Not good at games. A pugnacious but ineffectual fighter.

Temperament: He shows what might be called rat-terrier somatorosis. Incessantly somatorotic with much and loud to-do about little. He is active, noisy, mischievous, and assertive, but he is also viscerotonic. He is greedy for affection and approval, affectively extraverted. Fond of telling fantastic yarns, he can produce real tears in the midst of them and can make his listeners quake with emotion. Once he told so convincing a story of the wartime heroic death of a brother, and produced such realistic tears that some of the staff arranged a sort of sentimental funeral service at the Inn for the hero brother. Later it developed that there never had been such a brother. The staff is still a little sensitive on this point. ψ 3–2–1.

Delinquency: Persistent early truancy with remarkably refined mendacity concerning excuses and the like. At 8, regarded by teachers as unmanageable or incorrigible. Minor stealing at 10 and 12. Charge of "stubborn child" at 13. Bicycle stealing at 15. Refusal either to work or to go to school at 16 and 17.

Origins and Family: Third of fourteen, urban family. Father Scotch-Irish, short and muscular. He had a history of juvenile delinquency, is an alcoholic of long standing; court record of twenty-seven entries during twenty years, mostly for alcoholism with episodes of bastardy and adultery. Mother French-Canadian, called large and gynandroid. She died of cancer in her late thirties when this boy was 15. Both parents and all the siblings said to be of low or borderline IQ. Both parents were alcoholic and both had peptic ulcers of long standing. Boy reared in the home and he has been called the star of the family.

Mental History, Achievement: Finished the sixth grade after a poor record and many failures. IQ reports range from 78 to 89, here called 83. He gives a first impression of being brighter with his facile manner of speech and social address; he spins his yarns with eloquence. But he shows no sustained mental strength in any direction.

No vocational plan; no special abilities. The AMI is based on a bright, alert appearance. He has widely set, sparkling black eyes and seems to radiate enthusiasm. One social worker says "you cannot help wanting to mother him."

Medical: Normal birth and development history. Many hospital contacts but for the most part only the "luxury contacts" such as are enjoyed by the two ends of the economic distribution. Recurrent upper respiratory infections; trouble with ears and sinuses; the fashionable minor operations of the day; several hospitalizations for children's diseases; minor injuries and referrals for psychiatric study. He has received the common psychiatric diagnoses *psychoneurosis; behavior disorder;* and *without psychosis.* PX reveals no significant pathology except carious and ill-formed teeth.

Running Record: Keeping up with this boy at the Inn was like trying to house a flea circus in an open basket. He was in no sense vicious and committed no delinquency of violence. But he was elusive and resourceful as well as energetic in his defenses against doing work. He started numerous low-grade or dead-end jobs, always dropping them at the earliest reasonable moment. Minor medical complaints were of opportune occurrence whenever the work program threatened to catch up with him. In his personal relations he was like an untrained puppy, irresponsible with respect to time, place, person, and circumstance. After trying all of the meager bag of tricks which we had available and failing with these, we surrendered the boy back to the referring agency and gave ourselves a low grade on the undertaking.

Exempted from military service on

psychiatric grounds, he has done rather badly during the succeeding half-dozen years. For a year he vagabonded, traveling back and forth from coast to coast. Most of his nineteenth year was spent under detention in consequence of a series of robberies. Again he vagabonded for a year, then spent another year under detention for automobile stealing. At last report, a few months ago, he had grown heavier, and settled down to the extent of holding a job for three months.

Summary: Short, chunky mesomorph with brittle or slightly underdeveloped extremities. Possibly a trace of medical insufficiency. Mentality dull normal or a little less. Persistent somatorosis and long identification with minor delinquency.

ID 2–3–1 (6)
Insufficiencies:
    IQ 1
    Mop 1
Psychiatric:
    1st order ....

    2nd order 3
      Somatorotic (3–2–1)
    C-phobic ....
    G-phrenic ....
Residual D:
    Primary crim. 1

Comment: Prognosis perhaps not as bad as the recent history seems to indicate. His trouble may be merely that he has not yet developed his ulcer. Ulcer exerts a most mellifluous influence on somatorosis, and this youngster is of about the right physique and temperament for it, besides enjoying an ulcer history on both sides of his immediate heredity. The recent report that he has gained weight is also a favorable omen. In a case of somatorosis there is nothing like bringing up the endomorphic reserves, and if this can be accomplished without benefit of peptic ulcer, so much the better. The prognosis for delinquency is far from black, and he may soon quiet down. The outlook for his reflecting glory or major credit on man as a species is not very good.

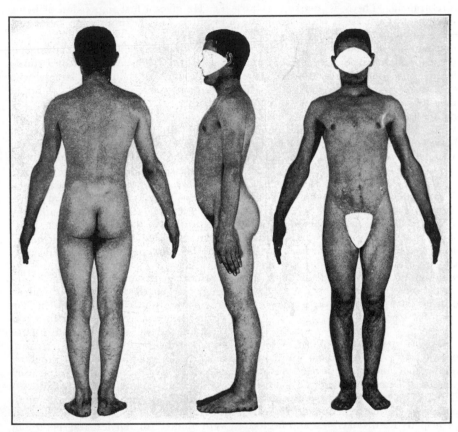

Description: Somatotype 3–5–2. A 17-year-old rather chunky mesomorph four inches under average stature. The trunk is sturdy, mesomorphically well developed, with deep chest and broad shoulders. Arms and legs a little less vigorously muscled although far from asthenic. Heavy bones throughout. Primary and secondary g±. Primary *t* 3, secondary *t* 3. Features large, strongly developed, of average molding; hands and feet coarse. This is a jaunty physique, typical of French-Canadian stock, although the comparative "muscular failure" of the extremities is not typical of that stock. General strength 3, hand strength 2. Coordination fair but jerky. He is overly energized, not athletic, and not good at fighting. Active like a rat terrier.

Temperament: Excessively active and boiling over with energy. He is hyper-motile. Violent outbursts occur with an apparently epileptoid rhythm, and the outbursts are always followed by a period of surly stubbornness. Somatotonia predominates with no manifest trace of cerebrotonia. There is marked extra-version of affect. He is energetic in the extreme, as boldly assertive as Douglas Fairbanks in an old-time movie, yet in the final analysis he is ineffectual and inept. The somatotonia always in the end turns to somatorosis. He loves to take long chances and despite an inabil-ity to fight is courageously pugnacious. When well fed and during the periods between his somatorotic episodes he is a smoothy, with infectious high energy. ψ 4–2–1.

Delinquency: Persistent early tru-ancy in school, first noted at 8. Periodic violence and defiance of authorities from this time to 14, when he left school. Persistent minor stealing be-tween 10 and 14. A famous breaker of windows at 10; breaking and entering at 14 and 15, and a chronic runaway during this period. Sent to state cor-rectional school at 16.

Origins and Family: Fifth of seven, urban family. Both parents Lithuanian immigrants and both sturdy, muscular people, the mother more so than the father. The latter had twelve court ap-pearances during a period of 15 years, principally for drunkenness and neglect. The mother, described as "ugly and dangerous when drunk," had twenty-three court appearances within a period of twenty years, mostly for charges as-sociated with alcoholism and morals difficulties. Although the two parents have remained together the children were taken over by agencies through court action and our boy was reared in foster homes from the age of 4. He had more than twenty foster home place-ments during a period of eleven years, proving incorrigible or uncontrollable in all of them.

Mental History, Achievement: Fin-ished the eighth grade after a long his-tory of unsatisfactory performance. IQ reports range from 81 to 90, here called 85. He gives a first impression of being brighter, but the impression fades rap-idly.

No vocational plan; no known spe-cial abilities. The AMI that of a sturdy little fellow of bounding energy who has sometimes been called a bright cherub.

Medical: Infancy history not known. No record of any serious illness or in-jury. Long list of minor infections with much hospital attention, but the in-fections have always readily cleared up. Enuresis to 14; none of record there-after. PX reveals no significant pathology except the very flat feet and a heart murmur which is probably "functional" —or without pathological significance.

Running Record: From the begin-ning this youth was obsessed with a craving for status as a delinquent. He virtually demanded to be sent to a cor-rectional school, as some youths have asked to be sent to college. He con-sistently sloughed off the work program, as well as various jobs that were secured for him, always with the defiant ex-planation that he wanted to be pun-ished. While at the Inn his interests were limited to movies and poolroom loafing. He stated with what may have been a wisdom beyond his years that he would be glad to behave in a just society but that since this is an unjust society he chose to do as he pleased and "you can all go to Hell." He proved incorrigible so far as our equipment was concerned, and yet we entertained a certain respect for his courage and de-fiance. While with us he laid claim to such heroic achievements as "rolling of fairies" and robbing of drunks.

After we gave up on him he continued in about the same pattern, was sent to correctional school for a year, then spent another year in civilian life just about as before, although now as a grown-up young man. Finally, after the war, he was inducted into military service. There the same old epileptoid pattern has seemed to hold. Within a few months he was in trouble because of drunken sprees, orgies of violence, spells of being AWOL. However, he has remained in the service for a year.

Summary: A squat, highly energized timberline mesomorph without athletic ability. Mentality dull normal. History of many infections and of enuresis to 14. Epileptoid temperament. Long and persistent flirtation with delinquency.

ID 2–3–1 (6)
Insufficiencies:
    IQ 1
    Mop 1
Psychiatric:
    1st order ....
    2nd order 3
      Epileptoid—somatorotic
      (4–2–1)
    C-phobic ....
    G-phrenic ....

Residual D:
    Primary crim. 1

Comment: Outlook considered dubious by local authorities. At an early age he made up his mind to try the delinquency experiment, and ever since has been demanding some proof of the wrongness of delinquency—proof that he can understand. None has yet been forthcoming. Perhaps the only proof that would be acceptable to him would be unanimously applied physical punishment. Such therapy not unanimously applied would of course be worthless, for if he could detect any *difference of opinion* on such a matter, he would be justified in rejecting the evidence as inconclusive. If we were to whip him, for example, and then somebody else not whip him for the same kind of performance, we would do him no good but would put ourselves in an almost indefensible position. This youth has probably for a long time entertained a sincere desire for what he could accept as justice. He possibly craves a just society as sincerely as anybody. But he is confused at finding no justice that he can understand, and this may be essentially the motivational outlook of many of the persistent delinquents—as well as of some of us who are less persistent.

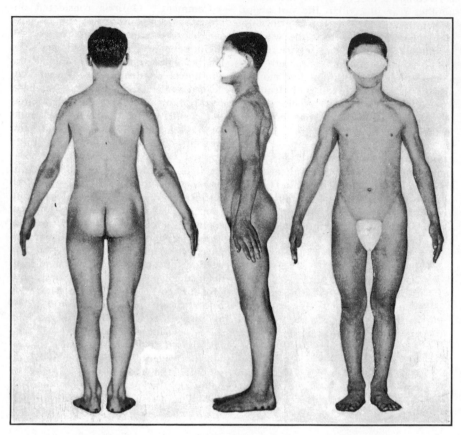

Description: Somatotype 2–5½–1½. A 16-year-old gnarled mesomorph three inches under average stature. Dysmorphic. A solid, chunky physique showing the arrested characteristic in all segments but most severely in the arms. Narrow straightened chest. Heavy bones; little indication of ectomorphy. The attention of the Potter seems to have wandered *badly* during the shaping of this one. Such a physique strongly suggests a dwarfed tree struggling at a mountain timberline (timberline mesomorphy). Primary $g\pm$; secondary g, no trace. Primary t 2, secondary t 2. Features crude although the face has a pleasant expression. He has level, steady eyes that can twinkle. Hands and feet very large and crude—at those points the Potter remembered what he had started out to make. Feet flat to an extreme degree (there the Potter forgot). General strength 4, hand strength 4, but coordination is poor and with his brittle arms he of course cannot fight effectively. Not good at any kind of athletics.

Temperament: Predominantly second component, with good and fairly well-integrated support from both the other components. He has humor. At PX he remarks, "Doc I've got one awful bad allergy—to keys and locks." He is a little too energetic for his somatotype, and perhaps too fond of risk. The reaction to alcohol is decidedly somatotonic, and he loves the ecstasy of thus getting rid of his inhibitory component. In his delinquency he always operated alone—called himself "the lone coyote." He is a romantic dreamer who is *also* breezy and aggressive. ψ 2–2–2.

Delinquency: Much early truancy. Persistent stealing between 8 and 15, at first from his home, later from stores and filling stations. To state correctional school at 14 for stealing. Went to work at 16 but lost several jobs because of persistent stealing. Dishonorable discharge from CCC for stealing. At 19, wandered off to a western state, later sent to correctional school there for stealing. Returned East at 20, soon involved in stealing, in breaking and entering, and in trouble for illegal possession of a revolver. He has left a long trail of cardiac wreckage, boasts of having "made" a hundred girls, and there is evidence that this is at least 2 per cent true.

Origins and Family: First of two, urban family. Father Irish and said to have been a nervous, alcoholic, and irresponsible youth. He married young but after a few years "got wanderlust" and deserted the family when this boy was 4. The Irish mother remarried and has since maintained a home. Her father was alcoholic. Her present husband is regarded as a well-established citizen and the family is respected. The boy lived with relatives for two years after the separation of the parents, then returned to the family.

Mental History, Achievement: Graduated from high school after a record of irregular attendance and of some failure. IQ reports fall almost uniformly between 115 and 120. There is no question that he has superior mentality. Also he has poise and humor and is a good conversationalist. One gathers the impression when talking with him that he is having a good time with life, that he has the situation in hand, and perhaps is delinquent only in the sense that slightly alcoholized college boys are delinquent when they go forth on nocturnal binges. But in his case it is a perpetual state.

No vocational plan; no special gifts. His identification has been mainly with having a good time. The AMI that of a tall, wide-shouldered, and handsome youth who loves to recite Freudian scripture with a twinkle in his eye. He was rejected, is a subconscious homosexual who sometimes carries a gun as a symbol of the male organ, and his delinquency is a consequence of seeking a father substitute—for punishment. He has awful guilt feelings and gets sexual satisfaction from punishing his father through his criminal activities. All this may not be orthodox, but it is "good." The boy has memorized it by rote and makes a gesture not unlike the sign of the cross after each recital, but with a twinkle in his eye.

Medical: Normal birth and development. Pyelitis several times recurrent between 4 and 9. Questionable tuberculosis at 19. Pneumonia at 20. He has been drinking pretty heavily since 16, smokes too much. PX reveals no significant pathology beyond flat feet and severe dental caries. He has a heart large to percussion and very large superficial blood vessels. This appears to be a cardiovascular system intended for extreme mesomorphy. Maybe the Potter made the cardiovascular system first.

Running Record:. During a relationship at the Inn which lasted nearly a year it was generally realized by members of

the staff that this boy had the better of us.
He usually seemed to enjoy himself, had
a remarkable supply of good stories,
successfully played off three or four different social agencies against one another, thereby making a reasonably
good living. He reflected the exuberance
of sexual intrigue judiciously blended
with alcohol. He borrowed, stole, and
begged freely, in general got by without
doing work. He started half a dozen
jobs but never remained past the first
payday. Several of our tougher mesomorphs hated him because of his undeniable success with the various girls
who more or less belonged to the circle.
On two or three occasions he thus became involved in altercations with the
real fighters of the House; on these occasions was badly whipped. Once he removed all the brass plumbing fixtures in
the House and sold them to a junk
dealer. This left us in a bad way.

Eventually his stealing became so
careless that he was given a sentence to
one of the correctional institutions.
There, after a few days, he developed
urgent somatic complaints and was
transferred to a hospital. When the
sentence was up he was again in good
condition, was soon involved in more
stealing, and presumably would have
continued in this pattern indefinitely
had not the war come along and driven
him into defense work. Thereupon he
married, started a family, and soon
there were agency contacts on the new
family. After a couple of years he
drifted away, has since wandered about
in various parts of the country. He has
had jobs of many sorts but always finds
them monotonous or tedious and moves
on after a few months. Says he gets
wanderlust. There have been brushes
with the law over alleged stealing, but
no further sentences. He drinks more
now, smokes excessively, seems a little
jumpy and nervous. He has lost some
of the youthful poise but retains the old
humor. He seems to be drifting and
degenerating.

Summary: Tall, handsome youth
with a dysplastic mixture of the second
and third components along with a trace
of primary *g*. Superior mentality; imperfect immunology. Persistent stealing and essential irresponsibility. Alcoholism. Second-order psychopathy.

ID 2-4-1 (7)
  Insufficiencies:
    IQ ....
    Mop 2
  Psychiatric:
    1st order ....
    2nd order 3
      *Somatorotic monotophobia
      (2-2-2)*
    C-phobic 1
    G-phrenic ....
  Residual D:
    Primary crim. 1

Comment: Outlook considered
doubtful at best. Now in his late twenties, he has deserted or neglected his
family and has seemed for several years
to be drifting toward derelict status. He
probably has put a finger on the primary
problem with the simple statement that
he cannot stand monotony. Despite an
undeniable wealth of the capacity to see
and enjoy the funny side of many
things, and despite a high-grade mentality and an attractive personality, there
is in him a restiveness which prevents
the development of ordinary personal
responsibility. The bugaboo against
which he can build no internal defense
is boredom, or routine. An instability
results which because of his personabil-
ity has already impaired half a dozen
other lives, and bids fair to render the
youth himself a derelict. This is the
kind of young man that gifted or privileged girls often marry impulsively. Perhaps he is a second cousin to the *DAMP
RATs,* and this essential instability may
possibly arise from a slight gynandroid
interference in an organism with a cardiovascular system intended for heroic
mesomorphy. The trouble with such

speculation is that so many variables are interacting that we have no statistical equipment for expressing and carrying these variables *as they interact*. To try to express them statistically *in vitro,* or as they do *not* interact, may be a fatal monkey trap and may lead only to the marshes of eventual academic confusion. In any event we still have on hand a hard problem in description before any statistical manipulation of these variables can be meaningful.

COMPANY B, PLATOON 1, SECTION 4
Second-Order Psychopathy; Multiple Complications: Nos. 144–164

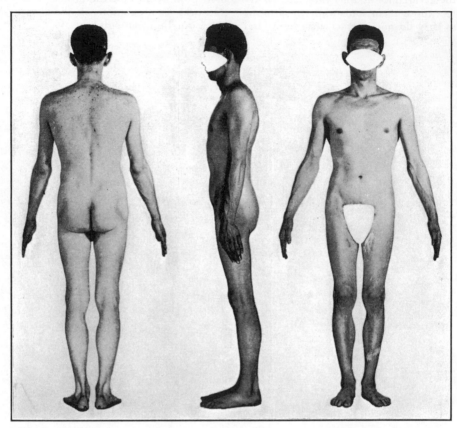

Description: Somatotype 3–4½–4. A 21-year-old ectomorphic mesomorph four inches above average stature. A straight-standing youth who presents a dysplastic mixture of the second and third components with the second strongly dominant above the diaphragm and the two about evenly matched below that landmark. There is a trace of primary g in the lower trunk. With his clothes on he looks large and powerful. Without clothing he is dysplastic with a trace of g. Primary g±—a trace; secondary g, no trace. Primary t 3, secondary t 4. This is a fine type of North Irish face. Features strong, well molded, and chiseled in a somewhat rough, masculine way. He has thick, curly hair with a high, strong forehead. Hands well formed, feet flat. General strength 3, hand strength 4. Coordination very good. He is good in a minor way at many athletic games but is not a successful fighter—the legs prevent that.

Temperament: He is vigorously and sustainedly somatorotic. There seems to be no straining in the role and no trace of cerebrotonic interference. He is loud, breezy, offhanded. When he is in the environment nothing can be done until he is in some manner attended to. The trait psychological callousness (see p. 26) is remarkably conspicuous. He is not manic, or even hypomanic, but is Dionysian. He seems to be overenergized and to lack the ability to express his great energy through conventionally accepted masculine channels. ψ 5–1–1.

Delinquency: A persistent truant from the first year of school. Long history of minor stealing, from 8 to 16. Described at 8 as having a violent, explosive temper and as being uncontrollable in school. He was larger than his contemporaries, fought with teachers, and was a "most disturbing influence." Repeatedly drunk at 15. Ten court appearances before 17. Sent to state correctional school mainly for drunkenness and larceny at 14; returned at 15 and 16. Morals charges apparently arising from sexual somatorosis at 15 and 16. Many times singled out by parole officers and others as "the promising one" among a group of young delinquents, and many times absolved from punishment. This attention he had come to regard as his natural due. He loved to flaunt his irresponsibility like a young millionaire on a spree. Liked to call himself "the Thief of Bagdad."

Origins and Family: Born extramaritally. Father a large, active Irishman of about the same physique as the boy. Said to have been alcoholic and reckless when young. Often involved in automobile accidents, and once in trouble on a charge of manslaughter with an automobile. He married the mother of this boy after the birth of the latter, became the father of two more, then deserted. Now known as "a common drunkard" and on agency support. The mother came from a populous Irish family, had a record of juvenile delinquency. Boy reared mainly in foster homes under agency management.

Mental History, Achievement: Quit school in the eighth grade with a record of fairly consistent failure. IQ reports fall between 90 and 95, here called 93. He gives a first impression of at least average intelligence, but this impression soon fades. He is chaotic, mentally unfocussable.

No vocational plans or special abilities. The AMI that of a breezy supersalesman. He towers over you and *assumes* you like him. Over six feet and well filled out, this great moon-faced boy exudes jovial energy. He is professionally good natured, a big man with a big smile. He has no need of the Freudian (or Christian) theology for a passport.

Medical: Birth and early history not known. No record of serious illnesses or injuries. Intermittent enuresis, at least to 14. Frequent heavy chest colds—no cerebrotonic head colds. PX reveals no significant pathology other than severe dental caries.

Running Record: At the Inn his *persona* was that of the millionaire playboy. The object of his life was to have a good time *every day,* and he could not be bothered by anything. We did not succeed in persuading him to enter upon the work program or any other program. So far as we were concerned he proved uncontrollable, and the Inn was not equipped to attempt to break him down or chasten him. For him life was a bowl of cherries. He was as devoid of morals and apparently of cerebrotonia as a porpoise. Yet he seemed to show traces of underlying intelligence in some of his conferences with members of the staff, and it was felt that he was capable of making an adjustment or adaptation, if and when a desire to do so should be born.

Within a year after leaving the House he was involved in bouts of drunkenness and larceny, was returned to correctional school. He promptly ran away, toured various parts of the country, was heard from in the Far West. A year after this he enlisted in military service under an alias, but soon deserted and was dishonorably discharged. He rollicked for another year, again enlisted —this time in another branch of the service. Within a few months he again deserted, was shortly thereafter picked up for automobile stealing and reckless driving; he served a sentence for this episode. At last report he seemed to have undergone no conversional experience.

Summary: A big endomorph-mesomorph with enough gynandromorphy to render him inept at fighting. Overenergized and somatorotic. Mentality nearly average; history of enuresis. Persistent Dionysian delinquency.

ID 1–4–2 (7)
Insufficiencies:
  IQ ....
  Mop 1
Psychiatric:
  1st order ....

  2nd order 3
  Dionysian (5–1–1)
  C-phobic 1
  G-phrenic ....
Residual D:
  Primary crim. 2

Comment: Outlook dubious, and local authorities consider it dark gray. He has many times been given the benefit of the doubt; has had scores of new deals and other chances. He was before the courts twice as many times as is usually the case before he was ever sentenced. Perhaps because of his great size and jovial extraversion, and because his delinquency has always been of a rollicking nature—there was never any evidence of "meanness" or of cerebrotonia in his misbehavior—he always attracted favorable attention and had friends at court. In the long run this may have been a misfortune. Perhaps he was spoiled in the courts as some youngsters get spoiled in the home.

This is one of the best examples of the nonpsychotic Dionysian personality to be found in the series, and one of the best I have seen anywhere. Whether such a personality is mainly born or made is a fascinating question. Some of us who have known him have wished he could be sent to sea in the "old navy"— just to see what would happen.

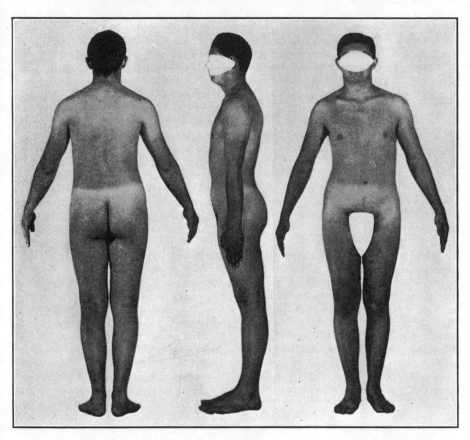

Description: Somatotype 4½–4½–2½. A 17-year-old endomorph-meso-morph six inches above average stature. Thick bull neck and massive head. Conspicuous primary *g* and a trace of asthenic failure in the chest and arms. Otherwise rather powerfully built, with good segmental development. Primary *g*+2, secondary *g*±. Primary *t* 3, secondary *t* 2. Heavy, coarse, ill-shaped features, with an enormous round face which at 17 is already fat. This boy has been told that he "looks exactly as Babe Ruth did at his age." General strength 4, hand strength 3—a very powerful boy with great strength in the back and legs. Coordination good but feminoid. He moves gracefully and lightly; cannot throw well and cannot fight. Uses his arms more or less as flippers, like a seal.

Temperament: Somatotonia predominates and is astonishingly sustained. He seems somatorotic *all* the time; has no patience, cannot sit still, talks too loudly and too rapidly, moves about jerkily and ineffectually. He always seems nervous in the expressive, somatotonic sense. When alcoholized he tends to seem more viscerotonic. I never saw him relaxed except when alcoholized. There is little indication of cerebrotonia. He has a seemingly Spartan indifference to pain—as shown at the Inn during an episode of acute appendicitis. The temperamental pattern appears to be that of frustrated somatotonia. The Potter clearly intended him to be a mesomorph but either the Potter forgot what he was doing or something went wrong afterward. The boy suggests a moth trying to fly with singed wings. ψ 2–2–1.

Delinquency: Early truancy and early stealing. Larceny, at 13, 14, and 15. Sent to correctional school at 13 and 15. After that he became something of a vagrant, wandering all over this and one or two other countries. He used aliases, was involved in numerous minor difficulties with the law, and fragments of his trail are to be found at scores of far-flung agencies. During this period he acquired the habit of periodic alcoholism.

Origins and Family: Only child, from a country town. Father Old American, tall and well educated; killed in an accident about the time this boy was born. Mother Old American, muscular and active although dysplastic; confined at least once in a mental hospital—diagnosis not known. She remarried and the boy was reared in her home until his delinquencies made it necessary to relinquish him to a correctional school.

Mental History, Achievement: Finished the eighth grade after repetitions and failures. IQ reports range between 70 and 92, here called 80. He gives an impression of mental alertness with poor attentional focus. He talks rapidly, uses language effectively, but his mind roams over a wide field of conversation without ever coming to a point. He talks the way an unbroken Irish setter hunts, ranging over the landscape like driven rain.

No vocational plans or special gifts. The AMI that of an unusual youth with an arresting face and a keen eye, who obviously has some good blood but seems mildly crazy.

Medical: Early history not known. Enuretic at least to 14, with episodes of somnambulism to 19. As a child and youth he lived in a middle class family, consequently had no benefit of medical consultation and no hospital or psychiatric referrals. No record of serious illnesses or injuries. PX reveals no significant pathology.

Running Record: His behavior at the Inn was not gladdening. He manifested a certain exploitative friendliness but looked upon the institution as a flophouse for his convenience (which perhaps it was). He had no more intention of being reformed or converted than does a buzzard of being converted by the dead rabbit he is about to consume. He was an avoider of reponsibilities, a good-natured liar, an intermittent drinker, and a titillator of the minds of our tender youths with excerpts of western brigandage. We were able to help see him successfully through a bout with appendicitis and shortly thereafter he left with the light of adventure in his eyes and with the announced intention of joining the Army.

He did join the Army but soon went AWOL, became involved in various episodes of vagrant delinquency, then enlisted in another branch of the service but after several months again deserted. Later he was picked up and given a medical discharge into the custody of a relative. Soon he eluded the relative and disappeared. A year later he reappeared and was inducted into military service for the third time, finally being given a psychiatric discharge within the course of another year. During the succeeding half-decade he has wandered about the country as of old, appearing in various places in various roles which range from bootblack to participant in radio programs. The general pattern seems unchanged.

Summary: Asthenic mesomorph very carelessly treated by the Potter. Mentality approaching borderline; enuretic and somnambulistic. Somatorotic. Mildly alcoholic and persistently vagrant.

ID 3-4-0 (7)
  Insufficiencies:
    IQ 1
    Mop 2
  Psychiatric:
    1st order ....
    2nd order 3
    Irish-setter somatorosis (2–2–1)

C-phobic 1
G-phrenic ....
Residual D:
  Primary crim. ....

Comment: Outlook doubtful from the standpoint of acceptability for Rotary Club membership. He will remain one of the peculiar ones, but before long there will be an appreciable blossoming of the first component and this will help the vagrancy no end. He may then relax and revert to the middle class morality within which he was born. There is at least one other favorable possibility, which we ought to have tried at the Inn but did not. For this youth alcohol may be a useful drug. It tends to bring out his relaxational reserves and to alleviate the somatorotic symptoms. Perhaps if alcohol were administered to him in controlled and moderate dosage—say a couple of gallons of good beer per diem—he might be content to stay home and plant potatoes. Then there would be the enuresis though.

159.

COMPANY B, PLATOON 1, SECTION 4
*Second-Order Psychopathy; Multiple Complications:
Nos. 144–164*

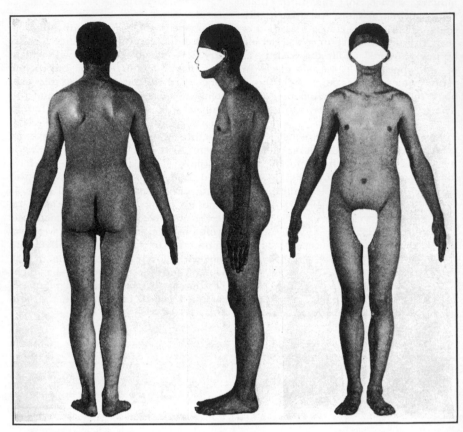

Description: Somatotype 3½–4½–3½. A 19-year-old asthenic mesomorph an inch above average stature. Very dysmorphic. All segments poorly
and disharmoniously developed. First region moderately mesomorphic. Legs
relatively heavy with an increment of both endomorphy and mesomorphy.
Arms and chest decidedly asthenic. Trunk short and dysmorphic—poorly
formed and poorly muscled. The facial skeleton is strongly developed and
when he scowls he has a fierce, almost predatory look. Primary $g\pm$; secondary g, no trace. Primary t 1, secondary t 3. Features well molded and suggestive of strength and courage. Hands and feet crude, asthenic. General
strength 2, hand strength 2. Coordination very poor. His awkward walk at-
tracts attention. At the Inn our humorists would look at him and ask, What
is it? His arms never seemed to swing properly with his legs. Inept at all
games and at combat.

Temperament: He expresses a tough *persona* in the highest degree. Persistent aggressive behavior without a smoothly sustaining somatotonia. He is *truculently* aggressive, harsh. But he is also irresponsibly Dionysian. His physical courage is well beyond his strength, which nevertheless is not to be despised. Fierce and strident vocalization is the hallmark of his presence. Alcohol makes him snarl and "show his meanness," but he loves it. The second component has the upper hand over the third. On psychiatric referral he has been called *psychoneurotic, paranoid trend.* ψ 2–4–2.

Delinquency: Early excessive truancy and incorrigibility. Stealing, running away, and vagrancy between 6 and 12. An insider and ringleader in a delinquent gang throughout this period and later. Charges of larceny between 12 and 15; breaking and entering at 16. At 18, he and two other boys, "beat a policeman unconscious."

Origins and Family: Second of three extramarital children. Father Irish with a long history of juvenile delinquency. He assumed no responsibility. Mother Irish and said to have lived promiscuously. She served a number of years in correctional institutions for juvenile delinquency and illegitimacy; frequently treated for alcoholism. Her IQ recorded as "in the 60's." Boy adopted but turned back to state agencies at 6 as incorrigible. Then sent to a long series of foster homes.

Mental History, Achievement: Left high school after completing about a year's work. IQ reports fall between 70 and 85, here put at 77. There is a certain practicality or hard realism about him which is refreshing.

No vocational plan or identification. His point of view is that society owes him a living and he's going to collect it. AMI based on a kind of coyotish defiance. He struts the *persona* of a predatory criminal, yet has much of the youthful ragamuffin in him and has Irish blue eyes. He is manly, talks no puerile slop about "rejections and that kind of stuff."

Medical: No early data. Many referrals to hospitals after age 6: Minor injuries, burns; dislocations of nasal, optical, and maxillary bones from fighting; tonsillectomy; impetigo, eczema, bronchitis, rhinitis, visual defects, upper respiratory infections. No serious illnesses or injuries. PX reveals no significant pathology beyond minor scars, defective vision, poor teeth, and flat feet.

Running Record: The Inn made many efforts to reach him but it was like trying to pet a coyote. We twice started him back to school. Each time he quit almost immediately. Several vocational and job programs came to naught. Through two years he was intermittently a corruptive element, instigating as much mischief and destruction of property, and as many minor headaches, as perhaps any boy ever to live at the Inn. He consistently maintained his *persona* of what he believed to be the typical criminal. When we first knew him he was a semi-habitual drinker. Two years later he was decidedly a drinker. Eight years later he is almost a chronic alcoholic. A cunning nuisance and an avowed destroyer of morality, he yet retained an element of Irish charm and forgivableness which almost counterbalanced his delinquency. He could never be called sneaky or crooked, or perhaps dishonest.

A year or so after our last contact with him he was inducted into military service. After spending somewhat more than two years in the service he was finally given a medical discharge. Since then he has been living an alcoholic life of intermittent larceny, automophilia, and police trouble—with detention now and again. He looks like a Zane Grey hero; is more entertaining than ever.

Summary: Hard Irish midranger but with dysmorphic brittleness. Mentality near borderline; health fairly good. Somatorotic or paranoid psychopathy of the second order; alcoholism; persistent appropriative delinquency.

ID 2–4–1 (7)
Insufficiencies:
IQ 2
Mop ....
Psychiatric:
1st order ....
2nd order 3
(2–4–2)
C-phobic 1
G-phrenic ....
Residual D:
Primary crim. 1

Comment: Prognosis dubious. It is even yet difficult to say whether the persistently delinquent and predatory outlook arises mainly from the psychopathy or from some motivational twist which may have been environmentally conditioned. On the one hand he presents all the common characteristics of a paranoid psychotic except the attentional (psychotic) disorientation. In facial expression, in his ordinary social address, and in most of his behavior he is as paranoidly hostile as a mastiff in a backyard. He seems far out on the same branch which at its tip produces the paranoid psychotics although his is clearly second- and not first-order psychopathy. On the other hand he was reared in an environment sufficiently reflecting his present outlook to make it seem very easy to blame the latter on the former. If a happy family life is to be taken as the goal and chief reward of human existence—as it is in the Freudian and to a degree in the Christian religion—then early nest relationships must indeed loom as of awful importance. The great difficulty with both of these religions is that the common current conceptions of family may be only incidental and ephemeral in the general development of human mentality. The few good minds may owe their emergence not to good family influence but to an escape from the current conception of family altogether. We might then have to say that this present youth had an unusually *good* early influence, rather than a bad one, in that he escaped the vulgarities of family influence. There is also the heartening possibility that early nest relationships are of relatively little importance to a personality already far enough along to get born. At birth a human being has millions of lifetimes and more likely billions of lifetimes of conditioning already behind him.

160. COMPANY B, PLATOON 1, SECTION 4
Second-Order Psychopathy; Multiple Complications: Nos. 144–164

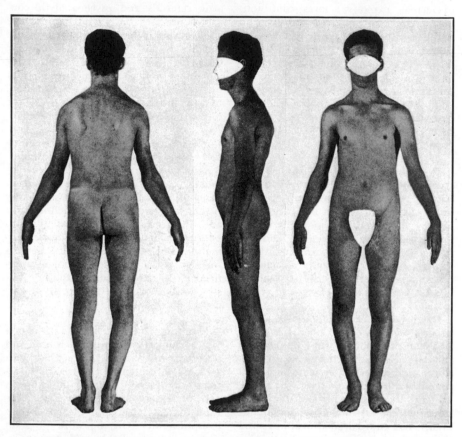

Description: Somatotype 3–4–4. A 19-year-old midranger two inches above average stature. Midrange somatotype throughout, with no particular dysplasia, but muscular development is poor in the distal segments and the whole physique is dysmorphic. Neck very heavy; chest somewhat asthenic. Primary $g\pm$; secondary g, no trace. Primary t 2, secondary t 3. Features large, regular, and hard in detail. The face and neck express a mastiff-like fierceness which the rest of the body is not able to support. Hands crude but heavily muscled; feet flat. General and hand strength 3. Coordination fairly good although movements are jerky. He is a quick and a hard hitter but has poorly sustained fighting power. Badly poised in the sense that a coyote might be badly poised at a dog show.

Temperament: He is constantly so-matorotic, appears *always* to have too much energy. The somatorosis is sustainedly hostile, but there is also flamboyant irresponsibility. He is noisy, overactive, explosive; loves confusion, action, and crowds. It is only in the night spots that he appears to find happiness and the sense of being at home. There he is literally a destroyer of pianos, a strident shouter and wailer, a thrashing machine of hysterical rhythm. Nightly he becomes alcoholized, and when he is alcoholic the second component is strainedly triumphant. He is a passionate destroyer of "peace." ψ 2–4–2.

Delinquency: Early uncontrollable truancy and unmanageability in school. Violent temper tantrums at all ages. At 12 he caused excitement but little damage by using a knife in fights. Occasional alcoholism between 16 and 20. Frequent drunkenness beginning at 20. Pattern of bumming and of being a hanger-on at night spots, from about age 18. Bastardy at 21.

Origins and Family: First of three, urban Negro family. Father a tall, active man of about the same physique as this boy. He has been a semi-alcoholic singer and entertainer, is regarded as unreliable and exploitative. The mother, more than half white and of average physique, comes from a nondelinquent family, has enjoyed good health, reared this youth in her own home after "giving up" on her husband and separating from him when the boy was 6.

Mental History, Achievement: Finished the eighth grade after a number of failures. IQ reports fall between 75 and 85, here called 80. He gives the impression of being scatterbrained. His conversation has been described as "a torrent of verbal debris."

The vocational identification is entirely with music and with night-club entertainment. He plays the piano in a wild, stiff-fingered manner which alcoholized night-club patrons find to their mood. The AMI is that of a rather handsome, broadshouldered Negro youth who is a veteran of many psychiatric referrals and psychoanalytic consultations, uses the Freudian language about the way barroom hangers-on use the Mr. G and JC concepts and other Christian language. His delinquency and shortcomings all stem directly from his rejections and early mishandling, but the intrafamilial expletives are for him principally a mode of profanity.

Medical: A rather small, five-and-a-half-pound baby, always called underweight but of normal early development. Occasional bouts of severe eczema from infancy. No other illnesses. Many psychiatric referrals for delinquency and incorrigibility. Labeled *psychopathic personality; psychoneurotic, primary behavior disorder;* etc. PX reveals no significant pathology. Large superficial blood vessels indicate the possibility of mesomorphic dysplasia in the cardiovascular system.

Running Record: Several efforts were made at the Inn to reach him, and we were intermittently in contact with him for three years. An attempt to return him to school failed within a week. Job placements were unsuccessful because of alcholism and of somatorotic irresponsibility. On the work program he was uncontrollable and unmanageable. He seemed to drift steadily toward more frequent alcoholism and toward greater disorganization. Finally he refused to participate in any kind of program and for a long time he lived by picking up such money as he needed at various night clubs. Many times he started regular jobs at these establishments but after the first payday tended to become too alcoholic and independent for further continuance.

Exempted from military service on psychiatric grounds, he has continued to drift for another five years; is still a semi-alcoholic night-club character who lives from hand to mouth, accepts no responsibility, and does not yet show overt indications of much physical deterioration.

Summary: Dysplastic ectomorph-mesomorph Negro with excessive energy. Mentality near borderline; good health. Somatorotic psychopathy. Early, persistent, and increasing alcoholism. Essential irresponsibility.

ID 1–6–0 (7)
Insufficiencies:
    IQ 1
    Mop . . . .
Psychiatric:
    1st order . . . .
    2nd order 4
    Somatorotic irresponsibility
    (2–4–2)
    C-phobic 2
    G-phrenic . . . .
Residual D:
    Primary crim. . . . .

Comment: Prognosis dark gray. Most of those who know this youth con- sider the outlook poor. He has been growing steadily more alcoholic, has never accepted responsibility of any kind or degree. Repeatedly he has been sent to psychiatrists, only to be returned with empty words. That he could be useful and perhaps happy in a disciplined environment is difficult to deny since no such environment is available or will be, and the power to prevent that is in a sense vested in his own hands. Meanwhile it may be that his behavior pattern ought to be called unsatisfactory only from a Utopian and impractical point of view. He gets enough to eat and to spare. Agencies see to it that he never misses a meal. He sleeps in a bed—and few can sleep in two beds. He is sexually popular and has reproduced his own flesh without constraint. He is more securely exempt from constraint or punishment than the majority of his ancestors have been, perhaps through countless generations. He has at his beck and call the most highly perfected medical and surgical services the world has ever known—and all of them without cost to him. Perhaps he is all right.

161. COMPANY B, PLATOON 1, SECTION 4
Second-Order Psychopathy; Multiple Complications: Nos. 144–164

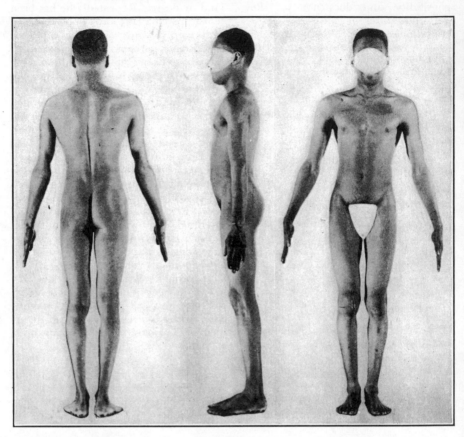

Description: Somatotype 1½–4½–4½. A 21-year-old ectomorph-meso-morph three inches above average stature. A slender, muscular Negro youth who is decidedly mesomorphic in the first two regions (head and neck and upper trunk) but equally ectomorphic in the arms and below the diaphragm. There is dramatic contrast between the mesomorphy of the upper regions of the body and the ectomorphy of the lower regions. This is a good example of the Nilotic physique (see p. 19) in contrast both with the thickset and muscular West Coast Negroes, and with the weaker, less energized and usually more mongrelized Negro stock which comes from the West Indies. Primary $g\pm$; secondary g, no trace. Primary t 4, secondary t 3. Features prominant and well formed. They show a not unpleasant blending of Caucasian and Negro characteristics. General strength 3, hand strength 3. Coordination ex-cellent. He is not athletic but has been a sort of semi-professional hot dancer or somatorotic contortionist in night clubs.

Temperament: He gives the uniform impression of both hostile and flamboyant somatorosis. Humorless, he seems to wear a perpetual snarl, like a small predatory animal in captivity. There is tremendous physical energy—sufficient to maintain his somatorotic aggression at a constant level. Speech is violent, strident, assertive. He seems always under pressure and often could be called hypomanic. No depression phase has been noted. He appears never to let down. Yet in him there is no true threat of physical aggression. One is constantly aware of an essential gynandroid weakness, or of inadequacy-at-combat. The inadequate hands and wrists define a striking contrast with the predatory facial expression. He seems to express a relentless malevolence, but also there are indications of cerebrotonic interference. The voice is always strained, poorly controlled, and there is a manifest hyperattentionality or watchfulness. It is as if he hated his own cerebrotonia and would try to snarl it down. ψ 5–3–1.

Delinquency: At 6, referred to a child-guidance clinic as destructive, violent, foul-mouthed. At 7, declared to be a behavior problem in the community and for the succeeding six years placed in various foster homes under agency management. Between 13 and 16 he lived largely in three different correctional schools, with intermittent visits to his own home. During this period there were about a dozen court charges for stealing, breaking and entering, burglary, stubborn child. Three times in court for assault and battery on the mother. In his court history, however, there is no other record of physical violence.

Origins and Family: Second of four, urban family. Father a Russian Jew of solid physique and short stature. A "medical and psychiatric delinquent." He has eighteen agency contacts over a period of twenty years, has been diagnosed *constitutional psychopathic inferior; psychoneurotic;* and *paranoid.* Also he has cardiac and renal trouble, and peptic ulcer. Several times in court on minor charges of larceny, receiving stolen goods, etc. The mother is a short 200-pound German Jewess with a somewhat similar history. She has frequently been in court because of "vicious fighting" with husband, children, and neighbors; has been diagnosed *psychoneurosis, mild, with paranoid trend.* There have been many medical complaints and numerous agency contacts. Boy reared in the home until seven, then principally in foster homes and correctional schools.

Mental History, Achievement: Finished the sixth grade, left school in the seventh after "biting, scratching and kicking" the teacher. IQ reports range from 80 to 88, here called 85. He gives the impression of somewhat better mentality than this, but his attitude is always harsh and defiant.

No vocational plan. Moderately gifted in music, fond of rhythm and jazz. The AMI is based on a fair mastery of current Freudian slang, resulting from long contact with psychiatrists. He recites that his difficulties emanate from rejections, that he has guilt feelings because of his father's shortcomings, that he has too much superego.

Medical: No data on birth. Growth and early development normal. No serious illnesses or injuries. Long history of referral to psychiatric clinics because of delinquency. Diagnosed variously as: *psychoneurotic; prepsychotic; psychopathic personality with borderline psychosis; primary behavior disorder; psychopathic personality without psychosis, with asocial and amoral trends.* PX reveals no significant pathology. Deep reflexes hyperactive.

Running Record: At the Inn he successfully defied all efforts aimed at persuading him to cooperate on the work program. He announced freely that he had no intention of working and cared little what anybody might try to do about it. In the end we failed to elicit cooperation from him on any kind of program. To efforts at consultation he responded with the sophisticated defiance of one who had been "consulted by experts." No one here succeeded in breaking through his hostility or in winning his confidence. In the end we gave ourselves F for failure with him.

Shortly after leaving the Inn he was apprehended at larceny and was returned to a state correctional school. From there he soon ran away and after vagabonding about the country for quite a long time he was inducted into military service. In the service he showed the same pattern of behavior as elsewhere—was hostile, defiant, and alcoholic. Within less than a year he was given a psychiatric discharge, and was soon again apprehended and returned to state supervision. During the succeeding three years he has spent about half the time under sentence for repeated larceny, has been involved in minor rackets, is now regarded as a sort of derelict. But if he is a derelict he is still a defiant and a rather undeteriorated one. There is temper in his metal.

Summary: Short, compact mesomorph with asthenic extremities. Good health; dull normal mentality. Somatorotic paranoid outlook. Long identification with minor stealing and exploitation.

ID 1–4–2 (7)
Insufficiencies:
  IQ 1
  Mop ....
Psychiatric:
  1st order ....
  2nd order 4
   Flamboyant—paranoid
   (5–3–1)
  C-phobic ....
  G-phrenic ....
Residual D:
  Primary crim. 2

Comment: Outlook generally regarded as dubious, but it should not be forgotten that the boy is a Jew, and I think that improves the prognosis so far as active delinquency is concerned. Despite recent hysterical propaganda to the contrary—and Jews themselves are in some degree responsible for this propaganda—there are clearly recognizable constellations of physical and temperamental characteristics among different human breeds. The general group of breeds collectively called Jewish is as clearly recognizable as any other group. It is possible that Jews just now have a better sense of agglutination, or of group loyalty, than any other white group. This may be one reason why they have a better *esprit de corps* and tend to look out for one another better than some other groups do. At any rate they do this, and from it arises a kind of patriotism which may be among the important human virtues. Being Jewish, this youth is probably more likely to "wake up and come out of it" than he would be if he were Irish or a nondescript mongrel.

COMPANY B, PLATOON 1, SECTION 4
Second-Order Psychopathy; Multiple Complications:
Nos. 144–164

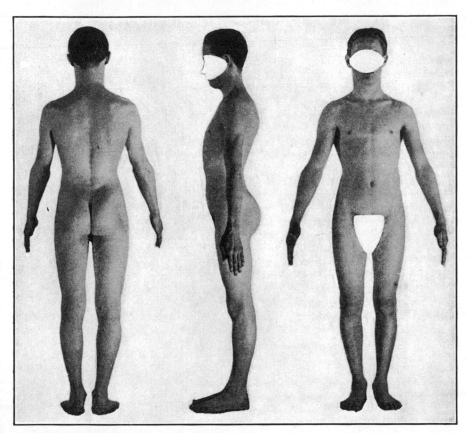

Description: Somatotype 3–5–2½. A 16-year-old mesomorph two inches under average stature. A short, compact, still immature physique with broad shoulders and arms showing asthenic inadequacy in both the proximal and the distal segments. There is a similar although lesser weakness in the upper chest and in the legs. Otherwise the boy is solidly built and in middle age will appear chunky and barrel-bodied. Primary g+1; secondary g, no trace. Primary t 3, secondary t 2. Features large, hard, and coarse. Hands and feet weak and badly formed. General strength 3, hand strength 2. Coordination good in that he moves gracefully and maintains an upright mesomorphic posture. No athletic ability. He cannot fight or throw well.

Temperament: Best described as epileptoid. He suggests a volcano which is always on the verge of eruption and at frequent intervals does erupt. Violent, threatening, pugnacious at all times, he is almost continually involved in altercation. The outstanding characteristics are courage, love of risk, and essential hardihood. He achieves a vocal violence rarely heard and has a seemingly continuous need for muscular action. There is little viscerotonic relaxation and never a sign of cerebrotonic restraint. He lives for the second component, is wholly indentified with hardness and toughness, expresses a constant and flamboyant somatorosis. Even so, the pressure seems to accumulate so that it becomes necessary to blow off steam violently at frequent intervals. Under alcohol he merely shows the same pattern more intensified. His life is a somatorotic episode with an epileptoid rhythm. ψ 5–3–1.

Delinquency: Incorrigible in school from the first day. Truancy, destructiveness, and violent fighting between 6 and 10. Sent to state correctional school at 10, where he remained intermittently for five years. Meanwhile and thereafter involved with a tough gang. Between 10 and 15, frequently apprehended in small robberies, acts of destruction, and vandalism. First arrested for assault and battery at 15. This offense later repeated several times, at 16 and 17. Between 12 and 17, numerous episodes of jack-rolling, robbing of drunks, luring and despoiling of homosexuals, etc. Regarded as the ringleader and the fighter for a delinquent gang. One of the three or four toughest youths of the series.

Origins and Family: Second of five, urban Irish family. Father of average muscular physique, delinquent from childhood, in and out of state correctional and penal institutions all his life: drunkenness, robbery, larceny, nonsupport. Diagnosed *alcoholic psychosis* and died in a state institution in his forties when the boy was 12. Paternal grandmother died in a state mental hospital. Paternal grandfather a state ward and later a chronic alcoholic. Mother, regarded as a mental defective, died in a state hospital in her late thirties after a history of epilepsy and obesity. She was one of a large family all of whom have been diagnosed as feebleminded or psychotic, and all have been under agency support at various times. Maternal grandfather died in a mental hospital after diagnosis of feeblemindedness and chronic alcoholism. He had been sterilized after siring twelve children. Of the four siblings of this boy three have died; the fourth diagnosed epileptic and feebleminded.

Mental History, Achievement: Quit school in the fifth grade after a history of tantrums and violence. IQ reports vary from 74 to 95, here put at 80.

No vocational plans although he comes close to being equipped for professional athletics. A terrific fighter who in routine quarrels has repeatedly knocked larger boys unconscious, he never entered boxing competitions or other organized athletics. His energies have been directed almost entirely into delinquent channels. The AMI that of a youthful and cocky buoyancy with a clear indication of underlying sturdiness or manliness. It is a very effective AMI and too much for any but the most hardened social workers. The boy has a sprightly manner of moving and of social address which catches and holds the attention even of the preoccupied.

Medical: No data on his birth and early development. To date he seems to have enjoyed vigorous health despite being virtually surrounded, in a hereditary sense, by the gravest sort of constitutional pathology (epilepsy, obesity, psychosis, feeblemindedness, alcoholism). From childhood he has been subject to violent tantrums and fits of rage, often without apparent provocation. Frequently called epileptoid. PX reveals no pathology beyond caries and acne. Moderately high blood pressure.

Running Record: Perhaps because of the irresistible AMI the Inn made numerous and persistent efforts to rehabilitate this youth. To these efforts he responded as the horsefly responds to the switching tail, making only such minor adjustments as were immediately necessary. He looked upon the Inn in precisely that light in which the horsefly regards the horse. He was altogether identified with his *persona* of delinquency or exploitation, but made himself respected and feared. He packed a tremendous punch, extracted protection money from other residents of the House, was frank and open in his methods. There was nothing underhanded, nothing crooked about him. While with us he was caseworked by numerous workers from various agencies whose mother-hearts went out to his frank Irish face. In his exploitation of these opportunities he had a logic-tight argument: "Why the hell shouldn't I get them hand-outs—they get paid too, don't they?" In the end he beat us a love set. He absorbed what we had to offer, but for this yielded up no part of his untamed soul.

Exempt from military service because of his record, he has followed essentially the same pattern for another half-dozen years and has gradually become more closely identified with the veteran criminal fraternity. Some of the irresistibility of the pristine AMI has now gone. He has found it necessary on at least two or three occasions to work, but to date such events have regularly been punctuated with episodes of robbery, breaking and entering, or assault and battery. During the six years he has been in jail about half the time, is at the present writing under detention for breaking and entering. He still carries an atmosphere of manly frankness, is still called a "square guy." That is something which no one can take away from a forthright mesomorph.

Summary: Powerful mesomorphic physique with almost first-rate athletic ability. IQ nearly borderline; history of vigorous health. Second-order psychopathy of both an epileptoid and somatorotic nature. Persistent criminality of violent appropriativeness.

ID 1–4–2 (7)
  Insufficiencies:
    IQ 1
    Mop . . . .
  Psychiatric:
    1st order . . . .
    2nd order 4
    Somatorotic, epileptoid
    (5–3–1)
    C-phobic . . . .
    G-phrenic . . . .
  Residual D:
    Primary crim. 2

Comment: The outlook is considered highly dubious, although he is not yet badly deteriorated to outward appearance and has not become an alcoholic. He has a rugged physique which has stood terrific punishment. Two or three years back, he is said to have slept in an alleyway all winter. Such hardihood commands a twinge of admiration. But the prognosis for long life is anything but good and in his middle twenties he is well into middle age.

His behavior almost smells of epilepsy. However he is not an epileptic by any clinical criteria and he has not yet given clear indication of any other specific physiological insufficiency. He is epileptoid but is also somatorotic over and above the epileptoid tantrums. That is to say, he is somatorotic *all* the time but *wildly* somatorotic only periodically. This is neither Dionysian nor paranoid somatorosis and he is not hebephrenic or schizoid at all. The psychopathy is not akin to any of the Kraepelinian "type entities" but is almost purely second-component psychopathy.

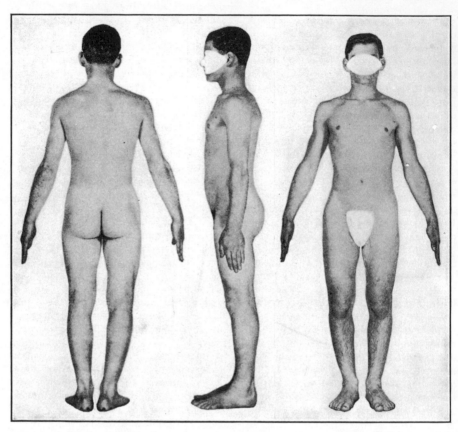

Description: Somatotype 3–5½–1½. A 17-year-old mesomorph an inch under average stature. A powerful and well-muscled physique except in the arms and distal segments of the legs, where muscular development has fallen behind the heavy skeletal structure. In these regions there is a suggestion of stunting or of scrub-oak mesomorphy, yet this remains a compact, resilient physique and one of great fighting power. Primary *g*±, secondary *g*, no trace. Primary *t* 4, secondary *t* 3. Features firm and well developed but a little crude. Square face, pug nose. General strength 5, hand strength 3—for his size one of the strongest boys in the series. Coordination excellent. He is a natural athlete and a fighter. Were it not for the slight stunting of the arms he might be a first-rate professional fighter. He is lightning quick and a straight hitter.

Temperament: The principal characteristic is harsh impatience frequently accentuated and reinforced with alcohol. Of tremendous energy, he seems to have a constant need for letting off steam in dangerous action. His unlimited courage, directness, psychological callousness, and lack of restraint define extreme somatotonia. No sign of cerebrotonic interference, no indication of conflict. He shows no cycloid tendency. He appears to enjoy the unlimited flow of energy necessary to maintain a high level of somatorotic behavior indefinitely. ψ 5–2–1.

Delinquency: Called by stepmother "an extremely bad boy as a child of 4." At 8 he would stay out all night, was defiant of authority, and was regarded as a terrific fighter. No record of truancy but called a chronic tough at 10. At 14 he had been charged with larceny, breaking and entering, drunkenness, use of aliases. At 16, panhandling, assault and battery, violation of parole, and "chronic" drunkenness had been added. Sent to state correctional institutions nine times between 12 and 17. Three times dishonorably discharged from the CCC, on the last occasion for attacking and beating a policeman. Repeatedly in trouble for alcoholism, larceny, and "unnatural sex practices" between 17 and 20. When alcoholized he has a tendency to commit active pederasty. However, he is normally heterosexual and his behavior in such instances seems to constitute an act of rollicking somatorotic aggression rather than one primarily of sexuality at all.

Origins and Family: Oldest of five, mill-city family. Father an athletic French mill worker who is described as a substantial, honest man. As a youth he was a professional athlete of national standing. Mother, French-Irish, died suddenly when this boy was less than 2. She had high blood pressure and had been under psychiatric observation. The father remarried and four more children were born. The stepmother has kept what is called a good home. None of her own children are delinquent. Boy reared at home until 12, then sent to correctional schools.

Mental History, Achievement: Finished the sixth grade. Quit in the seventh after fighting with the principal of the school, whom he says he gave a black eye. IQ reports range from 84 to 96, here called 90. At first he seems more intelligent than this, but he is so somatorotic and so ineducable in the ordinary social sense that the early impression is soon revised downward. No vocational plan other than a vague and general desire to be a professional fighter. The main achievement is pugilistic, but it is readily apparent that his ambition to be a heavyweight champion is to be disappointed. The AMI is based on physical exuberance and mesomorphic stalwartness, with a deep, wide chest and an atmosphere of superb physical competence.

Medical: No early data. Excellent medical history. Never sick a day in his life, so far as is known. PX reveals no significant pathology except evidence of minor injuries sustained in combat.

Running Record: A prolonged and vigorous effort was made with this boy. With so poor a history and so good a physical constitution he was considered a particular challenge to the Inn. Intermittently he seemed to show a favorable response. That is to say, he would remain sober for a week, meantime working with vigorous energy, and would use his great leadership ability to keep other boys in line and to handle such situations and quarrels as arose. During these periods he gave promise of being a success, but always after a week, or at most two, he would relapse into alcoholism. Several times he started to do well on heavy construction jobs, truck driving, and the like, but we failed to induce him to stay with anything of the sort for more than a few weeks. There was no response to educational or vocational influences. The alcoholism was always in the way.

After leaving the Inn he seems to have soon become as alcoholic as ever and to have identified himself with a thoroughly delinquent pattern. Exempted from military service because of his record, he has been confined in corrective or penal institutions for about two-thirds of the time during the past six years—mainly for episodes of robbery with violence.

Summary: Highly energized mesomorphy with nearly first-rate athletic ability. Excellent health; normal subaverage mentality. Persistent somatorotic delinquency from early childhood. An alcoholic of record from 14. Later delinquency of violence.

ID 0–6–2 (8)
Insufficiencies:
  IQ ....
  Mop ....
Psychiatric:
  1st order ....
  2nd order 4
    Somatorotic (5–2–1)
  C-phobic 2
  G-phrenic ....
Residual D:
  Primary crim. 2

Comment: Outlook considered poor. He has lived in a delinquent and alcoholic pattern long enough to be safely beyond the reach of cajolery or conversion. He seemingly wants to be and intends to remain what he is, and even as a delinquent drunkard he may be a better man than most of us. It is of interest to note that although he has the coordination and almost the power for first-rate athletic competition, he in this respect fell short of his father's and his own expectation. His whole career might be interpreted as a long sulk or protest, either against his father or against his own failure to grow to the proportions of a heavyweight champion. Yet if this were to be taken as "the reason for" his delinquency, then nearly all of us have good reason to commit murder.

In certain studies this youth has been listed as a homosexual, on the grounds of his occasional participation in pederasty when alcoholized. Yet his personality is not even distantly related to that of the homosexuals who seek and prefer sexual collaborators of their own sex. This boy was never *addicted* to homosexuality. When alcoholized he merely becomes sexually aggressive in the highest degree—seems to have no inhibitory component. If girls are not available he will seize upon whatever *is* available, and it can be almost anything. Extreme mesomorphs rarely masturbate, or rarely make a practice of masturbation. That practice seems to require a degree of cerebrotonia. Instead, extreme mesomorphs and somatotonic people tend to extravert their sexual energies, and when of nondiscriminative mentality they are likely to extravert it in almost any direction. If investigators of homosexuality would bear this general fact in mind, some of the confusion concerning that concept might clear up. This youth should never have been called homosexual, but if he *must* be so classified, it should be within a special sub-group such as *homosexualitas any-old-holibus.*

COMPANY B, PLATOON 1, SECTION 4
Second-Order Psychopathy; Multiple Complications:
Nos. 144–164

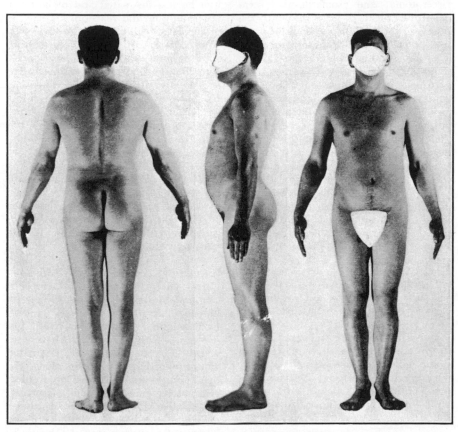

Description: Somatotype 4–5½–1½. A powerfully built 20-year-old endo-morphic mesomorph of average stature. The trunk, shoulders, and neck al-most reach heavyweight power but the arms fall short of that standard. How-ever, they are powerful arms and the physique as a whole is that of a poised athlete who in this photograph is about ten pounds overweight (he had spent a winter at the Inn, on the work program). Primary g±; secondary g, no trace. Primary t 3, secondary t 3. Features strongly developed and well molded although lacking in fineness. Hands and feet well formed. This boy stems back to good stock, and not very far back. General strength 5, hand strength 4. Coordination superb. One of the two or three best all-round ath-letes ever to live at the Inn, and possibly the best fighter. He is as quick as a cat and of lethal striking power.

Temperament: He has seemingly inexhaustible energy, yet always presents a relaxed, grinning exterior. This is an exasperatingly poised youth in whom viscerotonia and somatotonia seem beautifully blended. He is insolently deliberate, yet amiable, sociophilic, and tireless. One of those people with whom it is almost impossible to take a firm stand and make it stick. In consequence he usually does about as he pleases. Under the viscerotonia is a stubborn resolution to have his way and a ruthless persistence in getting it. One of our staff called him the soft-on-the-outside-hard-on-the-inside type. He is feminoid-tough, suggesting one of those padded, erect women whose realistically worldly eye is fixed unflinchingly on the immediate objective. If you have ever run up against one you need no further description. This boy's objective is always a carousal. One of the most alcoholic youths in the series. ψ 3–1–1.

Delinquency: Truancy and early stealing. Under arrest for stealing as early as 13. To state correctional school at 15 for larceny. Between 15 and 21, a long series of court appearances for drunkenness, reckless driving, fence for stolen goods, larceny, disorderly conduct, pimping, barroom loitering. For three or four years before our contact with the boy he had been "rarely seen sober."

Origins and Family: Only child, urban Irish family. Father stocky and rotund, a moderately alcoholic salesman for twenty years. He showed manic symptoms during the last four or five years of his life, died of apoplexy in the late forties when the boy was 17. Mother short and muscular with a long record of agency relationships and usually described as aggressive. In one five-year period she moved thirteen times. Boy reared at "home."

Mental History; Achievement: Finished a year of high school, quit in the second year with failing grades. IQ reports range between 85 and 100, here called 95. He gives an impression of being canny, although when we first saw him he was dissipated and of more or less cloudy mental reactions.

No vocational plans or special gifts. The AMI that of a relaxed, interesting youth whose teeth are almost entirely rotted out and who looks dissipated. He is generally called Baby Face, but he is no baby and beneath the soft exterior is a defiant independence which, one knows intuitively, nothing in this life will ever break down. In some fundamental sense he is unassailable.

Medical: Early history not known. No record of illnesses. History of soft, inadequate teeth in both the first and second dentitions. Numerous minor injuries from drunken brawling. PX reveals no pathology of significance.

Running Record: At the Inn noteworthy efforts were made to achieve a conquest of Baby Face and to convert him to something or other. He was offered a school program, started it but was drunk within two days. There were several job placements, all terminated almost immediately by drunkenness. On the work program he gave no trouble. He merely ignored it good naturedly. His single-minded objective was always carousal and he showed resourcefulness in smuggling liquor into the House as well as in corrupting others to do so. When not anaesthetized he was poignantly conscious of his feminoid softness and periodically he would start a course in muscle development at a local gymnasium. These courses did not seem to change his somatotype much. After a time the staff convinced itself of the difficulty of the undertaking and graduated the boy.

Exempted from military service because of his record, he has drifted during the intervening half-dozen years, occasionally working briefly as bartender or restaurant counterman. He has grown even more alcoholic, has been about a third of the time under detention for breaking and entering and larceny, and he still has the old complacent outlook. The real difficulty of the business is that when talking with this boy one always has the haunting fear that the boy may have the right outlook.

Summary: Well-energized PPJ physique with a strong complement of primary *g*. Relaxed outlook. Temperamentally complacent. Mentality normal; good health. Long identification with minor delinquency. A confirmed alcoholic at 21. Later a past master.

ID 0–5–2 (7)
Insufficiencies:
IQ ....
Mop ....
Psychiatric:
1st order ....
2nd order ....
C-phobic 4
G-phrenic 1
Residual D:
Primary crim. 2

Comment: Outlook generally considered poor, although he does not seem to have deteriorated much during the past half-dozen years. Perhaps he is one of those happily constituted organisms for whom alcohol acts only as a preservative. I can recall my grandmother standing in the front window of our village home, of a Sunday afternoon forty or more years ago, and gazing with indignant horror at old Ed Church as the latter beat his way with difficulty up the street, headed home from the village saloon. "Mark that man well," she said. "He is steering straight for a drunkard's grave." That he was, and still is. I saw him last summer, tacking heavily reefed on the same difficult course; about twenty paces to starboard to the big elm, then port to the telephone pole, starboard again to the corner of the old Rhodes house, and so home. Ed is said to have volunteered for service in the Civil War, but to have been rejected because he was too young.

Perhaps for another three quarters of a century this youth too will drink his way toward a drunkard's grave. He won't mind.

COMPANY B, PLATOON 1, SECTION 5
Alcoholics: Nos. 165–167

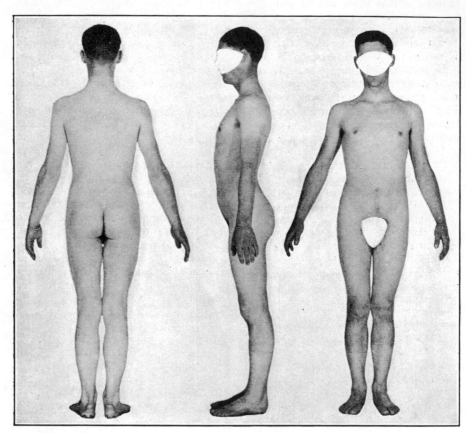

Description: Somatotype 4–4–2. A 21-year-old endomorph-mesomorph of average stature. Moderate ectomorphic dysplasia in the first region. Otherwise, even and harmonious development throughout. Good example of the PPJ pattern. A physique which will grow heavy—and easily very heavy in later life. Primary $g+1$; secondary g, no trace. Primary t 3, secondary t 2. Pudgy face with gross, nondescript features, although it is a comparatively strong face and has good symmetry. Strikingly coarse hands with fat, stubby fingers. Short, strong feet. General strength 3, hand strength 3. Coordination good. He handles himself like one of the felines in sleek condition, seems always relaxed. Too soft—insufficient snap—for fighting or for athletics.

Temperament: Both viscerotonically and somatotonically extraverted, with no sign of cerebrotonic restraint. He is so relaxed, amiable, and gluttonous, yet so aggressively sure of himself, that his presence in a group lifts the viscerotonic level by a notch or two. When fully under alcohol he becomes even more viscerotonic, embracing the universe in one comprehensive affection. When only partially alcoholized he is reckless, sexually aggressive, resourcefully profane. He tends to be energetic or somatotonic only *in the process* of becoming alcoholized and it is in this phase that he gets into trouble. He is "cycloid"; has periods of depression, has been called *prepsychotic, manic-depressive.* ψ 3–1–1.

Delinquency: Arrested for drunkenness as early as 15 and frequently thereafter. Known to have been alcoholic at an even earlier age and to have caused disturbances in school because of drinking. Arrested several times between 14 and 18 for stealing liquor. Associated with the alcoholism have been many arrests for vagrancy, disorderly conduct, and the like. Often in trouble for "irregular sex practices" which were carried on as a means of procuring alcohol. No history of stealing since 18 or of any delinquency except that associated with alcoholism. During the years between 18 and 24, several times institutionalized and subjected to "cures" but these had no effect.

Origins and Family: Youngest of four, urban family. Father Old American and of average build, at times a heavy drinker but otherwise reputable and responsible. Mother Portuguese and heavily built, described as "emotional, excitable, but of amiable disposition." She has "problems of high blood pressure." One maternal uncle confined in a mental hospital, diagnosis not known. Boy reared in the home but always looked upon as "the weak one."

Mental History, Achievement: Left school in the seventh grade after a series of episodes in which alcoholism played a part. IQ reports range from 80 to 106, here placed at 100. When sober he gives the impression of better than average intelligence. He has humor and a certain rich, eclectic insight into human frailties.

No vocational plan and no special abilities other than a good-natured geniality which renders him well liked and welcome in nearly all company. The AMI that of a natural actor with a salty commentative attitude. At his best he keeps up a running fire of comment on life and people which is faintly suggestive of Will Rogers. When drunk he does the same, with louder voice, less insight, and the comments are embowered in a language matrix of great richness.

Medical: Normal birth history but he presents a long record of childhood illnesses and hospital referrals. The question of congenital lues was frequently raised but no such diagnosis was made. He has a congenital visual defect and as the alcoholism developed this became worse. Now diagnosed *toxic amblyopia.* He had all the common children's diseases severely, several abscesses, two instances of septicemia from minor scratches; a number of episodes of venereal infection. He has been put through at least five different kinds of treatment for alcoholism, from attempted psychoanalysis to drug therapy; has spent more than two years under hospitalization in connection with this problem. PX reveals no additional pathology except moderately elevated blood pressure.

Running Record: For this youth the Inn offered a sort of hotel service and temporary parking place during the course of several years while various attempts at treatment of alcoholism were carried out. Psychiatric referral yielded the diagnoses, *alcoholic psychosis; psychopathic personality, with alcoholism.* We attempted such palliatives as temporary removal to the country, development of hobbies and of proposed intellectual interests, music therapy, and sedation. None of these had much effect. He always presented a difficult problem because of indiscriminate sexuality, or "perverse practices" associated with his alcoholism.

For two years following his last contact at the Inn the pattern remained about the same. He spent half of that time under hospitalization. Thereafter he was inducted into military service but was given a medical discharge within a year. Following this he was again institutionalized for a period and was then sent to the Merchant Marine, where he got along for nearly two years. He tells good naturedly of the assignment of one of his shipmates to accompany him on all shore leaves with a wheelbarrow in which to bring him back to the ship. After being discharged from the Merchant Marine he was once more committed to a mental hospital but more recently has been out again, drifting in the old pattern.

Summary: Mesomorphic endomorph with weak, asthenic arms and a gynandroid complication. Normal mentality. Some degree of immunological insufficiency. Chronic alcoholism from an unusually early age.

ID 2–6–o (8)
Insufficiencies:
   IQ ....
   Mop 2
Psychiatric:
   1st order ....
   2nd order 2
   (3–1–1)
   C-phobic 4
   G-phrenic ....
Residual D:
   Primary crim. ....

Comment: Outlook considered poor by those who have tried to cure his alcoholism, but from his point of view the outlook may be good. He seems to enjoy life. The cycloid psychopathy is sufficiently manifest, but this is characteristic of many people of his general somatotype and temperament and need not be regarded as premonitory of a manic-depressive psychosis. He has given no indication of any incipient disorder of attention which would point to first-order psychopathy.

This seems to be cycloid alcoholism, and it may be noted that cycloid Northwesterners are all-or-none people. When they go in for something, even alcoholism, they really go.

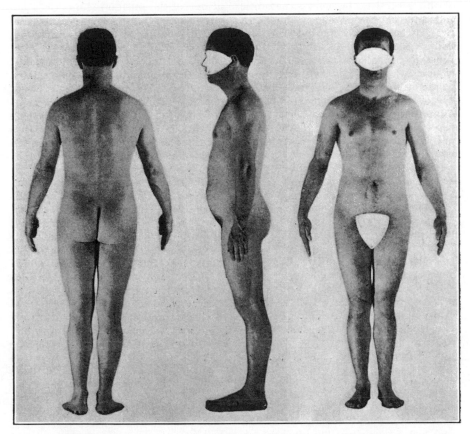

Description: Somatotype 5–4–1½. A 24-year-old mesomorphic endo-morph of average stature. Arms short, moderately asthenic, budlike. Trunk, neck, and thighs sturdy, well muscled. Primary g+2, secondary g+1. Primary t 3 despite the inadequate arms. Secondary t 2. Features coarsely formed, as if the Potter's mind had wandered. Hands strikingly small, hypoplastic. Large superficial veins. General strength 3, hand strength 2. Coordination good. He moves softly and gracefully, like a woman. Not good at athletic games, throws like a girl. Swims well.

Temperament: The temperament seems to belie the physique. He is normally quiet, with weak and almost rhythmic outbursts of futile rage. The total impression when he is not alcoholized is that of epileptoid weakness and perhaps of schizoid recession in all three components. However, he is frequently alcoholized and during the early stages of this process he becomes somatorotic and overriding. He then stands up straight, swells his tremendous chest, and gives the impression of feeling important or dominant. At such times he is generous, sociophilic, expansive to almost a hypomanic degree. With further advancement of the drug effect he becomes sleepy, seems viscerotonic. He is never ugly, has never been known to bully or take advantage of weaker boys, nor has he been known to fight, even when himself bullied. Combativeness apparently is not in him. ψ 3–2–2.

Delinquency: Early truancy and a long history of unsatisfactory school adjustment. He has been a disappointment to many people who have "taken an interest in him." Episodes of drunkenness at 16, and recurrent to the present time. When drunk he is addicted to reckless driving, on one such occasion caused a fatality. No history of stealing. His delinquency has been altogether associated with alcohol. Frequent question of "unnatural sex practices," usually in connection with the procurement of drinkables.

Origins and Family: Fifth of six, urban family. Father a large Irishman who had intermittent difficulty with alcohol, along with high blood pressure, and died in his forties when this boy was an infant, immediate cause unknown. Paternal grandfather was alcoholic and died young; paternal grandmother committed to mental hospital. Mother a Danish-French mill girl, described as "never strong," died of unknown cause when this boy was 8. She

had had a long sequence of illnesses. Boy then reared in foster homes under agency management.

Mental History, Achievement: Finished two years of high school although with low grades and an unsatisfactory record. IQ reports vary from 79 to 143, here put at 100. The 143 was achieved at one of the inflation clinics on a test which he had taken many times before and on which he had previously been coached. He gives the impression of about average mentality.

No vocational plan or special abilities. The AMI rests on the universal appeal of an apparently stalwart mesomorphy, and on a general atmosphere of manliness or virility, although this impression is not well sustained on closer acquaintance with the boy.

Medical: Early history not known. No record of illnesses except mild infections. For six or seven years, since he has been drinking, he has complained of dizziness and tremor. Psychiatric referral has yielded such diagnoses as *psychopathic personality, with alcoholism and paranoid ruminations.* PX reveals a conspicuous coarse tremor of the fingers, hyperactive tendon reflexes, and flat feet.

Running Record: At the Inn he was for the most part a gentlemanly person who identified himself largely with the *DAMP RAT* group, although he was never able to participate very actively in the arty conversations and interests of that group and was never regarded as basically a homosexual. He seemed feminoid without being quite effeminate, or quite arty. In general he was tolerated or respected, as all pronounced mesomorphs are respected, and was never ill treated except by two or three smaller and far tougher mesomorphs who singled him out for bullying. In the presence of these he showed an essential cowardice or weakness. Several efforts at treating his alcoholism were abortive. He made two or three false starts at a school program, and these soon resulted in boredom which required drowning. Outside the House he tended to agglutinate with the bums in the lowest dives, and to permit "degrading familiarities" for drinks.

After drifting for another two years in the pattern described he was inducted into military service. There he remained for three years, married, and became the father of children; but grew steadily more alcoholic and after spending some months in military hospitals was ultimately given a medical discharge. He is now regarded as a true alcoholic, with the outlook "not better than fair."

Summary: A physique approaching extreme mesomorphy, but with weak distal segments and a gynic complication. Normal mentality. Good health. Second-order psychopathy, alcoholism.

ID o–8–o (8)
   Insufficiencies:
      IQ ....
      Mop ....
   Psychiatric:
      1st order ....
      2nd order 2
        Epileptoid (3–2–2)
      C-phobic 4
      G-phrenic 2
      DAMP RAT
   Residual D:
      Primary crim. ....

Comment: This youth may have missed becoming a great athlete or successful politician by the narrowest of genealogical margins. Ontogenetically he certainly started out to be a powerful and athletic man, but something went wrong. The difficulty may have started in that delicate genetic mechanism controlling sexual differentiation, of which we know next to nothing. At any rate the difficulty progressed, and instead of becoming a happy and rollicking mesomorph he grew into an epileptoid, cerebrophobic gynandrophrene and carried an *almost* magnificent body to degradation in South End dives. He may have missed homosexuality by a margin as narrow as that by which he missed being an athlete.

The nature of the physiological deviation which gave such a powerfully built mesomorph a psychopathic trend offers one of the most dramatic mysteries in medicine. We do not even know whether the difficulty was in this case purely hereditary, purely postconceptional, or neither. Yet it would be comparatively easy to find out. If the history of all the immediate ancestors or descendants of this youth for three generations were to be known even as well as his history is known, which is not a very high standard to set, it is possible that a defensible hypothesis could be written. If all of the descendants of the known psychopaths in this series were to be followed that well, for a few generations, we might have an answer. The cost in money would be somewhat less than will be the cost of taking care of these descendants. And if meanwhile the compulsion toward promiscuous or universal reproduction could be controlled or inhibited, a psychotic might before long be a museum exhibit.

167. COMPANY B, PLATOON 1, SECTION 5
Alcoholics: Nos. 165–167

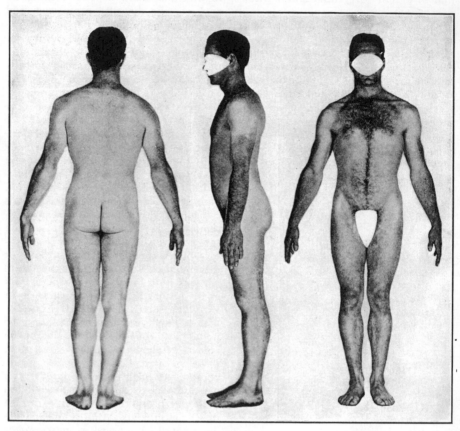

Description: Somatotype 3½–5½–2. A 21-year-old mesomorph two inches above average stature. The whole physique is powerfully developed except in the distal segments of arms and legs, which show a trace of the asthenic characteristic. At a glance he looks like a powerful man and a fighter, but he is not. Primary $g+1$, secondary $g+1$. Primary t 3, secondary t 3. Features well formed although too fine and delicate for the somatotype. General strength 3, hand strength 2. Coordination good. He moves gracefully but there is a strange, almost effeminate weakness in him. At handshake the hands are unresponsive, fishlike. They seem to have neither bones nor blood. Not good at athletic games and not a fighter.

Temperament: A womanly viscerotonia seems to predominate. His goodnature and wide-eyed ingenuousness put even ectomorphs at ease. He is markedly gynandrophrenic with no trace of the *DAMP RAT* syndrome. There is rather a fine femininity about him. He is easily expressive of feeling, cries and laughs too readily, and the principal "complaint" against him at camp was based on his gluttony and overfondness for food. He is vocally restrained and seemly; quietly careful not to attract attention. This is a viscerotonic-nice personality but cerebrotonia appears to be at least normally represented. He lacks aggression and lacks somatotonic energy in general, except for frequent brief moods of remarkable stubbornness. The temperamental pattern is probably normal to this somatotype, with an endomorphic control room matched against an ectomorphic boiler and driving machinery. ψ 2–1–1.

Delinquency: None until 17 when he was sent to a CCC camp against his desire. There he was unhappy, got drunk and was arrested, spending a term in jail. CCC officials state that his record was excellent up to the time of this episode. No later history of delinquency, and really no delinquency at all.

Origins and Family: Only child, urban family. Father a short, heavy Irish salesman who married the mother a few weeks before the boy was born and disappeared shortly afterward. He is described in agency records as "alcoholic, likeable, irresponsible." Mother Old American and described as "lively, pretty and vivacious" at 16 when she was married. A dozen years later she is described by one of the social agencies as "fat, drunken, gluttonous and degenerate." She was a PPJ. Between 17 and 30 her record shows a dozen court appearances, mostly on morals charges. She gave up her child after the father deserted and the boy was reared in foster homes, although his way was for the most part paid by relatives.

Mental History, Achievement: Finished the eighth grade, started vocational school, but after two years failed and quit. His record throughout grade school was good. He was always scored "excellent" in deportment. At vocational school he seems to have lost interest, neglected work, and truanted. IQ reports fall between 95 and 103, here called 100. He gives the impression of being normally intelligent but of lacking toughness in his mental fabric. He is alert and socially reponsive but all his interests are juvenile. He seems to be a boy who, at growing up time, is not quite ready to grow up.

No vocational plans or special gifts. The AMI that of a bright looking, round-faced, and warmhearted youth who calls out parental impulses.

Medical: Birth history and early development not known. No record of any illnesses and no hospital referrals—his way was paid privately, not by agencies. PX reveals no significant pathology.

Running Record: We took on this youth with a specific idea in mind. He had got negatively conditioned to school and had expressed what was called a "mulish stubbornness on the subject." We undertook to "bring him around" with the idea of putting him in high school. After three months we had to give it up as a bad job. At camp he did well, was considered weak and backward by the more somatotonic of the camp counsellors but to others was rather a source of delight. He was healthy, childlike, gluttonous, aquaphilic. In particular he was almost maternally kind and gentle with all sorts of living creatures. Therein he defined quite a contrast with the run of the camp mob. He seemed to have a flair for natural history. We used what cajolery we could muster to persuade him to accept a scholarship to the school plan; but school was the one thing he would not tolerate. Accepting failure at last, we were able only to send him to a poultry farm.

He did well at the poultry farm for about a year, probably would have stayed there for the rest of his life if the war had not interfered. The war took him from a $25-a-month rural job where he worked 60 hours a week to a $300-a-month urban job where he did infinitely less skilled work 40 hours a week. He didn't like the change, but after a time the situation was alleviated by induction into military service. He stayed in the service until the end of the war, added 20 or 30 pounds, brought back expensive habits and other signs of maturation, giving the impression of having been coarsened but of still lacking the underlying make-up to sustain a coarse way of life. He is one of the few in this series who refused the $20 per week unemployment dole that was distributed to ex-servicemen. During the years after discharge he has tried half a dozen jobs, finds them dissatisfying. He really wants to go back to the poultry farm but has expensive habits and has been spoiled for that by too much money. He is uncertain and unsettled.

Summary: Gynandroid midrange physique on the mesopenic side. Gynan-

drophrenia with no trace of the *DAMP RAT* syndrome. Mentality normal; excellent health. One brief flurry of delinquency, like a snowfall in June.

ID 0–1–0 (1)

  Insufficiencies:

    IQ ....

    Mop ....

  Psychiatric:

    1st order ....

    2nd order ....

    C-phobic ....

    G-phrenic   1

  Residual D:

    Primary crim. ....

Comment: Outlook very good so far as delinquency is concerned. He never was a delinquent and probably should not have been sentenced for his one alcoholic escapade. He may have been a victim of bad educational guidance. It seems a shame that he missed going to high school for he was equipped by nature to do well there and with his gynandrophrenia he was not equipped to do well at the vocational school that he attended. At the latter place he had a bad time, losing ground which he can never recover. Meanwhile the war has raised his standard of living tenfold, so far as dollar expenditure is concerned, and has probably spoiled him for the poultry farm which at $25 a month he loved. He seems to have been cheated all around.

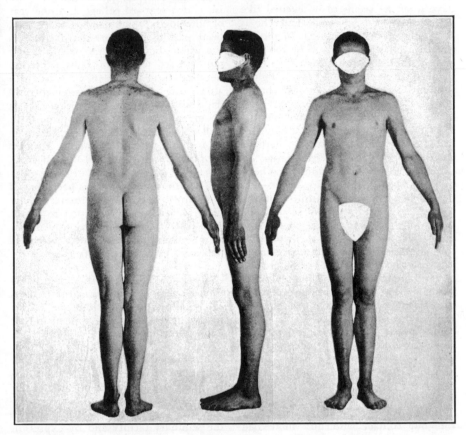

Description: Somatotype 4–3½–4. An 18-year-old dysplastic midrange physique, an inch above average stature. First region strongly endomorphic, with a short mesomorphic neck. Second and third regions—chest and arms—slightly mesomorphic. Below the diaphragm he is a mesopene, with strikingly dysplastic 4–2–5 legs. Excellent segmental development. No asthenic indications—this is regional dysplasia. Primary $g+1$, secondary $g+1$. Primary t 3, secondary t 3. Features well formed and well balanced, although a little pudgy. Hands and feet well formed but too large for this physique—a minor mesomorphic dysplasia. General strength 2, hand strength 3. General coordination poor but he has good secondary coordination; excellent finger dexterity and good eye-hand coordination. Poorly adapted to athletic games and to fighting; good swimmer.

Temperament: The predominant characteristic is that of a kind of intent fussiness. He shows a cycloid pattern, maintaining a high level of activity for days, when he seems to be excited like a bird dog on a hot trail. Later he is seen fatigued and depressed. In the hyperactive phase he tends to be too busy to be bothered. Cerebrotonia is strongly manifest in both phases. He is tightly restrained, particularly in the hands and face, and is hyperattentional. This is far from a manic-depressive picture. He falls short by half of possessing sufficient energy for that pattern. Perhaps we could call him a second-order, or possibly a third-order cycloid. Also he is apparently too gynandrophrenic—too honestly and simply feminine—for the *DAMP RAT* syndrome and in tastes he shows little overlapping with that group. His one contact with them is his love of music. It is important to remember that the *DAMP RATs* are not *extreme* gynandrophrenes—not honestly feminine. They are of another, perhaps mixed feather. With so much cerebrotonia and so much mesopenia this youth could never become a manic-depressive psychotic. But with so much gynandrophrenia he would be perhaps equally certain not to be a successful preacher. ψ 2–1–2.

Delinquency: Psychiatric only. Before our contact with him there had been signs of nervous breakdown, or of bewilderment and depression. A series of emotional outbursts had been called hysterical.

Origins and Family: First of two, village family. Father of German extraction and somewhat similar to the boy in physique but stronger. He is a minister who has lived happily in villages or small towns all his life. The mother, German-Old American, thrifty and healthy, seems to have done well by her family which has been a happy one

except for recent strain between the boy and his father.

Mental History, Achievement: Finished two years of college and one year of theological seminary. Grades had been passing and work satisfactory on the whole, but for a year or two before our contact with him signs of severe nervous strain had been manifest, with alternating episodes of excitement and depression. IQ reports agree closely at about 115. He gives the impression of well above average mentality, although he is impatient and querulous. He puts people ill at ease and is himself ill at ease.

The vocational plan has been that of the ministry. His real interests have been almost wholly confined to music. The AMI that of an obviously intelligent gynandroid youth who is baffled and manifestly needs a lift.

Medical: Normal birth and early history. No serious illnesses or injuries. PX reveals no significant pathology. Within his gynandroid limits he appears to have enjoyed first-rate health.

Running Record: For some time he had been doing poorly in seminary work and relations with the father had been growing more strained. He had come to the unfavorable attention of the seminary faculty and by expressing unorthodox opinions had elicited signs of alarm in that quarter. The father was concerned over the danger that the boy might prove delinquent in the fulfillment of his dedication to the ministry. The boy himself had given so many hostages to that profession that it had become difficult to think of making a sharp break. Yet it was clear that he wanted to make such a break, that in fact he already knew he was going to do it, and that his interest was elsewhere. Moreover he presented a good temperamental pattern for the teaching of music and for the arty way of life, a poor one for the practice of a ministry. After a few consultations he responded with enthusiasm to his own idea of giving up the seminary and shifting to a college of music with the goal in mind of teaching. Our role was merely that of the physician who writes the prescription for the trip to the seashore that the patient demanded. It proved not difficult to find scholarship aid to help the boy accomplish the shift, and he spent two years on the school program in music training.

He then got a job as a teacher of music, did well at it for a time until he was inducted into military service. There he served in a band until the end of the war, had a good time, saved money, got married, and started a family. Following his separation from the service he took advantage of the opportunity of furthering his musical education on the GI Bill; now has a good teaching job and is called "a very good influence indeed."

Summary: Gynandroid mesopene of very low physical strength. Feminine personality, excellent health, about college average mentality. Mildly cycloid history. Vocational maladaptation.

ID 0–2–0 (2)
  Insufficiencies:
    IQ . . . .
    Mop . . . .
  Psychiatric:
    1st order . . . .
    2nd order 1
      (2–1–2)
    C-phobic . . . .
    G-phrenic 1
  Residual D:
    Primary crim. . . . .

Comment: Outlook excellent. He is well adapted to his chosen work, is happy and now prosperous in it. He will of course continue to have his emotional ups and downs, will remain mildly cycloid. This does not mean that he is a psychopath, but merely that he has a cycloid temperament. His case should further emphasize the point that the principal problem in psychiatric diagnosis remains that of describing temperaments. The term cycloid overlaps normal and pathological behavior. It does not delineate a psychiatric entity.

This is the kind of case that might be written up as a success with the implication that we "did something." In fact, we did nothing except let the boy talk out his problem without theological or emotional obstruction. He knew well enough what he wanted to do, but he didn't know that he knew, and of course he lacked a semantically sound vocabulary for describing himself. There may be only two elements of value in the whole fabric of what has been called psychotherapy or analytic therapy. First, the matter of supplying an operational vocabulary with which to think, and the consequent removal of theological hangovers that lurk in loaded words. Second, emergence from the sense of being blocked, or achievement of a sense of emotional one-directionality. All religious movements of history, from the ancient mind-body dualism which gave rise to Christianity and to other thousands of similar sects, to the latter-day mind-body dualism which gave rise to Freudianity and to the tautological concept of psychosomatics—all these religions have supplied the second element at the price of selling out the first. That is to say, they have offered emotional one-directionality at the price of swallowing a mess of theological verbiage. The problem of psychiatry, and of psychology, is to build a descriptive edifice *starting from the organism* so patiently and so semantically that the hysterical flight to a mind-body dualism will be *manifestly* childish and absurd in all its guises. When we have done that, the dark ages will be at an end.

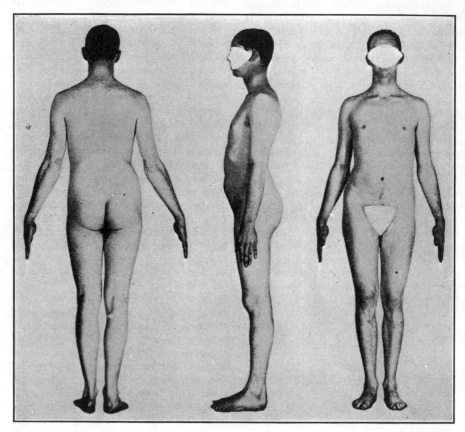

Description: Somatotype 5–2½–4. A 22-year-old ectomorphic endomorph of average stature. A mesopenic and gynandroid physique with no marked dysplasias. A rarity in this series because of the pronounced mesopenia. Head extraordinarily small. Primary $g+3$, secondary $g+2$. Primary t 2, secondary t 3. The body as a whole is of fine texture, with delicate skin. Features small, stubby, rather poorly molded. Hair fine. Hands and feet delicately and finely formed. General strength 1, hand strength 1. Coordination very good but altogether feminine. He moves, acts, and speaks like a woman. No competitive or athletic ability.

Temperament: He showed a minor somatorosis, which is to say that he was maladaptively overactive but for the most part inconsequentially so. His mind and most of his energy had got stuck, or focussed, on the subject of sex. He had a "sexual obsession," said one psychiatrist. Friendly and sociable in a superficial sort of way, he seemed to have a new set of friends every few days. He touched all things lightly. Only when cornered and faced with the necessity of accepting some temporary responsibility did he show signs of cerebrosis. Then he would become momentarily tense, apparently apprehensive, and clearly unhappy. There was no masculine pugnacity in him. Although often faced down or squelched by smaller boys, he would never fight and he expressed no truculence. He was airy, a trifle gynandrophrenic yet not quite arty. He bordered on *DAMP RAT* territory but was not quite a *DAMP RAT* and was certainly not homosexual. He had none of that peculiarly affected "Oxford" speech which is often the password among *DAMP RAT*s of the polite stratum. ψ 1–2–1.

Delinquency: Minor stealing between 12 and 15. No other positive delinquency. He has consistently shown what seems to be essential or general irresponsibility. Quit high school at 15 and thereafter refused to "take anything seriously."

Origins and Family: Extramarital, urban parents, father unknown. Mother a healthy Scotch-Irish woman of average physique, from a family of low economic status but of good general standing. She seems well respected by those who know her. Boy reared by relatives with no agency help.

Mental History, Achievement: Finished one year of high school with several failures which teachers called "unnecessary." IQ reports fall between 95 and 106, here called 100. He seems brighter than average but appears to have poor mental stamina, and the focus of attention fluctuates rapidly.

No vocational plan. Now entirely out of sympathy with school. He is convinced that he cannot learn mathematics and can pass no courses "with math in them." He may be right. This is a common failing with gynandrophrenes. The AMI that of a tall and straight good-looking youth who expresses an easy friendliness but on second look gives the impression of a certain shoddiness of moral fiber.

Medical: Normal birth. Walked and talked at about 1 year. No serious illnesses or injuries. PX reveals no significant pathology. He has good teeth, normal vision, good arches and foot structure.

Running Record: With us intermittently through a period of nearly two years, he made many false starts at work programs, always quitting within a week or two. Three times he started a school program but could not follow through. He would do well at first and would make a good impression, but would soon forget all about it and would be off on another scent. We called him the setter puppy. When closely supervised he was all right. When the supervision relaxed he relaxed. At camp and elsewhere he proved perfectly honest in money matters, seemed to pay no attention to opportunities to steal but was irresponsible in the execution of duties of every sort. Throughout our acquaintanceship with him he was sex crazy. His energies and attention appeared to be focussed on sexuality to such a degree that no other interest could for long hold the stage of attention. At dusk he would take off, apparently to prowl about in more or less timorous pursuit of sexual adventure through the evening, and sometimes through a large part of the night. In this one matter he was defiant of rules. Girls, or even the thought of girls, seemed to disorganize him and to put all other thoughts to flight. He seemed to have a sexual somatorosis, but at the end of our contact with him we were reasonably sure that he was not actively delinquent in any other sense.

Fortunately the war came along at just the time when he needed it most. He was inducted into military service and the uniform in wartime gave him exactly what he needed, especially abroad. It was, as he later put it, a passport to sexuality. He "got along" in the service, although with a good deal of hospitalization; married and started a family. Back in civilian life for another two years now, he doesn't like it as well as he liked the military adventure and has been showing signs of the old irresponsibility. He has picked up the popular point of view of getting as much as possible without working too hard, but there have been no indications of active delinquency.

Summary: Tall, barely mesomorphic youth with some gynandroid interference. Average mentality and excellent health. History of irresponsibility with almost irrelevant minor delinquency. Problem of sexual somatorosis.

ID 0–3–0 (3)
  Insufficiencies:
    IQ ....
    Mop ....
  Psychiatric:
    1st order ....
    2nd order 1

Trace of Dionysian irresponsibility (1–2–1)
  C-phobic ....
  G-phrenic 2
Residual D:
  Primary crim. ....

Comment: Outlook probably good in the sense that he is not a criminal or likely to require institutional care. Outlook poor in the sense that he will fail to make the most of his natural endowment. He is likely to become an intermittently employed taxicab driver in South Boston. That is his present ambition. Probably he just barely escaped homosexuality, although having missed that road he missed it cleanly. He has *the sort of* gynandrophrenia that the most persistent and incurable homosexuals show, *but less of it.* There may have been a period in his development when the balance between homosexuality and heterosexuality was a fine one. It may have been good fortune, or some accidental meeting, that sent him to the right instead of to the left. Or it may be that this problem is almost wholly one of constitutional endowment. The only way to get at such a problem, so far as I can see, is to describe and follow a series of individuals in the way that the boys of this series have been described and followed, but more thoroughly. It is necessary to do a great deal of intensive research, particularly physiological research, on perhaps a relatively small number of cases. There is urgent need for coordination of expensive techniques in biochemistry and physiological chemistry with the constitutional frame of reference.

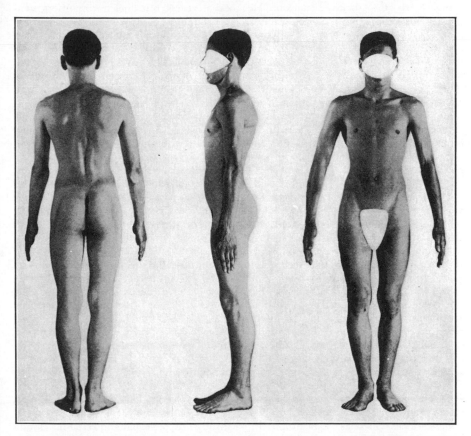

Description: Somatotype 2½–4–4. A 16-year-old ectomorph-mesomorph three inches above average stature. Wide shoulders. Bones comparatively heavier than muscles. High, peculiarly slender waist—gynandroid lower trunk. Primary $g+1$, secondary $g+1$. Primary t 3, secondary t 3. Features well developed and sharply chiseled but a little asymmetrical or irregular. The face has an overly keen, birdlike appearance. Hands and feet well formed. General strength 3, hand strength 4. Coordination good although somewhat feminoid. He moves quickly and gracefully but with a feminine hip sway. Good at minor athletics and fairly good at baseball pitching. Not good at the contact games like football and basketball. He is no fighter.

Temperament: Superficially he gives an impression of smooth adaptability, but he is in fact inordinately stubborn, resistive, and given to violent temper outbursts or rage tantrums. The posture is erect, alert, and he is sensitively responsive to the social situation. He dresses with the utmost meticulousness, looks like an Arrow collar boy. There are indications of strain, or of cerebrotonic interference, yet there seems also to be a good supportive viscerotonia. The picture suggests temperamental overloading. The temper tantrums resemble feminine rage and frustration rather than the epileptoid pattern. He is markedly gynandrophrenic but has no trace of the *DAMP RAT* syndrome or of homosexuality. ψ 2–2–1.

Delinquency: Some early truancy and several episodes of minor stealing before age 12. History of ungovernable temper and of violent outbursts of rage at all ages, although with no epileptoid rhythm or prodromality. He seems simply to go all out to get his own way, and usually in very minor matters. He has no balance or perspective, tends to "throw away everything" in the Olympian fury of the moment. Two episodes of larceny between 15 and 17. Automobile stealing at 17. To state correctional school at 17.

Origins and Family: Second of two, urban family. Father a slender Old American, described as "a fastidious introverted man of aesthetic leanings." After some years of vocational confusion he went into industrial work which he didn't like, and committed suicide when the boy was 14. The mother is a heavy and muscular French-Irish woman, described as "coarse, excitable, paranoid." She came from a large family which has produced several psychiatric and delinquent personalities. Boy remained at home until 14, then to foster homes under agency management.

Mental History, Achievement: Graduated from high school with good grades, although weak in mathematics and science. IQ reports vary from 119 to 134, here called 125. He gives an impression of quick intelligence and of mental alertness, but does not manifest mental stamina.

No vocational plans. He has been called promising and is a sort of Beau Brummell. The AMI is based on his energetic alertness, excellent appearance, and high secondary *t* component. There is an atmosphere of unspoiled or unsophisticated eagerness about him, and the unsophisticated trait sets off a sharp contrast with the *DAMP RAT persona*.

Medical: Birth and early history called normal. No serious illnesses or injuries of consequence. He never got along very well with other children; now considered something of a "sissy." PX reveals no significant pathology.

Running Record: He had been overcaseworked, having been referred to at least four different psychiatrists and thereby picking up a mess of Freudian slang. In his first interview at the Inn he explained that he had been rejected by his mother, felt a need of atoning for his father's guilt, was a sort of sadomasochistic martyr. He had first-rate verbal alacrity and had written an autobiography loaded with Freudian symbolism. Our problem was to break through these verbal and religious clouds and to try to get his feet back on the ground. Although he did poorly both at the work programs within the house and at outside jobs, we tried to persuade him to enter college on a school program. We had no success. Instead he wasted his time for several months, then was apprehended at larceny and was returned to state correctional school. Six months later he reappeared, and this time manifested a degree of curiosity about himself. A trace of insight into his constitutional nature seemed abruptly to change his point of view. But he declined the college program and took an outside job. There he did well for a year, was inducted into military service, and got along until the end of the war. In postwar civilian life he has kept out of trouble and has earned his way. He is called a "success" but he probably will not "make anything of himself."

Summary: A well-grown and handsome mesomorphic youth with a *g* component. Superior mentality and excellent health. Persistent early delinquency which seems to have stopped abruptly at 19.

ID 0–3–0 (3)
  Insufficiencies:
    IQ ....
    Mop ....
  Psychiatric:
    1st order ....
    2nd order 1
    (2–2–1)
    C-phobic ....
    G-phrenic 2
  Residual D:
    Primary crim. ....

Comment: Outlook considered good. He is one of the most intelligent youths in the series, and although there no longer seems to be any hope that he will develop his mental potentialities he has apparently found himself to such a degree that he can keep out of trouble.

There is no way of assessing whether the happy emergence is a result of a trace of constitutional insight, of treatment at the state correctional school, of experience in the Army, or of all three. Of the three factors I think that the military institution played the most important role. This youth somehow had too high a secondary *t* for the kind of life into which he was born. He had a Cinderella complex, or the frustrating sense that he belonged to something better and that he should have this better life *suddenly*, without having to earn it step by step. The Army coarsened him a little, and fattened him. Both changes helped. The Army did not stimulate him mentally but then, we can't have everything.

In dealing with this youth we felt poignantly the tragedy of the almost. He was *almost* a good personality. He had the brains, the sensitivity, and the romantic vision necessary for first-rate achievement. Perhaps the early influence of a person well oriented to time might have done much for him. That was his difficulty—orientation to time, or religion. Too intelligent or too honest for the supernatural theologies, he seized eagerly upon Freudian theology during his adolescent years. But Freudian theology has nothing of nobility or fine aspiration in it, and does not induce first-rate achievement. Perhaps the unavailability of a first-rate religion was the real tragedy of this life.

171. *COMPANY B, PLATOON 1, SECTION 6*
Gynandrophrenes: Nos. 168–184

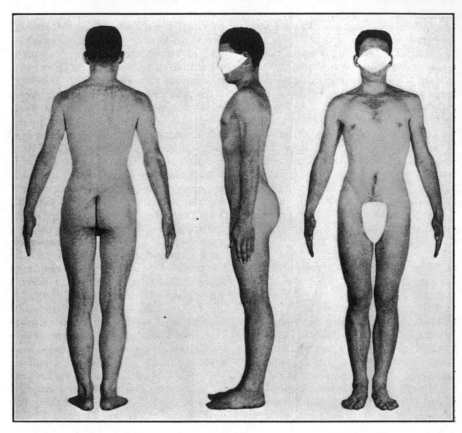

Description: Somatotype 3½–4½–3. An 18-year-old moderately meso-morphic youth, three inches above average stature. No particular dysplasias and excellent segmental development, but there is a notable primary *g* in the lower trunk and there are secondary gynandroid traces throughout the phy-sique. Long eyelashes, fine hair, feminine subcutaneous finish. Primary *g*+1, secondary *g*+1. Primary *t* 3, secondary *t* 4. Features delicately molded and sharply chiseled but they suggest feminine, not masculine beauty. Hands and feet well shaped. General strength 3, hand strength 3. Coordination ex-cellent for dancing and for general bodily grace, but he is not good at games, cannot fight, and is unhappy in the gymnasium.

Temperament: The outstanding characteristic is his long history of hysterical tantrums, occurring for the most part in connection with guerilla warfare with the mother. He is extremely stubborn, overbearing if crossed, and is direct or rather businesslike in going after what he wants. The hysterical tantrums seem to be of gynandroid, not epileptoid pattern. He has had many slap-fights with the mother, but does no fighting with boys. No indication of cerebrotonic interference. When happy, or when given what he wants, he is manifestly viscerotonic. There is much affability and old-fashioned YMCA laying on of hands; in fact, a laying all over of hands. He has a strong trace of *DAMP RAT* but on the whole is more YMCA than *DAMP RAT.* ψ 3–2–1.

Delinquency: His delinquency is associated almost entirely with the warfare mentioned above. There were several complaints of "stubborn child," and also of minor stealing, but nearly all of the stealing was from his own home.

Origins and Family: Second of three, urban Negro family. The father, about half white, is a professional man of good education. He has done well but long since retired from active service in the intrafamilial wars. The mother, also about half white and a rugged gynandroid woman, is described by one agency as "an energetic and paranoid go-getter who gets in on whatever there is to get." She has made a number of agency contacts although she is in fact a rather well-situated person. Boy brought up in the home, with much manifest sibling rivalry and general rejection all around, each member of the family rejecting the others. One source of difficulty appears to lie in the gradient of their color. This boy is really high yellow; the mother and one sibling are nearer to white; the father and another sibling are much darker.

Mental History, Achievement: Finished high school with a fairly good record. IQ reports fall consistently between 110 and 120, here called 115. He gives the impression of mental alertness, together with a certain canny materialistic or perhaps only viscerotonic outlook.

His vocational plan and ambition is, if possible, to go to college. The AMI is based on viscerotonic bigness and on his nice YMCA laying on of hands. He is vital, and both somatotonically and viscerotonically filled with Christian fellowship.

Medical: Normal birth and development history. "Born large and always large." No serious illnesses or injuries. PX reveals no significant pathology.

Running Record: His relations here were on the whole good. He was regarded as a "sissy" or homosexual and was unappreciated by some of our mesomorphs who, being vulgar, misunderstood the laying on of hands. It developed that one important factor in the earlier history of delinquency and confusion had been "a too vigorous expression of sexuality." The mother had got in on some of the repercussions, had concerned herself vigorously therewith. The boy liked white girls and some of them had taken to him. A good deal of confusion and frustration had resulted from the boy's persistent efforts to pass as white. The Inn encouraged him to forget it and instead to try to grow a mind. The Inn was able to put him on a school program which gave him an opportunity to go to college.

He finally finished college on the school program and immediately entered a professional school, where he has now spent three years with a satisfactory record. There is no doubt as to his competence to finish, and he seems to be a credit to himself. He was exempted from military service because of educational and professional school identification. There has been no further indication of delinquency. He has grown heavier, no doubt will be a "very big man."

Summary: Tall, gynandroid endomorphic mesomorph, half Caucasian and half Negro. Excellent health, IQ about college average. History of stubbornness and intrafamilial warfare, with hysterical tantrums.

ID 0–3–0 (3)
　Insufficiencies:
　　IQ . . . .
　　Mop . . . .
　Psychiatric:
　　' 1st order . . . .
　　2nd order . . . .　1
　　　Hysterical tantrums (3–2–1)
　　C-phobic . . . .
　　G-phrenic . . . .　2
　　　Trace of DAMP RAT
　Residual D:
　　Primary crim. . . . .

Comment: Outlook presumably good. When the long-range health factor is good such a physique may be in some respects an excellent one. With good motivation and freedom from homosexuality, a personality with this kind of foundation can sometimes turn out a prodigious amount of work. There is no distraction from athletic interests or from "masculine participations," and there is little need or taste for physical exercise. Such individuals do not become hunters, explorers, or out of doors enthusiasts. They often become dilettantes, lounge lizards, arty degenerates and the like, but they are protected from one of the greatest dangers to human full development—the danger from the somatotonic monkey trap of perpetual muscular adolescence. The price of such protection, of course, is to be exposed to grave dangers from other directions.

In this case the mother and son, about equally gynandroid, enjoyed a hilarious running battle for years, and if it is permissible to rest a generalization on the evidence of one case, here may be the ideal family setting. This boy must have been given just the right impetus, in his early conditioning, for he has now gone well beyond his expectation and may become a distinguished man. We at last have an answer to the question as to what is the ideal family, for in modern life it is results that count.

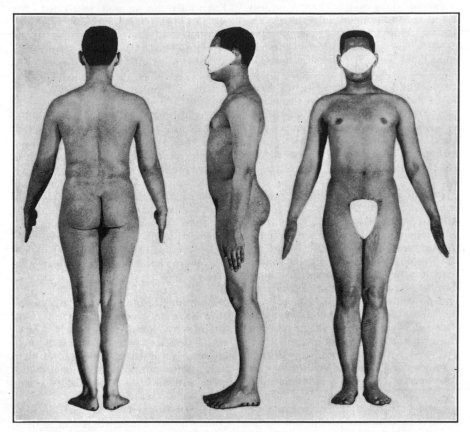

Description: Somatotype 4½–5–2. An 18-year-old endomorphic meso-morph five inches above average stature. A tall, well-developed light-skinned Negro youth with no dysplasias but with conspicuous g in the lower body. He is also diffusely gynandroid throughout the body. Primary g+2, second-ary g+1. Primary t 3, secondary t 2. Structurally the features fall about half-way between Negroid and Caucasian modeling. Face often described as las-civious. Mouth voluptuously or almost flaccidly viscerotonic. Hands com-paratively small and weak. General strength 3, hand strength 2. Coordina-tion smooth but he is too gynandroid for any kind of athletics. He cannot throw or hit with his fists, but he can slap.

Temperament: The outstanding characteristic is lack of humor. He is a determined youth and austerely stubborn, but at the same time brittle and tense. He gives the impression of being under great strain; is generally referred to by psychiatrists and others as "that paranoid young man." There is no leaven of amiability or of vulgarity in him. He is seclusive, secretive, yet develops *DAMP RAT* crushes on other boys and then shows great dependence upon the whim or good will of the object of his crush. The temperamental picture seems to be that of overloading in the second and third components, or of an odd entanglement between these components, with a heavy gynandrophrenic complication. He is a severe or austere *DAMP RAT*. ψ 1–5–2.

Delinquency: Long history of tantrums and destructiveness, beginning at least as early as age 5. Extreme stubbornness and violent temper outbursts throughout childhood. This tendency continued to the time of our contact with him, giving rise to spirited intrafamilial warfare. No history of stealing, and no court record. Twice referred to psychiatric clinics. Diagnoses: *Diagnosis deferred, paranoid tendency; psychoneurosis, reactive depression.*

Origins and Family: First of two, urban family. Father Old American. A tall, slender man described as "always shy and introverted and from a fine old family." He inherited wealth but lost it, and during the past twenty years appears to have rather given up on life. Mother Old American and of tall, athletic build. Described as a "practical, managing and rather domineering person." Both parents have good medical histories. Boy brought up in the home until at 16 he became altogether unmanageable.

Mental History, Achievement: Finished a year of high school although with great difficulty because of personality problems. IQ reports range from 113 to 128, here called 120. He gives the impression of superior general intelligence, despite a shocking lack of humor.

Vocational plan: To get through high school and if possible to go to college. Essentially, he is well motivated. No special gifts. Great interest in things aesthetic and sharp distaste for things athletic. The AMI that of a towering, well-set-up youth who is excessively proper and has an expressed cultural interest in music and art.

Medical: Normal birth and early history. No serious illnesses or injuries. Always lonely or seclusive as a child, and jumpy or oversensitive to pain and touch. From infancy he had a harsh or suspicious outlook on life, with periodic tantrums of violence. At 15, out of school a year because of "mental depression." Called prepsychotic by one psychiatrist. PX reveals moderately defective vision, extreme deviation of the septum, moderately elevated blood pressure.

Running Record: Within the limits of a seemingly paranoid distrust and intermittent hostility to nearly everybody, his behavior at the Inn was good. He was rigorously honest in money matters, carried out work assignments and other duties with a responsibility as dependable as that of anybody.

He was entered on the school program with some misgivings and against the advice of psychiatrists who regarded him as prepsychotic. He lived at the House intermittently during three years, finally finishing high school with fairly good grades. During his first year at the Inn there were two attempts at suicide, both in connection with crushes on other boys. Both attempts were questionable; may have been theatrical. There were occasional, almost periodic temper tantrums or spasms of rage, when his face would twitch in a peculiar manner and he would seem to be on the verge of going berserk. But these episodes always passed quickly and it was felt that they became less violent and less frequent as he grew older. His crushes seemed to be more of an idealistic or romantic nature than homosexual. If he was ever overtly homosexual we didn't know about it. His identification was with the *DAMP RATs* but even toward them there seemed to be a final barrier of paranoid asperity.

A scholarship was found for him on which to start his college career, and he succeeded in finishing a year of college with passing grades before being inducted into military service. In the service he had an unpleasant time and was extensively hospitalized, but he stayed in grimly until the end of the war, then returned to college on the GI Bill, and now gives every indication of being able to see it through to graduation.

ID 0–4–0 (4)
Insufficiencies:
  IQ ....
  Mop ....
Psychiatric:
  1st order ....
  2nd order 2
  Possibly epileptoid (1–5–2)
  C-phobic ....
  G-phrenic 2
  DAMP RAT

Residual D:
  Primary crim. ....

Comment: Outlook probably good. He has passed the most dangerous reefs and may now find smoother sailing. The *DAMP RAT* identification, while it may have been nearly fatal, was incomplete. He has now shown signs of being able to pilot his ship and if he succeeds in getting a first-rate education under his belt his early confusion and *DAMP RAT* flirtations may get translated into material that will fertilize a mind. This youth might develop into a useful personality and might even be the outstanding person in the series. Much will depend on the choice he makes after graduating from college. It is usually during the first five years after college that an education begins or the hope of it fades. If within that period he does not enter upon one of the common opportunisms or professions, he may grow up.

It is of interest to note that of the two parents the mother was physically the dominant one, the more mesomorphic, and gynandroid. In a long series of observations on the *DAMP RAT* syndrome this has turned out frequently to be the case. There may be some direct relationship between gynandrophrenia and parental dominance. Gynandrophrenic males seem often to have mesomorphic and gynandroid mothers. There is a good Ph.D. problem here for somebody.

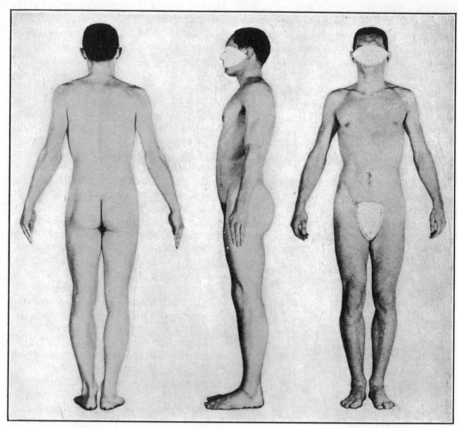

Description: Somatotype 2–5–3. A 17-year-old mesomorph six inches above average stature. All segments well formed, with no conspicuous dysplasia. Arms a little weaker than the rest of the body but not asthenic. Waist a trifle too high, and just a trace of primary g in the lower trunk. Diffuse secondary g throughout the body, particularly in the face. Primary $g\pm$— a trace; secondary $g+1$. Primary t 3, secondary t 3. Features fine and sharply chiseled but the face shows too much feminoid delicacy and is markedly asymmetrical. Hands and feet well formed. General strength 3, hand strength 3. Coordination rather poor. He is awkward or ungainly although he maintains dignity by standing stiff and straight. He is most unhappy in the gymnasium, abhors "things physical," does not know how to use his body at games or at fighting. The face suggests brittleness and dessication.

Temperament: A conspicuous *DAMP RAT* with strong underlying somatotonia. He is supremely stubborn and determined to have his way, yet most of the common characteristics of manifest somatotonia are absent. The voice is quiet and meticulously modulated. He moves as noiselessly as a mother cat on the prowl, although on occasion he is capable of the wildest kind of exotic dancing and contortioning. He loves to gamble and is quite a shrewd gambler. He is physically relaxed, a gourmet, shows childlike greed for affection and approval under some circumstances. Highly dependent on people when troubled. He is arty-perverse and no other term fits the pattern quite so well. He has great physical energy—is often hard put to it to get rid of it. He has been called both paranoid and cycloid by psychiatrists. ψ 3–3–1.

Delinquency: Moderate degree of early truancy, and unmanageable in school. Always a "difficult and peculiar child" but never a very actively troublesome one. No history of stealing, and no court record of any kind. Throughout adolescence and later he was subject to what seemed to be deep depressions, or periods of emotional viscerosis; twice referred to a psychiatric clinic at 18 for attempted suicide. Diagnosis, *psychopathic personality with depression.* The question of a prepsychotic condition had several times been raised, although there was never any evidence of disorientation or attentional difficulty.

Origins and Family: Tenth of twelve, urban family, both parents immigrant from Poland. The father, of average physique, came to this country as a boy, married young, was several times before the courts because of alcoholism and neglect of family; died of apoplexy in his late forties when the boy was 17. The mother, Polish and said to have had some Jewish blood, died of a malignancy when the boy was 2. The father re-married and the stepmother is said to have been abusive. The family as a whole show nearly fifty agency contacts during a period of twenty years. Boy lived in the family for ten years, then with various relatives. He disagreed with the stepmother on a number of more or less abstract questions.

Mental History, Achievement: Finished the eighth grade after a number of failures. IQ reports range from 85 to 104, here called 95. He gives an impression of better than average mentality and in his gynandroid way is alert. Yet he has disappointed several people by failing to develop mental stamina or sustained intellectuality.

No vocational plans. He has excellent rhythm and is a first-rate dancer; has been an entertainer with his contortions at this art. No other known special gifts. The AMI is based on the arty *persona*. He is coy like a girl, has arty enunciation, identifies closely with the *DAMP RAT* group.

Medical: Birth history and early development not known. No history of serious illnesses or injuries. Psychiatric referrals as noted. PX reveals no significant pathology.

Running Record: Through several years of association with the Inn he was essentially well behaved and free from delinquency. Although affected and theatrical, he did work assignments well and after being placed on the school program stuck doggedly to the task of getting through high school—finally accomplished it. He did poorly in mathematics and science but very well in art, literature, and design. At camp in the summer he developed into a good cook. Despite the *DAMP RAT* characteristic he was never, so far as we know, accused of homosexuality. In money matters he turned out to be thrifty and responsible. By rigorous self-sacrifice, shrewd lending, gambling, and the practice of petty rackets he built up a savings account while at the Inn and is one of the very few to have accomplished that. He was a combination of shy boy-girl and realistic, thrifty businessman. He seemed to be overtly Dionysian only in his dancing, had periods of profound depression in which real emotional suffering was apparent. One psychiatrist tagged him as a potential *manic-depressive, depressive*.

He was exempted from military service on psychiatric grounds and for two or three more years was unhappily at loose ends. Too thrifty and realistic for loafing or for prolonged agency symbiosis, he was too *DAMP RAT* for any work he seemed able to find. Finally he decided to be a cook, and at this work he appears to have done well and to have saved money. He has kept out of trouble. The depressions seem to be less severe than when we first knew him. He is heavier, more relaxed, has continued his habit of saving, is now contemplating a business enterprise of his own.

Summary: Overenergized mesomorphy with secondary *g*. Average mentality; good health. *DAMP RAT* syndrome. History of severe depressions. No problem of active delinquency.

ID o–4–o (4)
Insufficiencies:
  IQ ....
  Mop ....
Psychiatric:
  1st order ....
  2nd order 2
  (3–3–1)
  C-phobic ....
  G-phrenic 2
  DAMP RAT
Residual D:
  Primary crim. ....

Comment: Outlook probably good, and it has improved during the past three years. He finally succeeded in solving his difficult vocational problem by doing something at which he is *naturally* good, thereby joining a rather small circle of what may be the human elect. As a cook or restaurant operator he is potentially first rate. At any calling which would not make use of his excellent gynandrophrenia he might be a most unhappy failure, and with his depressional history the outlook would then be poor. Here the vocational problem was closely identified with the problem of constitutional insight, and the boy deserves credit for having found this out or thought it through.

174. COMPANY B, PLATOON 1, SECTION 6
Gynandrophrenes: Nos. 168–184

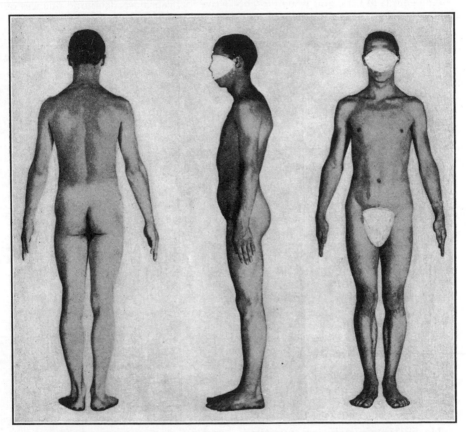

Description: Somatotype 3-4-3. An 18-year-old slighty asthenic mesomorph of average stature. The neck and the regions below the diaphragm
show good mesomorphic development. Face, chest, and arms moderately asthenic. Primary $g\pm$, secondary $g+2$. Strongly feminine atmosphere. Primary
t 3, secondary t 3. Features lack sharp molding but have a trace of fineness
especially about the eyes. General strength 3, hand strength 3. Coordination
excellent, but it is feminine coordination—not that of the fighter. He is
smooth, lithe or sinuous in his bodily movements, and is a good runner.

Temperament: He is moderately *DAMP RAT* and the general impression is that of feminine perverseness. However, he is usually quiet, relaxed, self-effacive. There are frequent brief and minor tantrums or flashes of spirit. Also there is a love of the occasional bout of Dionysian revelry. He can flare up like a summer storm but the explosion amounts to little and is soon forgotten. Afterward he is inclined to sulk. The pattern is possibly epileptoid but with only weak, token-like explosions. Perhaps we could call him petit mal epileptoid. He is dependent and jealous, gets crushes on other boys, then suffers from jealousy. This youth is a clinging vine; the other boy is always the dominant one, in the homosexual attachment. ψ 2–2–2.

Delinquency: No delinquency of record. He was for several years in great conflict over homosexuality, before finally accepting that pattern. The upheaval seems to have interfered with his achievement of educational ambitions. For two or three years before our contact with him he had been moderately alcoholic.

Origins and Family: Second of four, urban family. Father Irish and of slender or light build. He has always been regularly employed and is well regarded. Mother also Irish and a massive or burly woman but never known to be delinquent. She is described as gynandroid. Boy reared in the home with no agency help.

Mental History, Achievement: Graduated from high school with good grades but did not enter college. Two IQ reports agree closely at 110. He is of better than average mentality but not brilliant. He gives the impression of honesty and reliability but also of a great need to lean on others. He has what might possibly have been a good feminine mentality.

No particular vocational plan. He has done well for several years at clerical work, does not like it but has no alternative in mind. Gifted at drawing and at music. His interests and desires seem all to be centered on symphonic music and on art. The AMI that of a shy, sincere youth with wide, starry eyes and long eyelashes; red, parted lips; a sensitive, delicate nose; feminine nuances of expression.

Medical: Normal birth and early development. No serious illnesses or injuries. He has always been more girl than boy. As a child he played alone, was easily delighted with simple things. He had the same periodic brief, weak tantrums that he still shows. Never made any successful contact with other boys. Could not play the games or talk the language of boys. He is easily fatigued, has low blood pressure. There have been occasional fainting spells, frequent crying spells. He has always had periodic headaches and spells of "hypochondria." During adolescence he was called "hysterical," but these symptoms seem to have disappeared. He smokes too much and drinks too much. PX reveals no significant pathology.

Running Record: At the Inn for brief visits only, he seemed a shy and kindly youth who ought to be a teacher of English or of one of the arts or humanities. He was courteous, considerate, thoughtful of others, retiring, and overly modest. He talked and behaved as one unaware of the rough and seamy side of life. He appeared to derive insight and satisfaction from a brief constitutional examination of himself; gave promise of developing humorous understanding of some of the vicissitudes of the human species on this pellet, including homosexuality. He had already decided that he must somehow make peace with this phenomenon. When relaxed and sure of his environment or when partially anaesthetized by alcohol he was capable of quite spirited expression of the attitudes and clichés of the *DAMP RAT* fraternity. In conversing with strangers or new acquaintances he seemed merely delicate minded and meticulous of speech. The bait of a chance to go to college and to become a teacher in the field of his greatest interest stirred up in him a weak flare of initial enthusiasm. For a time he seemed to build around this plan as if he might carry it out. However, he put off the endeavor and during the interim the storm of war broke.

He forgot the academic plan, escaped from his old clerical job, and went into a defense industry. After a time he did not like that very well either but stuck to it through the war; saved money. Now, half a dozen years after our first contact with him, he has settled back and has given up all thought of academic ambition. He is thrifty, rigorously honest and reliable, and is only mildly *DAMP RAT*. He is about as alcoholic and about as arty as when we first knew him. The pattern seems to be permanently formed.

Summary: Asthenic or imperfectly developed mesomorphy with pronounced secondary *g*. Mentality above average; good but not robust health. *DAMP RAT* syndrome. No delinquency.

ID 1–3–0 (4)
   Insufficiencies:
      IQ . . . .
      Mop   1
   Psychiatric:
      1st order . . . .
      2nd order   1
         Petit mal epileptoid (2–2–2)
      C-phobic . . . .
      G-phrenic   2
         DAMP RAT
   Residual D:
      Primary crim. . . . .

Comment: Outlook good except for the primary complaint, and he seems to have a better time as he grows older. The effort to rehabilitate him to an academic plane of life failed but that may have been a fool's idea in the first place. Perhaps it would only have degraded him to have taught sociology at Princeton, or music appreciation at Wabash. He has now given up the conflict over "going to college," and can ecstasize over Beethoven's thirteenth sonata with the greater delight.

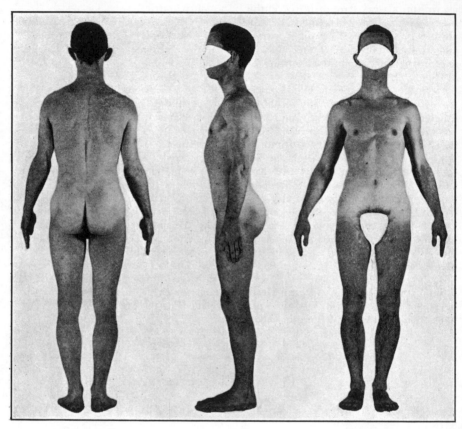

Description: Somatotype 2½–4½–3. A 20-year-old moderately mesomorphic youth an inch above average stature. There is a strong trace of asthenic failure in the face and in the distal segments of the arms—fainter traces throughout the body. High waist and narrow chest. Comparatively heavy bones. Primary $g\pm$—a trace; secondary $g+2$ and especially conspicuous in the face. Primary t 3, secondary t 3. Features fine and delicate but sharply asymmetrical. Hands stubby and crude. General strength 2, hand strength 3. Coordination excellent in that he is graceful and light on his feet. He is helpless in a combative or athletic sense.

Temperament: Almost cerebrotically shy, hyperattentional. At first impression the third component seems strongly to predominate. On further observation it is seen that he is also, in his way, aggressive, stubborn, determined. His approach to people is a delicate and apologetic one but he *does approach,* and he often gains the reward of successful social aggression. He has good push but delicate contact. Also he has a good viscerotonia; is physically relaxed, tremendously loves sociophilic eating, is hungry like a puppy for approval and affection, gets emotional crushes on other boys. The temperamental pattern appears to be that of generous endowment in all three primary components. But the most conspicuous characteristic is gynandrophrenia. He seems female and all his mannerisms and habits suggest feminity. He is coy, blushes constantly, shows feminine confusion, sways his hips and flutters his eyelids in ordinary conversation. In his relations with other gynandrophrenes he wears a female *persona* and is a sort of feminine tyrant—very intuitive, willful, and romantic. He has deep depressions; on psychiatric referral has been called hypochondriacal and suicidal. The primary identification is *DAMP RAT* but he is always in conflict over it. ψ 3-2-4.

Delinquency: No delinquency of record except a few episodes of vagrancy and periodic bouts of drunkenness. He has had a number of brushes with police for drunkenness in night clubs. We have but one report on his earlier life in foster homes and that a favorable one. He is there described as shy, quiet, and lonely.

Origins and Family: Born extramaritally, father unknown. Mother said to have been a large buxomly built Russian Jewess who abandoned the boy at birth. He was taken over by agencies and placed in foster homes, later living for a time with maternal relatives. His early life was one of much shifting about in various places. He finally found a relative with whom he lived long enough to finish three years of high school, then after further Odyssean wonderings turned up in Boston.

Mental History, Achievement: Finished three years of high school with satisfactory grades. IQ reports vary from 105 to 122, here called 115. He gives the impression of superior mentality but of excessive dependency and of viscerotic or gynandrophrenic need for leaning on others.

No vocational plans or special gifts. He expresses an identification with the usual artistic and musical fields of *DAMP RAT* interests, but these do not seem to be deep indentifications. In contrast with many *DAMP RAT*s of this series he has a sense of responsibility and a desire to earn his way. The AMI that of a tall, shy cerebrotic youth of unquestioned sincerity and affective warmth.

Medical: Birth and developmental history not known. No serious illnesses or injuries of record. He has been a psychiatric delinquent, often seeking reassurance regarding his inferiority, his "weak mind," his fears and emotional depressions. There have been periods of very deep depression, numerous intimations of suicide. PX reveals no pathology other than dental caries.

Running Record: At the Inn he was one of our most satisfactory boys. Scrupulously honest in money matters, responsible and dependable on work assignments, he established himself high in the confidence of the staff. He presented only two problems—periodic alcoholism, and the embarrassments attendent upon excessive gynandrophrenia together with his persistent problem as to whether or not to be a homosexual. This latter question seemed never to get quite settled. He loved the night clubs, loved rich food and drink, was a jitterbug devotee, and naturally enough exhibited great interest and concern over sexuality. On the school program he finished high school and then two years of a vocational school with good grades —an accomplishment which in itself exerted a favorable influence in the House.

For a year after leaving us he was unhappy and unsettled. His fondness for alcoholic anaesthetics, the problem of homosexuality, and his peculiar vulnerablility to the dangers of night life seemed to keep him in a turmoil. Yet he worked and earned his way. Then he was inducted into military service, where he struggled along for somewhat more than two years before being given a psychiatric discharge. For another two years now, in civilian life, he has made his way and has been self-supportive, although he is still subject to profound depressions and is still caught in the old conflicting entanglements.

Summary: Tall gynandroid youth with graceful coordination but without combative strength. Mentality about college level; good health. Hypochondriacal, depressive, and partially *DAMP RAT*. Periodic alcoholism.

ID 0–5–0 (5)
Insufficiencies:
   IQ ....
   Mop ....
Psychiatric:
   1st order ....
   2nd order 2
      Hypochondriac-cycloid
        (3–2–4)

   C-phobic 1
   G-phrenic 2
      Trace of DAMP RAT
Residual D:
   Primary crim. ....

Comment: Outlook still uncertain. He has no criminal propensities but borders on psychiatric and suicidal delinquency, with sufficient mentality to understand what is going on and to suffer from a sense of cosmic conflict. At times it seems to him that alcoholism and Dionysian revelry offer the only solution. But he lacks the mesomorphy and the energy to outride the physiological havoc wrought by the Dionysian orgy, and almost every indulgence is followed by profound depression and thought of suicide. Then he gets ennobling impulses and he feels a desire to rise above his entanglements. There follows a period of struggle in which the outcome always seems in doubt, as when a junebug struggles in a spider's web. Tired out, he rests from the struggle and his energies rise again. With the energy the Dionysian impulse returns, borne on a rising flood of sexuality.

In this youth's favor is his endomorphy. Within the ensuing decade he should begin to grow heavy, and then the choppy agitation of postadolescent sexuality will give over gradually to the rolling smoothness of the open sea. He is sailing in a dangerous channel, and so far as I know neither psychiatry nor medicine has anything to offer him but a confused theology and a bed.

176. *COMPANY B, PLATOON 1, SECTION 6*
Gynandrophrenes: Nos. 168–184

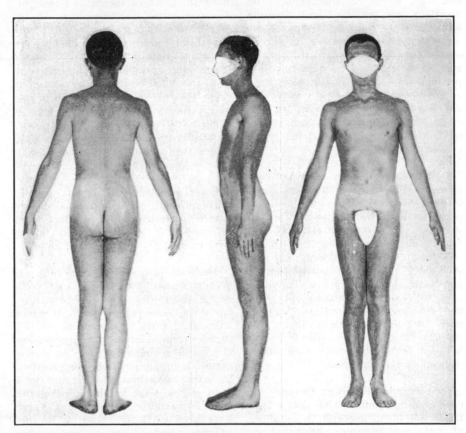

Description: Somatotype 4–3–4½. A 21-year-old youth of nearly mid-range somatotype four inches above average stature. Asthenic chest and arms. Otherwise of 4–4–4 structure. Heavier and stronger below the diaphragm than above it. Conspicuous primary *g* in the lower trunk and diffuse secondary *g* throughout the body. A physique which in mid-life will easily become fat and heavy. Primary *g*+2, secondary *g*+2. Primary *t* 3, secondary *t* 3. Features finer than average but the face is asymmetrical. Hands small, asthenic. Feet well formed. General strength 2, hand strength 2. Coordination exceptionally good but gynandroid. He moves with a lithe, lemur-like grace, loves swimming. Noted for effortless, willowy dancing. A physical personality very similar to that of Vernon Castle, famous dancer of thirty years ago. He is helpless in the athletic or combative sense.

Temperament: The outstanding characteristic is an almost rhythmic mood swing. At one time he is harsh, sarcastic, spits forth aggressive cynicism and high scorn. At another time he manifests an amiable and friendly warmth. At all times he is somatotonic —posturally assertive, active and direct, overly mature in manner and appearance. The second component is always predominant, with a mood swing from apparently paranoid hostility to a tolerant and friendly viscerotonia. In both moods he is feminoid; in the former strident and harsh, in the latter warm and motherly. ψ 4–2–1.

Delinquency: Violent tantrums and incorrigibility in foster homes at least as early as age 5. Between 5 and 12, petty stealing, mendacity, fits of destructive rage, a frequent runaway, episodes of fire setting. At one foster home he "fought, clawed, chewed, bit, and smashed things in his tantrums of rage." His foster home history is well punctuated with violent tantrums. Breaking and entering at 14 and 15. Sent to state correctional school at 15 on this charge. Periodic bouts of alcoholism between 16 and 19, often with orgies of hostility and somatorosis.

Origins and Family: Eleventh of twelve, rural family. The father is a tall, well-built mesomorph. A foundling of unknown paternity, he has been "thought perhaps to be" a mixture of Spanish, Negro, Portugese, and Indian. Said to be moderately alcoholic but not otherwise delinquent. The mother was a large and muscular woman who died of cardiovascular disease in her late thirties when our boy was 5. Said to have been part Negro, part Indian, and part white—possibly Portugese. After her death the boy was taken over by agencies and reared in a long series of foster homes. Five of the siblings died in early childhood; three more have records of delinquency.

Mental History, Achievement: He had finished the eighth grade with a spotty record. IQ reports vary from 113 to 128, here called 120. He is alert, intelligent, quick of speech and thought. His mentality lacks discipline. All reactions seem at first to be too quick and superficial, but on talking with him one gathers an impression that the necessary ingredients of mental growth may be present. Whatever the IQ measures, it does not seem to do full justice to this youth's potentialities.

No vocational plans. He is poetic, moderately gifted in music, draws well, writes with a fine rapid hand, is considered artistic, and identifies himself with art and aesthetics. The AMI that of an obviously intelligent, usually gracious youth of great physical energy who is interested in things cultural and although a *DAMP RAT,* is in conflict over it.

Medical: Birth history and early development not known. No serious illnesses or injuries. He is an "upper respiratory delinquent" with frequent colds that settle on the chest and incapacitate him for varying periods. Furunculosis is recurrent and on a few occasions minor scratches have resulted in severe infections. He presents to a mild degree what has been called the infectious syndrome (see p. 255). There have been psychiatric referrals because of the periodic tantrums, and he has been called *epileptoid.* PX reveals no significant pathology. The septum is sharply deviated.

Running Record: He was placed on the school program with a plan to go through high school. For four years there were many false starts, tempestuous episodes, triumphs, and disappointments. During this time he finished about two years of high school. In one year he started the sophomore course at three different schools but in each instance lost patience with the "stupid fatheads" who ran the school, and dropped out. There were short periods of job placement. He showed real ability at cooking and in the care of children. He did well at camp, was a central figure there. Throughout his association with the Inn he was something of a center for both intellectual life and cultural interests. He became a prodigious reader with an insatiable appetite for ideas, for new cultural patterns, and for forms of art. Always he shied off from any rigorous training. He would undertake no mental discipline but roamed in many of the available fields of artistic and literary expression. He was a center and the mental spark for the *DAMP RAT* group. Like many other *DAMP RAT*s he was at various times accused of homosexuality and was in conflict over that problem. He frequently participated in Dionysian alcoholic orgies.

When the war broke he was inducted into military service and after about two years was given a discharge on psychiatric grounds. Upon returning to civilian life he made use of the GI Bill of Rights to return to school; got into college and stayed for more than a year before alcoholism and the epileptoid tendency got the upper hand. At last report he was still in vigorous doubt as to which really did have the upper hand—the Dionysian desire or the educational ambition.

Summary: Powerful mesomorphy with good *t* and secondary *g*. Superior mental ability; epileptoid history. Juvenile delinquency. Alcoholism. *DAMP RAT* identification.

ID 1–5–0 (6)
Insufficiencies:
  IQ ....
  Mop 1
Psychiatric:
  1st order ....
  2nd order 2
    Epileptoid (4–2–1)
  C-phobic 1
  G-phrenic 2
  DAMP RAT
Residual D:
  Primary crim. ....

Comment: Outlook still uncertain but he has come a long way. He has an alert, active mind and now has a rich background of experience. He cannot tolerate monotony and is easily bored. It is fortunate that he was not born an ant. He is a *DAMP RAT* but one of the most vigorous and dynamic personalities we have encountered with that agglutination. He has the physical energy of a heavyweight champion, but whirs with it like a powerful and complex engine which cannot be thrown into gear. At bottom, his real problem is what to do with the energy. Time will always take care of such a problem as this, but the question is—will it do so before the onset of catastrophe or old age? Old age seems to come early to one who has this degree of mesomorphy.

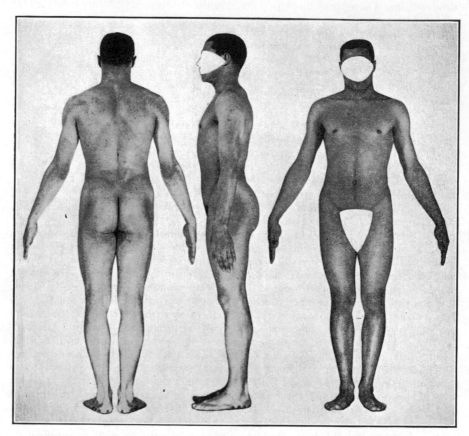

Description: Somatotype 3–5½–2½. A 19-year-old Caucasian-Negroid mesomorph two inches above average stature. The neck shows extreme mesomorphy and the Potter may have had that ideal in mind when he started. The trunk falls away only a little from extreme mesomorphy but the arms and legs—especially in the distal segments—show Nilotic brittleness or ectomorphic dysplasia. Primary *g*±, secondary *g*+1, especially in the face. Primary *t* 4, secondary *t* 3. Features comparatively fine, well chiseled, although asymmetrical. There is a sharp alertness and a suggestion of brittleness about the face which defines an odd contrast with the short muscular neck. Hands delicately formed and well molded. General strength 4, hand strength 4. He is powerful, with excellent coordination. He moves with brisk effectiveness and economy of effort, although with a certain swish like that of an efficient mesomorphic woman. He is a good dancer, disdains athletics. With his great strength he can fight when pressed, although he is not a puncher.

Temperament: The two outstanding characteristics are sparkling vivacity and monotophobia. He cannot stand routines. He seems to have too much energy—is restless, overly active, strives to dominate other persons and soon succeeds or gives up the relationship. Yet cerebrotonic interference is always apparent. Although gifted with a good singing voice and excellent pitch he is unable to sing in public. There appears to be too much self-consciousness for that. He has poor sleep habits, has been unable to routinize his life in any respect or to form work habits. His stumbling block is the periodic Dionysian festival. He has a particularly bad time with alcohol; he goes on frequent alcoholic orgies but for days afterward he seems to be torn to pieces. He is a dyed-in-the-wool *DAMP RAT,* with both somatorotic and cerebrotic complications. ψ 2–3–2.

Delinquency: Early persistent truancy during the first years of school. History of repeated running away between 7 and 15. To correctional school at 9 for running away. Between 10 and 15 he several times wandered about the country, was frequently picked up as a juvenile vagrant. To correctional school at 13 as a vagrant and stubborn child. Incorrigibility and unmanageability in foster homes at all ages to 16. No history of stealing or of personal violence.

Origins and Family: Extramarital. Nothing known of the father except that he was Irish and "a man of good education." The mother is a short muscular Russian Jewess who is said to have been violent and willful as a girl. She was institutionalized as feebleminded and manic after producing three illegitimate children. History of cardiovascular disease. One maternal grandparent died in a state mental hospital and the maternal siblings are described in agency records as a "defective lot."

Boy reared in foster homes under agency control.

Mental History, Achievement: Finished the eighth grade, then quit "for the road." IQ reports range from 106 to 121, here called 115. He gives an impression of possessing superior mentality which is undisciplined or perhaps largely undeveloped. He talks too easily, is too readily persuasive, exploits by using the vulgar clichés of the day—in short fails to use his mentality.

No vocational plan. Excellent general ability in music. The AMI that of an obviously intelligent, fine-looking youth who is *DAMP RAT* and has botched up his school career, yet gives an impression of underlying ability and "ought to be salvaged."

Medical: Early history not known. Long series of medical referrals for minor ailments but no serious illnesses or injuries. His health has been on the whole good although there have been periods of unexplained general fatigue. PX reveals no significant pathology.

Running Record: The history of his relations at the Inn was a disappointing one since we failed to return him successfully to school. Five different times the school program was started but we could not hold him to it. His inability to stand routine and his penchant for the periodic alcoholic and homosexual orgy were too strong. It was clear to him as well as to us that he would have a chance if he could once get past the bugaboo of high school and could embark on a college course, where discipline and routines are less exacting. About half the time he was hopeful, full of zest and new resolution, but the high peaks of hopefulness were always followed shortly by blowouts of alcoholic and sexual Dionysianism—then by somatic complaints and by what two local psychiatric clinics called *neurasthenia.* He seemed to carry on a struggle between integrative and disintegrative impulses that was painful to watch. He felt the need of orientation in time, in his good moments discussed life with insight, saw only too clearly his need for identification with the academic field. He met two or three successful academicians with personality patterns and problems similar to his own. After such a meeting he would for a few days address himself eagerly to the task of overcoming time-wasting habits, but he always yielded again to what seemed to be a tidal wave of Dionysian somatorosis, and then he would go on a bender. In about a week he would recover and would start over again. For his debauchery and alcoholism he always disappeared from the Inn, turning up later as bedraggled as an Irish setter straggling home from one of his September moon-runs.

After leaving us he struggled with his problem through a series of other agency contacts but never changed the pattern. Psychoanalytic therapy was attempted and the boy is credited with this statement: "Analysis is like sweeping all the dirt into the middle of the floor but leaves you with no dustpan and brush." Exempted from military service on psychiatric grounds he has drifted for another five years, holding many jobs briefly and vagabonding about the country, with intermittent orgies. He has not deteriorated noticeably, and when rested he looks like a bright and intelligent youth who ought to have a good future. But more often he looks fatigued and old and drawn.

Summary: Asthenic mesomorphy with weak chest and arms. Mentality

about college average; health good in a fragile way; *DAMP RAT* syndrome with monotophobia of such a degree as to reach second-order psychopathy. A wanderer.

ID 1–5–0 (6)
  Insufficiencies:
    IQ . . . .
    Mop   1
  Psychiatric:
    1st order . . . .
    2nd order   2
      Somatorotic monotophobia
      (2–3–2)
    C-phobic   1
    G-phrenic   2
    DAMP RAT
  Residual D:
    Primary Crim. . . . .

Comment: Outlook dubious. The prognosis has probably worsened during the intervening half-dozen years. Yet many who have been associated with him have had a haunting feeling that he is *almost* a good person. He seems just barely to fall short of mastering the fatal monotophobia which is the *bête noire* of the *DAMP RAT* syndrome. Meanwhile his strength wanes. Like nearly all *DAMP RAT*s he seems at times to have the energy of a higher degree of mesomorphy than his physique shows, and this phenomenon may contain the nucleus of an explanation of the seemingly strange antics of a strange fraternity. Possibly some of these people are almost heroes or supermen, by-products of an abortive but recurrent Potterian impulse to create something extra special and *really* in His own image.

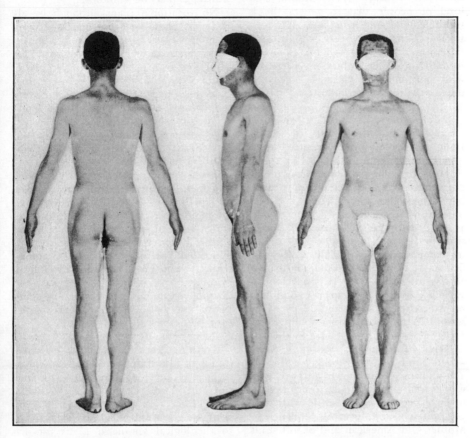

Description: Somatotype 2½–3½–4½. A 21-year-old mesomorphic ecto-morph an inch above average stature. General suggestion of arrested meso-morphy. Mesomorphic first region. Long trunk with high waist, and narrow or asthenic chest. Moderately asthenic arms. The legs are finely molded, showing higher *t* than the rest of the body. Primary *g*±—a trace; secondary *g*+1. Primary *t* 3, secondary *t* 3. Features well formed and clean-cut but the face is badly asymmetrical. Hands crude; feet well formed. General strength 2, hand strength 3. Coordination excellent but feminoid. All bodily move-ments are executed with a delicate grace. No athletic or combative ability.

Temperament: *DAMP RAT* pattern, with monotophobia the predominant characteristic. He bubbles with energy; seems to boil over too easily, like a tea kettle at high altitude. There is no discipline or restraint. Yet despite the feminoid somatorosis he is so amiable and socialized, so sincerely viscerotonic and fond of people that in general he is welcome, pleasing company. His *persona* is that of a breezy sophisticated saleswoman. He runs a gamut of moods in which gushing enthusiasm alternates with pouting perversity. He is always theatrical, restive, dilettante. ψ 5–1–1.

Delinquency: Early truancy and restlessness or uncontrollability in school. Long history of minor or near delinquency throughout the early teens. From 10 or 12 he associated with "moral degenerates," was a peddler of contraband goods like spicy pictures and sexually associated articles. Between 15 and 17, frequently in difficulty over homosexuality. At 17, in trouble with police for impersonating a female. Rolling of drunks at 18. Several episodes of drunkenness at 17 and 18. Participation in various panhandler enterprises and confidence schemes at 17 and 18. No very serious charges; borderline delinquency.

Origins and Family: Second of three, urban family. Father strongly built and a foundling of unknown ancestry who was reared under agency control. Said to have been a difficult child with temper tantrums and "neurotic tendencies." Mother Old American and of soft stout build; described as a somatotonic and mannish woman who despite outward difficulties "did pretty well to keep a home together." Boy reared in the home.

Mental History, Achievement: Finished two years of high school. IQ reports range between 105 and 133, here called 120. He is bright and gives the impression of being one who with aca-demic training might develop an adequately good nonsemantic or nonscientific mind. He is good at literature and at cultural subjects, poor at mathematics or at anything requiring a quantitative orientation. He is mentally active, seethes like a boiling stew with schemes which tend to be grandiose.

No vocational plans although he always has plans for acquiring large sums of money quickly. He is gifted in music and is an acclaimer for all the arts. The AMI that of a personable *DAMP RAT* youth who at first gives the impression of being a born salesman but soon oversells himself and then resorts to feminoid distress signs.

Medical: Birth and early development normal. Violent, possibly epileptoid tantrums appeared in early infancy and have continued to the present. He has spells of what he calls red fury. Frequent upper respiratory infections which settle in the chest and leave him with a cough that seems to be present about half the time. Addiction to homosexuality and bouts of acute alcoholism from age 15. Psychiatric referrals with diagnoses translating the primary complaint into Latin. PX reveals no significant pathology.

Running Record: Keeping up with him was like trying to keep track of a colony of ants. He brought forth possibly three wild schemes a week—plans for getting rich; for reorganizing the Inn; for going to college, to law school, to theological seminary; plans for organizing a chain-store system, also a string of saloons and of red light oases. He is *almost* the promotional type of personality. He has great momentary energy, tremendous enthusiasm, quick mentality; but lacks the sustained drive for carrying through. He is not quite hard enough coal and the somatotonia burns off too quickly. In spurts he did well on work assignments but on outside jobs he would succumb to boredom within a week and would get drunk. He did not quite fit in with the *DAMP RAT*s at the Inn. His arty interests like all others were superficial and would not withstand sharp probing. He was considerate in that he always went elsewhere for his orgies and alcoholic bouts. Once he fell in with a religious foundation and they offered him a scholarship that would send him through theological seminary. This tempted him for quite a while but at last he turned it down with the comment that he didn't think he could get through algebra.

Exempt from military service on psychiatric grounds, he remained in the community for another year, became more alcoholic, was referred to more psychiatric clinics. Then he drifted to another eastern city where for four years he seems to have indulged in a prolonged spree. But he still has periods of reform and recovery. As late as three months before the present writing he announced a plan for going to college, almost sounded as if he meant it.

Summary: Gynandroid endomorph with too much energy. *DAMP RAT* pattern. Mentality college level; a trace of medical insufficiency. Epileptoid history. Alcoholism.

ID 1–5–0 (6)
  Insufficiencies:
    IQ ....
    Mop 1
  Psychiatric:
    1st order ....
    2nd order 1
      Epileptoid (5–1–1)
    C-phobic 2
    G-phrenic 2
      DAMP RAT
  Residual D:
    Primary crim. ....

Comment: Outlook still uncertain. As yet he has neither deteriorated nor climbed out of the marsh. If you are going to be amoral you have to be so good at something that society will tolerate your idiosyncrasy and will let you get away with it. This youth knows all that, so periodically decides to be "a great preacher or something." He may come through. He still has intelligence and a winning personality, has many times seemed on the verge of applying himself. But so far, the monotophobia has always got him. Probably even now his best hope lies with the academic ship. He could be a very successful instructor in the romance languages. For preaching, his IQ is wrong by a third.

179.

COMPANY B, PLATOON 1, SECTION 6
Gynandrophrenes: Nos. 168–184

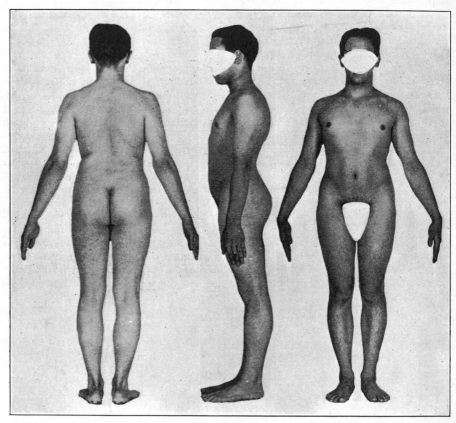

Description: Somatotype 4½–4–2. An 18-year-old mesomorphic endomorph an inch under average stature. Trunk a little short. High gynandroid
waist, but otherwise all segments well developed. No dysplasias. Primary
g+1, secondary *g*+2. Primary *t* 3, secondary *t* 3. Delicate features of average
molding. Some facial asymmetry; bright, alert eyes. General strength 2, hand
strength 2. Coordination good in a feminine sense. He moves gracefully although like a girl with a swish and hip sway. No athletic or combative
ability.

Temperament: He is gynandrophrenic and shows the *DAMP RAT* syndrome, but in a very restrained manner. The *persona* seems to be that of a shy, mousy woman who is nice. For the most part he is like a clinging vine, with viscerotonic dependency and with an inconstant extraversion of affect. Yet now and then, at periodic intervals, the second component takes over vigorously. The long suffering "urge to masculine assertiveness" then seems to waken from its slumber and to have its hour—in a weak, poorly sustained temper tantrum or in an alcoholic festival. After the explosion or spree he feels better, is relaxed and even amiable or solicitous. He compares the after-affect of the somatorotic spasm to that of the sexual orgasm. ψ 2–1–2.

Delinquency: None. Problem of homosexuality. He has never smoked or used alcohol, has never been suspected of untoward behavior of any kind, except involvement in homosexual episodes. He was quiet and well behaved throughout his school life, although considered shy and girl-like. In reviewing his criminal career he says he "once rang a doorbell at Hallowe'en." Sent to a boy's camp at 16, very much against his will, "in order to bring him out." He returned addicted to an overt sexual practice which has continued.

Origins and Family: Second of five, urban family. Father Old American, called "tall, loose-jointed, honest, ineffectual." He comes from a rundown family, has always been sickly, has never been quite able to make a living. Mother also Old American, described as "a tall, somewhat bewildered woman who does her best and is well considered." Boy reared at home. Other siblings "all right, although not outstanding."

Mental History, Achievement: Finished high school with fairly good marks and excellent behavioral record. Poor in mathematics; main interests: music, art, literature. IQ reports run from 104 to 117, here called 110. High achievement level at verbal and language tests; poor at tests of dexterity and at math. He gives an impression of possessing an alert intellect but his thought is undisciplined and butterfly-like. In discussing Bach, Beethoven, the theater, and the current crop of artists he is pretty well at home. Otherwise pretty well at sea.

No vocational plan and no special abilities. Can play two or three musical instruments passably but too shy and insecure to do so in public. Visualizes himself as a Shakespearian actor but lacks the somatotonic address to carry any kind of part on any kind of stage. The AMI that of a weak and sincere youth who is confused; he seems caught in the web of a *DAMP RAT* dream.

Medical: No serious illnesses or injuries. As an infant, shy, isolated, unable to play successfully with other children. From early childhood he tended to develop deep emotional attachments of a dependent nature, usually to some weak and isolated boy like himself. A lonely creature in high school but apparently lighthearted and happy in his fantasies. He seems always to have been essentially happy and his history shows no indication of disorientation of any kind, at any time. In this he appears to depart sharply from the schizophrenic track. PX reveals low blood pressure and feminoid behavioral tendencies; nothing else. The conspicuous primary *g* without any marked secondary *g* is striking.

Running Record: In his relations with us he was quiet, considerate, courteous in every way. Overtly he was bewildered by a world not at all adapted to his needs. Yet he seemed in some almost mystic way to be having a good time and to be enjoying his *DAMP RAT* role in the play. To him life was certainly just that—a play—and he was flouncing through it. He regarded himself as a total failure but it didn't seem to matter much. Even about that he had decided to be a good sport. It would perhaps not be quite accurate to credit him with humor but he had internal peace, which is one of the prerequisites of humor.

He had been struggling along in a course in business accounting and was doing badly at it. His mentality appeared to be "too light," he said, for that kind of work, and we had to agree that the situation seemed a little like trying to cut firewood with a jeweler's saw. We wanted to see him attempt a liberal arts college, offered to back him if he would try, but he demurred. He seemed to feel that he didn't quite have the mentality for the undertaking, and he may have been right. His IQ is high enough to carry an athletic mesomorph through college with honors; but for such a person as this youth a *really* high IQ may be needed, in order to take up the slack.

During the six or seven years since our first contact with him he seems scarcely to have changed at all. He has kept out of trouble, has now held a clerical job for several years, lives the narrowest sort of life, overtly at least. He loves his few books and furniture, caresses his collection of music records as a mother would a child, probably has very little sex life and certainly has no heterosexual outlook. He has no abiding interests beyond the theater and art; even these interests seem thin and remote. Yet in some indefinable way he gives the impression of having a good time. Or perhaps that is only my fancy. The *DAMP RAT* mentality somehow fascinates me. Something in it that is probably essential seems to elude me, and I feel toward it as a mud turtle must feel toward a blue heron.

Summary: Asthenic mesomorphy with a conspicuous gynandroid influence. Good general health. Mentality near college average. *DAMP RAT* syndrome.

ID 0–3–0 (3)
Insufficiencies:
  IQ ....
  Mop ....
Psychiatric:
  1st order ....
  2nd order ....
  C-phobic ....
  G-phrenic 3
  DAMP RAT
Residual D:
  Primary crim. ....

Comment: Outlook excellent so far as criminality or the need for institutional care is concerned. The boy is at least as certain as the reader not to commit any crimes of theft or violence, and is perhaps even more certain not to be guilty of the arrogance of his own reproduction. The case raises one question which I think is important to those who in any capacity take the responsibility of prescribing for youth. This has to do with boys' camps and with forced group gatherings of all sorts. There are some youngsters who should be protected from "being brought out" in this manner as from smallpox. A later generation of human life will some day emerge from the fatal *enantiodromia* or fashion swings between introversional and extraversional education. The present "progressive" fad is for "extraversion," which is as bad for about half the population as was the Christian evil of "ten commandment introversion" for the other half. We need to mix a little diagnosis, or cogent description, with educational policy.

180.

COMPANY B, PLATOON 1, SECTION 6
Gynandrophrenes: Nos. 168–184

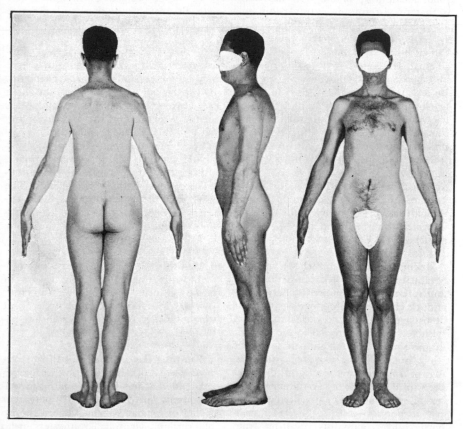

Description: Somatotype 3½–4–3. A 23-year-old asthenic midrange physique two inches above average stature. All segments but the legs are asthenic and show arrested development. Face, neck, and chest weakest. Arms very heavy boned but poorly muscled. There was a peculiar failure of the bud to exfoliate properly. Narrow chest, high gynandroid waist. Primary *g*+2, secondary *g*+1. Primary *t* 1, secondary *t* 2. Features irregular, uneven, and asymmetrical. Eyes dull, lusterless. General strength 1, hand strength 3 —quite unusual. Coordination fair in a feminine sense. He moves gingerly although a little clumsily. It is as if he were fearful of disturbing a sleeping infant. Helpless at any kind of athletics or at fighting.

Temperament: Viscerotonia predominates but there is also a strong somatotonic drive and some evidence of cerebrotonia. He is as relaxed and poised as a well-fed tomcat. An enormous eater and a great appreciator of food; sociophilic, affable. The hallmark is that of viscerotonic extraversion but also he has great physical energy and is aggressive in a quiet, ceremonious way. Cerebrotonia is manifest only in his singing. He has a rich baritone voice but becomes self-conscious in public. Before an audience his voice is strained, breaks, misses notes. A cycloid trend is conspicuous. There are almost rhythmic somatorotic outbursts in which he is hysterically loud and creates a disturbance. Referred to psychiatric clinics, diagnosed *hysterical*. But he does not seem to show depression. The energy level appears to oscillate between high and normal, not between high and low. He is gynandrophrenic and arty to an extreme degree. ψ 4-2-2.

Delinquency: Early school unmanageability. There called temperamental and referred to psychiatrists. Between 8 and 12, frequent episodes or sprees of destructiveness, window-breaking, fire-setting. At all ages from 8 to the present he has shown a minor sadistic tendency —pinching, poking, twisting, and hurting of smaller children, and this has been observed to be accompanied by sexual excitement. On psychiatric referral, diagnosed *sadistic*. Several "stubborn child" complaints resulting from violent temper outbursts and from guerrilla warfare with the mother. Frequently in trouble through complaints of "unnatural sex practices."

Origins and Family: Only child, urban family. Both parents seem to present about an even mixture of white and Negro blood. Father well educated, left the family shortly after this boy was born. Mother heavily built and always an active, aggressive person. Regarded as a social leader among the Negro élite. She has tremendous energy with a manifest manic component. Hospitalized at least once with diagnosis "manic behavior." Boy reared partly at home, partly with relatives. His manic or hysterical phase never seemed to integrate well with that of his mother and the two fought violently.

Mental History, Achievement: Finished the eighth grade, then quit school because of personality maladjustments. IQ reports fall between 90 and 110, here put at 100. It is difficult to gauge his mentality because of the gynandrophrenia and the artistic *persona*.

Vocational interest, singing and music. He wants to be a professional singer, although the trace of cerebrotonic interference makes that impossible. The AMI that of a gifted genius, with the laying-on-of-hands habit and a relaxation seldom achieved outside the feline kingdom except by Negroes.

Medical: Birth and early development called uneventful. No record of serious injuries or illnesses. Numerous psychiatric referrals without any cogent diagnoses. PX reveals no significant pathology.

Running Record: At the Inn he was a problem both because of the hysterical tendency and because of the gynandrophrenic psychopathy. His persistent laying on of hands brought him the ire of certain vigorous youngsters who named him "the goose." But he maintained his *persona* of the rising artist and was imperturbable both in his Oxford accent and in his contempt for the "vulgar," except when the hysterical phase was on. At such times he would express excited rage for perhaps a quarter of an hour and would slap or pinch like an infuriated wench. Among the *DAMP RATs* he was a fringer or visiting cousin, never an insider. Frequently accused of homosexuality, he certainly never "got much" at the Inn. Several efforts were made to send him to school for vocal training but he would soon discover that the teachers were humbugs. When the hysterical mood was dominant he would demand recognition of his greatness *now,* would brook no postponement and no intermediate period of humiliation. Job placement was tried with even worse success. Work was foreign to his nature.

After his stay with us he toyed with other programs of training in music, under the aegis of other agencies, and was finally inducted into military service. There he was hospitalized for many months with complaints of fainting spells and hysterical behavior, being finally given a medical discharge on grounds of "psychoneurosis." But after peace was declared he decided he liked the service and was permitted to reenlist. For a time he was a chaplain's assistant, in charge of music. During one six-month period he was hospitalized four times with complaints of nervousness and fainting spells. Recently, following a particularly spirited series of "hysterical episodes," he was once more given a psychiatric discharge.

Summary: A midrange Negro physique which will become very heavy in later life. Normal mentality and good health. Second-order psychopathy with gynandrophrenia. YMCA disease.

ID 0–5–0 (5)
　Insufficiencies:
　　IQ ....
　　Mop ....

Psychiatric:
　1st order ....
　2nd order 2
　(4–2–2)
　C-phobic ....
　G-phrenic 3
　DAMP RAT
Residual D:
　Primary crim. ....

Comment: Outlook probably good both from the standpoint of criminality and from that of the boy's enjoyment of life. From the point of view of useful citizenship it is anything but good. Whether or not a psychotic component is present is controversial. He is believed by at least one psychiatrist to be prepsychotic, but by our criteria the psychopathy seems to be of the second order. He is what we have sometimes called a minor cycloid, as distinguished from the major, or psychotic cycloid.

The gynandrophrenia is in this case regarded as a pathological factor, since it has repeatedly brought the boy into trouble and since he has failed, hitherto, to adopt a pattern of life into which the gynandrophrenia can be acceptably incorporated. It does not necessarily follow that he is a homosexual. Homosexuality is one concomitant of gynandrophrenia, but it seems to be only a potential concomitant. Possibly certain kinds of ability and genius are associated only with gynandrophrenia. But this boy has not yet found a way to harness that difficult and recalcitrant horse into his team.

181. COMPANY B, PLATOON 1, SECTION 6
Gynandrophrenes: Nos. 168–184

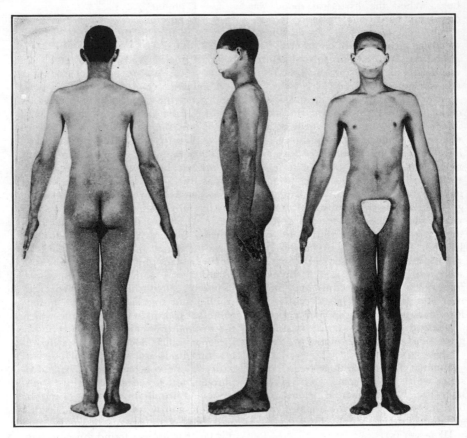

Description: Somatotype 4–4–4. A 17-year-old Negro youth of midrange somatotype possibly a little on the endomorphic side, and seven inches above average stature. A towering physique, more endomorphic and mesomorphic below than above the diaphragm. Heavy bones throughout. Small head, slender neck, and a trace of asthenic influence in the chest and arms. Primary $g+2$, secondary $g+2$. He reeks faintly with secondary g, recalling to a nostalgic memory the YMCA secretary of a period now happily fading into twilight. Primary t 3, secondary t 3. Features Negroid but fine and relatively delicate. Hair comparatively fine. Skin of soft, feminoid texture throughout the body. General strength 2, hand strength 2. Coordination excellent although feminine. Every movement is smooth and seemingly made with a studied grace, as if he were a professional draper.

Temperament: This is a hysterical personality. His life suggests a prolonged tempest in a teapot. He has spasms of rage or of hysterical emotionality when he seems to be in danger of not getting his way. Overenergized, extraordinarily active; always into things and troublesome in a minor way. Diagnosis by one psychiatrist *manic-depressive, prepsychotic*. We did not concur in that diagnosis. His second component is not strong enough for manic behavior. He is hyperactive, almost hypomanic, but with this physical endowment a full-blown manic psychosis is probably impossible. His mannerisms and gestures are effeminate, as is his speech, but he seems to be merely a confused gynandrophrene and in no sense a *DAMP RAT* or homosexual. He is overloaded with somatotonia and viscerotonia, yet is incapable of achieving the relief or satisfaction which comes from athletic expression. As one of our social workers remarked, it is as if he had perpetual sexual excitement without being able to do anything about it. ψ 4–1–1.

Delinquency: Early truancy and unmanageability in school. Persistent minor stealing between 6 and 12. Ran away several times at 11 and 12, also at 13 and 14. Frequent petty stealing between 12 and 16, although no court charges pressed on this score. "Stubborn child" complaints at 15 and 16. His real delinquency, during the two years before our contact with him, consisted in open warfare with the mother, who is a powerful gynandroid woman. At 16 he was under police surveillance for identification with a delinquent gang. His outlook has been more delinquent than his achievement. He is always about to have somebody shot or taken for a ride by his gang. He has a loud although not entirely malevolent bark; little if any bite.

Origins and Family: Oldest of five, urban family. The father, German-Irish, is a heavy man of about the same physique as the boy. He has been a successful tradesman of good general standing. The mother, French-Irish, is a gynandroid mesomorph who has been called "excitable, quarrelsome, a poor disciplinarian." She suffers from high blood pressure and gall bladder trouble. The maternal grandfather and grandmother died young, of apoplexy and cholelithiasis respectively. Boy reared at home until 15, then transferred to foster homes under agency control. His relationship to his family had been normal in the sense that there has been comprehensive and enthusiastic all-around rejection.

Mental History, Achievement: Finished a year of high school with poor grades. IQ reports cluster at 100, with only slight variation. He gives a first impression of better intelligence than this because of the effective way in which he has learned to tell his story, but on further acquaintance the early good impression does not hold up.

No vocational plans or special abilities. He has become violently estranged from scholastic ambition. The AMI is based on his mastery of the family rejection story. He knows the catechisms and can bring delight to the hearts of agency people and social workers who have been sprayed with that theology. He is jealous of his father (he says), has fears and ambivalences and guilt feelings, was rejected by the mother, is a sublimated homosexual. He also has sufficient first and second component to fix the listener with a moistening eye and to hold her enthralled.

Medical: Normal birth and early development. No serious illnesses or injuries. Always ineffectual and gynandroid, with a history of poor social adaptation. Seriously defective vision from infancy. PX reveals no significant pathology except severe dental caries and poor vision.

Running Record: Working with this lad was like trying to train a puppy over the telephone. It seemed impossible to get at him. He had a good time at the Inn except on the rare occasions when he was constrained to fulfill a work assignment, and he laughed off every effort to lure him into a constructive program. His standard response to pressure of any kind was an outburst of loud yelling—so loud and so gesturally reinforced that he seemed "hysterically disoriented," but he was not disoriented. He continued to give the social workers a run for their money. Requiring a special type of glasses, which of course were paid for by one of the agencies, he succeeded in losing or breaking six pairs within two months. He was mildly alcoholic at the Inn and in the end we scored ourselves a failure on the case and turned him back to the referring agency.

For another year or more he avoided the humilitation of work but finally was inducted into military service. There he seems to have been regarded as hopelessly incorrigible and eventually was given a psychiatric discharge. During the succeeding two years he had rather a bad time of it and was led to accept a number of jobs although he kept none for more than a few weeks. Meanwhile there was no delinquency of record but he began to look rundown and blowsy. He was frequently observed to be alcoholic. About a year before the present writing he reenlisted in another branch of the service. He is still in.

Summary: A soft endomorph-mesomorph, gynandroid enough to be almost a weakling, yet heavily energized. Somatorotic and "hysterical." Mentality average. Good health, poor vision. Rather feeble efforts at delinquency.

ID 1–4–0 (5)
Insufficiencies:
   IQ ....
   Mop 1
Psychiatric:
   1st order ....
   2nd order 1
     Dionysian trend (4–1–1)
   C-phobic ....
   G-phrenic 3
Residual D:
   Primary crim. ....

Comment: Outlook probably good for an "adaptation"; poor from the standpoint of mental development or achievement. He should soon grow fat in the Army and this will dampen the Dionysian or hysterical trend. He has no major problem of sexuality. He probably has learned permanently to avoid the discomfort of being caught at stealing. His dangerousness, or violence, is about that of a barnyard goose. With that personality and an IQ five points higher, he might have had a happy and successful academic career. Many such personalities are to be found in the college pastures but they have to work hard and keep quiet while getting their Ph.D's.

For those interested in the study of interpersonal relations, particularly within the family, this is a beautiful case. Both the boy and the mother are gynandroid. That is to say, the boy is a soft "sissy"; the mother hard and masculine. The *g* component just about wipes out the natural differential, with respect to fighting power, so the two are well matched. Result: joyous jousting.

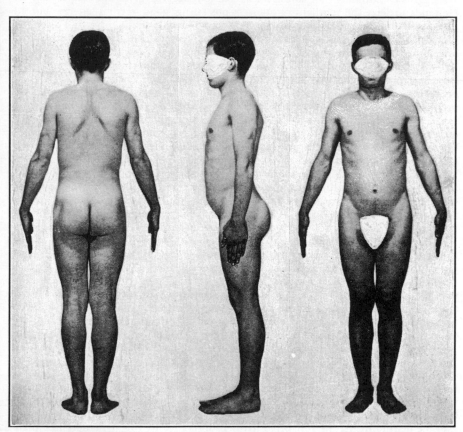

Description: Somatotype 4–4–3. A 17-year-old midrange youth two inches above average stature. A large plethoric physique which in middle life will be tall and perhaps very heavy, but not very muscular. Rather poor muscular development throughout. The chest and arms are the weakest segments. Primary $g\pm$—just a good trace; secondary $g+2$. There is diffuse secondary g throughout the body, and moderate hypogenitalism. He is soft all over, like a girl, and has feminine subcutaneous finish. Primary t 2, secondary t 3. Features regular but small and delicately chiseled; too delicate for a male. Face broad and a little doughy. Hands and feet weak, delicately formed. General strength 2, hand strength 2. Coordination good in the sense that he has an airy feminine grace. Worthless at games, unable to throw or fight. Not quite an out-and-out "sissy" in his physical presentation but distinctly gynandroid.

Temperament: Somatotonia seems to predominate. He is ceaselessly active and aggressive although not courageous. He tends to seize the spotlight of attention and to hold it; yet there is no more physical combativeness in him than in a large, buzzing fly. He is theatrical, meretricious, perverse. The term which seems most succinctly to describe him would be breezy affectation. He gives the impression of a certain underlying effeminacy, or sissification, along with a kind of arty sophistication at a comparatively low intellectual level. He is well energized, poorly intellectualized. This is the *DAMP RAT* syndrome without the first-rate mentality which such a pattern subsumes and, for success, requires. ψ 2–1–1.

Delinquency: Early unmanageability in school. Truancy, tantrums, mendacity, minor stealing, all before age 12. Between 12 and 16, vigorous warfare with the mother, violent quarreling with teachers, refusal to go to school or to work. Also minor stealing, and concern on the part of social workers over reported homosexuality.

Origins and Family: Oldest of three, urban family. Father Lithuanian, described in social agency records as violent and neglectful. On his part, however, he maintains that he supported his family adequately until "social agencies began to monkey with them." Mother a heavily built 200-pounder of German origins, described in harsh terms by social workers. "Low mentality, unstable, aggressive, quarrelsome, greedy, dominating"—in short, a perfect Freudian mother. Boy reared at home with much agency help. One of the siblings obese and mentally retarded. Family considered partly Jewish on both sides although there is no profession of Jewish religion.

Mental History, Achievement: Quit school in the ninth grade after a history of failure and unsatisfactory behavior. IQ reports range from 75 to 96, here called 85. He gives the impression of possessing good mental energy but of being entirely undisciplined. This is the sort of case which gives one the feeling that the IQ "might have turned up "higher" if the child had been reared in a disciplined environment.

No vocational plan; no special abilities. The AMI based on virtually a rote recital of Freudian syndromes. He was rejected by both parents, he says, is jealous of the father and is ambivalent toward the mother. He has had an Oedipus complex since 4. Recently he has suffered from a castration complex and has had sublimated homosexual yearnings which have resulted in "polyeidetic identifications." This is not bad for a 16-year-old with IQ 85, although I have known even younger children with even lower IQ's to recite prayers in Latin.

Medical: Infancy history not available. No serious illnesses or injuries. Several hospital referrals for minor illnesses. PX reveals gross dental caries and flat feet. He is skittish or ticklish, coy at PX.

Running Record: Throughout his stay here he disregarded rather than disobeyed rules, maintained a kind of airy indifference to vulgar matters like planning for the future or earning money, occupied himself now and then with the preliminaries of composing a perfect poem. He seemed to visualize himself as essentially an artist, although his choice of a field of artistic expression had not yet crystallized. Sometimes it would be poetry, sometimes the drama, sometimes just art in general. But he was not seriously interested in art, even "in general." There seemed to be surplus mental energy for many sorts of dilettante discussion; none for serious participation in anything. He failed to agglutinate with the *DAMP RAT* fraternity despite an unmistakable temperamental affinity in that direction and an apparent desire to be one of the group. They failed to take to him, repeatedly shooed him off as a flock of geese will shoo off a stray puppy. He was perhaps offensive to them intellectually, and not sufficiently attractive physically. He seemed to want to be a homosexual. Whether or not he actually achieved that kind of adaptation we never knew.

After our contact with him, which we felt had led nowhere, he drifted in the environment, had a few odd jobs, maintained contact with social agencies, was exempted from military service on psychiatric grounds—*psychopathic personality*. For five years he has kept out of the hands of police except for a couple of alcoholic episodes. Within the past two years he has twice held clerical jobs for several months, but in the end was considered unsatisfactory because of persistent "pretense of illness." He is reported to be drinking immoderately.

Summary: A large feminoid youth of midrange somatotype and mesomorphic first region. Mentality dull normal; health good. *DAMP RAT* psychopathy without a *DAMP RAT* adaptation. Probably borderline homosexuality.

ID 1–4–0 (5)
Insufficiencies:
  IQ 1
  Mop ....
Psychiatric:
  1st order ....
2nd order ....
C-phobic 1
G-phrenic 3
  DAMP RAT
Residual D:
Primary crim. ....

Comment: Outlook uncertain, although now more likely to be good than bad. He has arrived in the twenties without any very dramatic mishaps and has not shown alcoholic or general deterioration, although he has been known to be an episodal drunkard. He is a pronounced gynandrophrene and a good example of the *DAMP RAT* pattern—a syndrome which includes homosexuality as a frequently occurring secondary characteristic. But it cannot be too often pointed out that homosexual practice is not a constant or primary accompaniment of this syndrome. Possibly such a practice is the most identifying and dramatic symptom of the syndrome but it is one of the least constant symptoms, and to indicate that a youth has constitutional affiliation with the *DAMP RATs* does not identify him with homosexual practice any more than web feet identify a bird as a duck. Perhaps a distinction should be made between homosexuality and homosexual practice. If the former be taken to mean only a *tendency toward* the practice, then the *DAMP RAT* syndrome and homosexuality would have a closer identification.

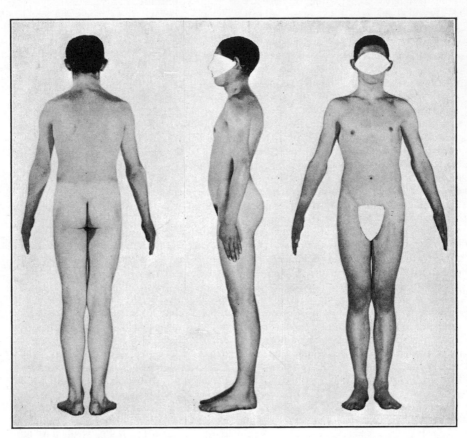

Description: Somatotype 4–4½–3½. A 16-year-old youth with a slight mesomorphic predominance, four inches above average stature. An overgrown, soft, loosely built physique. Large head, enormous face, prominent features. Neck strongly mesomorphic. Arms and chest comparatively undeveloped or asthenic in comparison with the rest of the body. This is not ectomorphic dysplasia but some kind of developmental failure. Primary $g\pm$, secondary $g+2$. He has a strongly feminine atmosphere and the entire body is soft, with feminoid subcutaneous padding. Primary t 3 despite the weak arms; secondary t 2. Features coarse, pasty, lacking in "character." Hands flabby, feet poorly formed and flat. General strength 2, hand strength 2. Coordination fair but feminoid. He moves with a swish and with feminine rolling of the hips. Entirely foreign to the gymnasium and to athletic games but fond of swimming. No combative ability.

Temperament: Predominantly viscerotonic. Fond of food, comfort, and company; emotionally extraverted to a remarkable degree. But also weakly demanding, like a nagging woman. The somatotonic mood, or impulse, seems to appear with a wavelike rhythm but viscerotonia is steadily manifest in his affective extraversion. He has a cycloid tendency and there is a dreamy unreality about him. He seems to be not closer than third cousin to the manic-depressive psychotics—not enough energy for that. ψ 3–1–2.

Delinquency: No truancy, and a good deportment record in school prior to age 12 when he began to get into difficulties arising from "homosexuality." Never a thief, he began to be alcoholic at 15; between 15 and 20 was often in trouble for panhandling, petty swindling, and for alleged homosexuality. At 22, known by many aliases and looked upon by police and social agencies as a degenerating bum. Yet in a way respected for his intelligence and good humor, and never considered quite a criminal. Numerous little panhandling rackets, which he himself never takes seriously but conducts with the friendly jocosity of a politician passing out a daily column of slop for the local newspapers.

Origins and Family: Third of five, urban family. Father of Irish-American extraction and a colorful alcoholic. A former juvenile delinquent, later a migrant drunkard, he was an illegitimate son of a similarly colorful Irishman by a daughter of a "fine old Boston family." The mother of our boy, Irish, called mentally defective and physically inadequate, became very obese, died in her early fifties of what was reported as a chronic aortic infection. Of the other four siblings three, all illegitimate, hospitalized as mental defectives. Boy reared at home, although with constant agency management of varying degree,

and with nearly annual migration from one slum district to another.

Mental History, Achievement: Finished the eighth grade, started high school but dropped out in the first year. Record called good. Efforts were made by several teachers and social workers to persuade him to go back to school. Instead he went "on the bum." IQ reports range from 102 to 118, here called 115. He gives an impression of superior intelligence and has a rich, salty humor. An excellent *raconteur*.

No real vocational ambition although he is interested in music and art, and has a sort of half desire to write. He plays one or two musical instruments, has written poetry in some quantity. He gently extracts a living by his delightful conversational ability. The AMI that of a tall, relaxed, Dionysian youth who is of superior intelligence, has his tongue in his cheek, and is fun to talk with. He has a ridiculously cultured voice, a Harvard accent, smokes an English pipe with graceful deliberation, talks entertainingly of social foibles and of his own delinquency.

Medical: No record of illnesses or injuries. No indication of any serious physiological insufficiency. PX reveals no significant pathology. He has a bleary, dissipated appearance; already looks a little like a chronic alcoholic.

Running Record: At the Inn his intelligence and especially his humor rendered him a welcome guest, and during his viscerotonic or rather nonsomatorotic periods he was a useful assistant in the House. He could be trusted with statistical and other work requiring accuracy and mental responsibility. Often a plan for returning to school was outlined with him and arrangements for such a move were several times made. But before the plan could be matured two or three days of submanic euphoria would intervene and then would follow an alcoholic debauch which would terminate in the lowest South End dives. In two or three months he would return for a fresh start. In the House his behavior was above reproach, at least so for as alcohol and homosexuality were concerned—he was too intelligent to mix his lives. But when it came to *a choice between* the life suggested at the Inn and that of the periodic bout of debauchery the latter always won. Even at his best or soberest moments he predicted that the way of the bum must in the end be *his* way and we never entertained any very sanguine expectation that he would prove himself mistaken. In dealing with this youth we lacked "faith." Perhaps that is why we failed. But then perhaps the reason we lacked faith was because there was no ground for it.

He drifted and bummed for another two years, degenerating conspicuously, then was inducted into military service. There he spent several months before being given a medical discharge, and returned immediately to the old haunts and the old way. At last report he looked middle aged and had given up all contact with "respectability." But the old salty humor remained. He expressed no regrets and voiced no complaints.

Summary: A large, gynandroid endomorph with weak arms and with essential physical incompetence. College level mentality with humor—a rare enough occurrence. *DAMP RAT* psychopathy and alcoholism.

ID 0–7–0 (7)
Insufficiencies:
 IQ ....
 Mop ....
Psychiatric:
 1st order ....

2nd order 1
(3–1–2)
C-phobic 2
G-phrenic 4
 DAMP RAT (but not arty)
Residual D:
Primary crim. ....

Comment: Prognosis generally regarded as poor although he may never need institutional care. He seems to know what he is doing and he set out on his present course of life as a first choice at about the age when most youngsters begin to think about what college to attend. He has never deviated from his primary loyalty to the pattern. He *seems* to be having a good time. The *DAMP RATs* of the series, taken as a group, seem in a way to be a happy lot of people. They appear to go through life as through a play, very much as the psychotics seem to live out a dream, and they are almost as devoted to the dramatic theme as the schizoid psychotics are to the dream theme. It is just about as difficult to get a *DAMP RAT* to abandon his theatrical role, too, as to awaken a schizophrene from his dream. I am not sure that I have ever seen one of either pattern change, in any fundamental sense. But I think that overt homosexuality can be regarded as a variable which in its expression is somewhat independent of the *DAMP RAT* pattern. There are some homosexuals, in the technical or legal sense, who are not *DAMP RATs* (see No. 164), and among the *DAMP RATs* there are many who would be as shocked as your aunt Priscilla at the thought of homosexual practice.

From the standpoint of abandonment of his bad habits, perhaps the darkest feature in the present case is the youth's excellent health. If his health holds out for another decade there will be little hope of any dramatic recovery.

COMPANY B, PLATOON 1, SECTION 6
Gynandrophrenes: Nos. 168–184

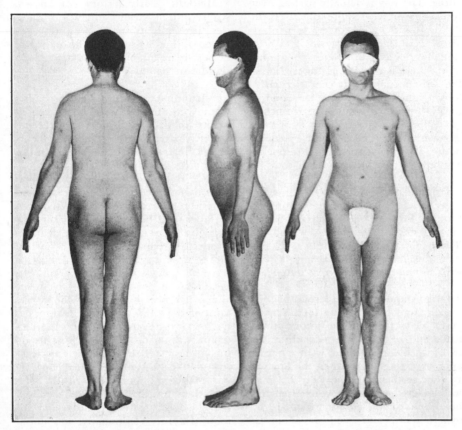

Description: Somatotype 5–4–3. A 22-year-old mesomorphic endomorph, four inches above average stature. Good development except in the face, neck and arms, all of which segments are moderately asthenic. Arms particularly weak, but they do not show the flaccidity and the lack of the power of extension seen in schizoid personalities. Primary $g+1$, secondary $g+1$. Primary t 3, secondary t 3. Fine texture throughout the whole surface of the body; features too small, nose stubby and weak; face large, broad, and pasty. Hands and feet delicately but finely formed; feet well arched. General strength 2, hand strength 2. Coordination good in the feminoid sense. He moves with studied grace. No physical combativeness or ability at games; no real physical competence.

Temperament: He shows the pattern sometimes called "sleeping tomcat somatotonia." For the most part he is relaxed, placid, apparently content, but an eye is always open for anything exciting. The boy is actually tireless, overly energized. He requires relatively little sleep and loves danger, particularly after dark. He is courageous and occasionally tries to fight although he cannot fight—there is no hitting power. He has the second component characteristic of looking older than he is. There is no indication of cerebrotonic interference or of temperamental strain of any kind. Temperament: Somatotonic predominance. Possibly a trace of visceropenic-cerebropenic pathology. ψ 2–2–1.

Delinquency: Moderate degree of early truancy and of minor stealing before 12. Two episodes of larceny and of bicycle stealing between 13 and 15. Twice found carrying a knife at 15. History of vigorous quarreling and fighting with the mother between 15 and 17.

Origins and Family: Second of four. Urban family. Father Scotch-Irish and a short, heavy man with a history of violence and of moderate alcoholism. He had high blood pressure, went out with apoplexy at about 50 when the boy was 15. The mother was a heavy Irishwoman who suffered for many years from diabetes and complications, together with hypertension, and died at about 40 when the boy was 17. Boy reared in the home.

Mental History, Achievement: Finished the sixth grade after a history of truancy and failure. IQ reports fall between 81 and 92, here called 85. He gives just about that impression—dull normality.

No vocational plan. He has some musical ability, can play several instruments, but has never been inclined to develop the gift to vocational proportions. The AMI is that of a broad-faced and wide-eyed youngster who smiles easily and looks as if he surely would do well if somebody would just give him a chance.

Medical: Early history not known. No record of serious illnesses or injuries. Intermittent spells of enuresis between 12 and 17 although no record of it before or after that. PX reveals no significant pathlogy.

Running Record: Before coming to the Inn this youth had been exposed to the influence of at least three Freudian psychiatrists, had learned fragments of the lingo in which all things arrange themselves around the concepts of mother rejection and the intrafamilial mess. One psychiatrist had diagnosed him a repressed homosexual and had been treating him with that as the central idea. The boy had remained indifferent to psychiatrists although he had picked up enough ideas to deal more or less effectively with social workers. In the House he evaded work assignments and other responsibilities without friction, merely slipping out of them quietly like a cat out the back door. If an attempt was made to force him to do something he became vigorously resistive and surly. With very small boys he was pugnacious but was pitifully helpless when his challenge was taken up. He steadfastly refused to develop his musical ability vocationally, announced the plan of living off social agencies for the remainder of his life. He was known to pick up quarters, beers, cigarettes, and the like by "pederastic prostitution." But we never saw any signs of what we would call homosexuality in him. He maintained the upper hand over us in the sense that he effectively blocked all efforts either to reform or to reeducate him.

For a year or more after our contact with him he drifted and bummed, seemed to deteriorate. There was minor delinquency of appropriation. Then the military institution picked him up and for well over two years now he has at least stayed in. He has gained 40 pounds, looks as if he might burst.

Summary: A short, endomorphic mesomorph with asthenic arms and not good at fighting. Dull normal mentality. Cerebropenia and history of enuresis. Persistent identification with minor delinquency.

ID 2–1–2 (5)
  Insufficiencies:
    IQ 1
    Mop 1
  Psychiatric:
    1st order ....
    2nd order 1
      C-penia (2–2–1)
    C-phobic ....
    G-phrenic ....
  Residual D:
    Primary crim. 2

Comment: Prognosis guarded, although recent developments are favorable. The full blossoming of the first component usually exerts a beneficent influence on delinquency. The fire of somatotonia is best extinguished with a blanket of fat. Nothing seems to take the edge off misbehavior like an expansion of the waistline, and the effect is often so dramatic that I should not be surprised to see fattening diet and inactivity some day used as a treatment of choice for somatorotic delinquency.

This youth had developed a stubborn identification with the exploitative pattern. He seemed to have been very deeply offended by life. The usual psychiatric diagnoses of mother trouble, rejections, rivalries, and the like explain none of the essential aspects of such a picture. These are nearly meaningless generalities applying more or less to most of us, and are scarcely more than names for vague universals or archetypes in human experience. The boy was resenting something more specific, and closer to his present life than mothers, siblings, or childhood events. Probably his trace of gynandromorphy was one thing he resented, although I never heard him express any verbalization of the fact. Perhaps the reason for such verbal dereliction was that the popular language to which he had been repetitiously exposed had not got back to things so organic and operational as gynandromorphy.

185. COMPANY B, PLATOON 2
Primary Criminality: Nos. 185–200

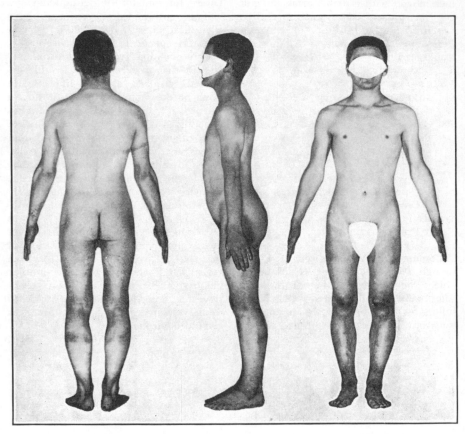

Description: Somatotype 3–5½–1½. A 17-year-old endomorphic meso-morph three inches under average stature. A squat, chunky, sturdily built youth with arrested or asthenic arms. He is destined to be barrel-shaped in middle life. Arms strikingly weak for the somatotype. The buds of these segments seem to have failed to develop properly, or the Potter got tired at the end. Primary $g\pm$—just a trace; secondary g, no trace. Primary t 2, secondary t 2. Short, sturdy legs; long trunk; head nearly spherical. Features stubby, underdeveloped, poorly molded, asymmetrical. General strength 4, hand strength 2. Coordination fairly good in the sense that he moves smoothly, but he is not good at games; throws weakly, cannot fight.

Temperament: He has a tough *persona* and hostile somatotonia is predominant although manifested more by eager following of delinquent leaders than by independent aggression on his own account. A surly stubbornness of manner which is almost a truculence characterizes his relations with people in authority. He is courageous, loves risk and danger, but he is incompetent at fighting and therefore always plays second fiddle to some delinquent but more competent mesomorph. He brings up the delinquent rear. Good relaxation; no outward indications of cerebrotonic restraint or of internal conflict. ψ 2–2–1.

Delinquency: Early truancy and troublesomeness in school although always as a follower of older boys. As a juvenile he attached himself to the tough element in a highly delinquent environment and from the beginning appears to have been a hanger-on, not one of the really potent personalities. Persistent minor stealing from 8. Larceny, breaking and entering, racketeering—numerous charges of stealing between 10 and 18. To correctional school at 16. Robbery and holdup at 19. In every instance of his apprehension he was associated with stronger and more competent youths, and it was his clumsiness or lack of resolute wit that often resulted in the capture.

Origins and Family: Oldest of four, urban family. Father German-Swedish. Long regarded as a semi-alcoholic ne'er-do-well; numerous court appearances on minor charges. Mother Swedish. She has a court record for drunkenness, larceny, neglect of children; and a history of social agency symbiosis. She finally deserted the family when this boy was 5, and the children were reared mainly in foster homes under agency management.

Mental History, Achievement: Finished the eighth grade with a poor record. IQ reports fall between 76 and 89, here called 83. He gives an impression of being stupid. Called by his associates "the dumb Swede." After nightfall he seems to become more alert and active, like an only moderately feebleminded tomcat. Of dependent mentality, he seems never to have ideas of his own but reflects the opinions and clichés of the dominant "left-wingers" in his immediate environment.

No vocational plan: no special abilities. The AMI that of a big broad-shouldered youth with honest blue eyes that stare straight into your face when he talks to you. There is a certain generous breeziness about him, and an impatience with all things mean. He is a liberal.

Medical: No early data. He has had essentially good health despite a number of clinical referrals for infections and for a recurrent, almost chronic skin disease. A number of teeth have been abscessed and nearly all of his teeth are carious or gone. PX reveals nothing more except moderately defective vision, flat feet with badly formed arches, very bad breath. This is a case of slight or incipient medical insufficiency. He is about on the borderline between good health and insufficiency.

Running Record: At the Inn he responded in healthy manner, absorbing with alacrity what was offered in the way of service and maintenance while quietly rejecting what was offered in the way of spiritual medication just as a discriminating dog quietly picks out the meat from the stew and leaves the parsnips and carrots. He was inconspicuous in the House, yet was nearly always peripherally involved in whatever rowdyism or mischief was afoot. For weeks he followed after one of our really tough boys like a shadow but since he was good at neither fighting, running, nor talking, and was not a clever thief, he turned out to be only an encumbrance to the latter and was finally forced to select another leader. This pattern was repeated several times in the course of a few months. In the end we felt that we had accomplished nothing with the boy that could be considered boastworthy. At the Inn he was a drinker but not quite a drunkard.

During the succeeding half-decade he has continued in about the same pattern. Inducted into military service, he was finally discharged on medical or psychiatric grounds. A series of defense jobs followed but even the romance of $80 a week for leisurely pushing a dust mop to the accompanying blare of radio noise could not hold him for more than a month. He tried the maritime service but soon deserted. For a couple of years now he has maintained close association with a barroom group, living from month to month and happily making the rounds of agencies. He is becoming decidedly more alcoholic.

Summary: Solidly but disharmoniously built mesomorph with poor fighting ability and with a trace of medical insufficiency. Dull normal mentality. No demonstrable first- or serious second-order psychopathy but persistent identification with the delinquency of indigence. Developing alcoholism.

ID 2–2–2 (6)
Insufficiencies:
　　IQ 1
　　Mop 1
Psychiatric:
　　1st order ....
　　2nd order .... (?)
　　(2–2–1)
　　C-phobic 2
　　G-phrenic ....

Residual D:
　　Primary crim. 2

Comment: Prognosis guarded. He remains a hanger-on of criminality and now in his middle twenties identifies strongly in that direction. The usual resources of social agencies, psychiatric clinics, and correctional institutions have had no more apparent effect on him than water on a duck's back. But what *kind* of delinquency is this? It is one thing to label it "environmental" or "constitutional," quite another thing to throw any real light on its nature. That a perfect environment would in the beginning have prevented most delinquency may be safely granted, or that perfect constitutional endowment would survive with integrity the most atrocious influences is perhaps axiomatic. However, nearly all cases of delinquency present mixtures of endogenous and exogenous ineptitude. So far as this youth's innate endowment is concerned there can be no question that he could work if the ruling power in his world were to press him to do so or were to punish him (in a way he could understand) for not doing so. But the ruling power in the present social arrangement is really an abstraction of the boy himself and is committed not to use pressure in this sense. The boy, with an IQ around 80, knows enough to know that, but doesn't know enough to see beyond it. So the prognosis is guarded. If we were sure that the social picture would remain for the next thirty years exactly as it is now we could say almost with certainty that the prognosis is poor. But changes may take place before this youth grows too old to work.

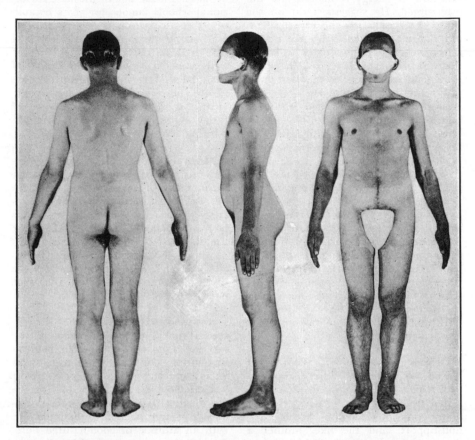

Description: Somatotype 4–4½–2½. A 19-year-old endomorphic mesomorph two inches above average stature. A somewhat dysmorphic physique with many traces of asthenic underdevelopment above the diaphragm. Much heavier below the diaphragm than above it. Yet no signs of primary component dysplasia. The bony structure appears to be equally heavy throughout. This seems to be arrested mesomophy. Primary and secondary $g\pm$. Primary t 2, secondary t 2. Features broad and coarse with no suggestion of fine molding. Hands and feet crude. Skin blotchy with very coarse pores. General and hand strength 3. Coordination rather poor. He slouches or lurches, handles himself only fairly well in the gymnasium, not very good at games or at fighting.

Temperament: Sustained somatotonia with good relaxation. Vigorous health, abundant energy, and no trace of the epileptoid unevenness of temper. His flow of energy is smooth and uninterrupted. He suggests a cat on the prowl; sly, predatory, and rather silent, but dangerously competent. He thrives on physical action, dominates his immediate environment, loves risk, is courageous and free from any manifest trace of cerebrotonic restraint. His aggression is overt and direct, not veiled behind an inferiority complex. Under alcohol he tends to become a swaggering bully, but he is not a drunkard. ψ 3–2–1.

Delinquency: Early truancy and persistent stealing before 12. Long identified with delinquent juvenile gangs. Between 14 and 18, sentenced many times to correctional school for stealing and for breaking and entering. Ran away from one state correctional school fifteen times. At 16 and 17, arrested four times for automobile stealing. At 18, most of his delinquency had been stealing but there were three or four instances of assault and police considered him a dangerous boy.

Origins and Family: Fourth of twelve, urban family. Father Old American with a long delinquent history. Arrested twenty times over a period of as many years for alcoholism, bootlegging, nonsupport, and the like. Mother a "large-soft" mentally weak Irishwoman who was always sickly and died of tuberculosis when this boy was 11. Children taken over by agencies and reared in foster homes. Ten of the siblings have been involved in delinquency; nine have IQ's recorded as below 70; three known to be epileptic. This boy considered the flower of the family.

Mental History, Achievement: Left school in the sixth grade after repeated failure and intractability. IQ reports all fall between 70 and 80, here put at 75.

No vocational plan although he has marked athletic ability and is gifted in music. He plays several instruments by ear with some proficiency. His prowess at football made one of the state correctional schools famous for years because of its football team. His feats still re-echo along the ancient corridors and cloistered walks. The AMI is that of well-composed mesomorphy and of what passes for modest taciturnity. He is quietly composed, like one of the great cats, and shows little change of facial expression. Also he is straight, tall, and physically competent.

Medical: A very large baby, with apparently normal early history. Although his mother had active tuberculosis when he was born and throughout his infancy, repeated examinations of this boy have failed to reveal evidence of the disease. No history of serious illness or injury. PX reveals severe dental caries and high blood pressure. He is a youth of robust health and abundant energy.

Running Record: At the Inn he seemed quiet and modest except on the rare occasions when he became involved in fighting. He was then a tornado of energy and one of the four or five most lethal fighters ever to live at the Inn. In his relations with the staff he was cat-like, accepting shelter or maintenance with an attitude of good-natured boredom. He was not impressed by efforts to interest him in his own future or in the paths of righteousness. To try to convert him in such a direction was like trying to convert the tomcat to vegetarianism. To him we were just another social agency with something to hand out and with some hot air to be tolerated. In the course of time he was caught at robbery and at automobile stealing and was returned to one of the correctional schools.

This is a boy for whom the war seems to have brought success and glory. After another year of the customary delinquent pattern, spent mainly under detention, he was inducted into military service. There he had a good time, married in one of the European countries, now has a family. His service record is good, so far as we can determine, and he indicates a desire to stay in the service permanently if he can.

Summary: Well-developed mesomorphic physique with good athletic ability. IQ nearly borderline; health excellent. No indication of first- or of serious second-order psychopathy. Persistent criminality but apparently he is doing well in military service.

ID 2–0–3 (5)
Insufficiencies:
   IQ   2
   Mop . . . .
Psychiatric:
   1st order . . . .
   2nd order . . . . (?)
   (3–2–1)
   C-phobic . . . .
   G-phrenic . . . .
Residual D:
   Primary crim.   3

Comment: The outlook may be good. On purely constitutional grounds, except for the borderline IQ, he seems to be an adequate person. In general physical competency he would fall among the upper three or four per cent of the male population, and no good evidence can be made out that any kind of first- or second-order psychopathy exists. What we can say is, (1) that this youth has been a singularly persistent thief, and (2) that there are no overt constitutional findings which seem to "explain" it. Perhaps the only answer is, he *wanted* to be a thief. There appear to be personalities in whom a certain flair for *direct* predation, or possibly in some cases a too keen awareness of unpunished predation all about them, exerts the predominant influence in their motivation. This may be what we shall in the end have to mean by *primary criminality*. But then there will remain all sorts of different kinds of primary criminality. Some will clear up spontaneously with maturation or with passage of time. Some will be curable by exhortation and example; some by an opportunity for vigorous participation in a war or something—as will possibly be the case with this boy; some only by the rod, and some will be as persistent as life.

187. COMPANY B, PLATOON 2
Primary Criminality: Nos. 185–200

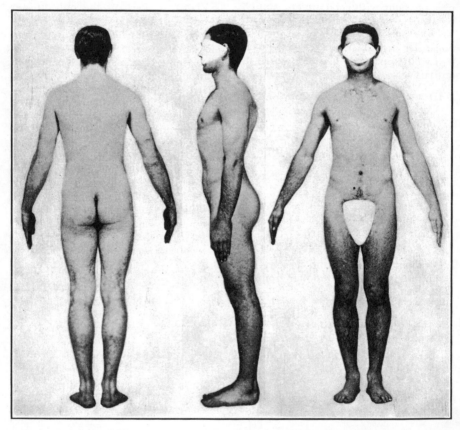

Description: Somatotype 3–5½–2½. An 18-year-old mesomorph three inches above average stature. Strong and harmonious development throughout the physique. Primary g±; secondary g, no trace. Primary t 4 despite a slight kyphosis. Secondary t 2. Features coarse, stubby, ill-defined. Low receding brow. Hands and feet well formed. General and hand strength 4—one of the strongest boys in the series. Coordination excellent. He is an athlete, a first-rate amateur boxer, and a star football player.

Temperament: He is misleading unless you have the habit of looking beyond superficial appearances—beyond the manifest pattern. He looks like a scowly weakling, and he at first seems viscerotonically adaptive to the expressed attitudes of others. Yet underneath he is stubbornly somatotonic and is ready to take long chances. He is primarily interested in adventure and activity, not in adaptation or in viscerotonic satisfactions. To casual observation he seems more viscerotonic than somatotonic. He is misleading in the way that an emasculated tomcat is misleading in the daytime. His supply of latent energy is remarkable. This boy was able to carry on fairly good outward relations at the Inn through the day while spending most of his night trailing around with a tough gang, and was able to do this for long periods without breakdown or apparent fatigue. Temperament: Predominant somatotonia well supported by viscerotonia. The aggression against "society" is overt and viscerotonic, not covert; there is little third component in it. ψ 3–2–1.

Delinquency: Extensive truancy during the first years of school, and persistent stealing during the same period. Numerous court appearances between 10 and 16 for larceny, breaking and entering, use of dangerous weapons, robbery. Between 16 and 19, five appearances for automobile stealing. No record of delinquency of violence although several times caught with weapons, and once caught with a revolver.

Origins and Family: Fourth of four, Irish urban family. The father was a teamster of average physique with a long delinquency record: Drunkenness, assault and battery, idleness and disorderly conduct, desertion. He left the family when this boy was an infant, died of pneumonia and alcoholism at about 40. Mother a truant and "stubborn child" as a girl. She had at least two illegitimate children and was always considered irresponsible. This boy remained with her until 14, then to foster homes under agency management. One sibling died in childhood, one is an epileptic, one has a long record of major delinquency.

Mental History, Achievement: Finished the sixth grade after many failures. IQ reports center at 85 with very slight variation. He gives just about that impression although he has bright blue eyes and there is the feeling that "somehow this boy has good in him and ought to be smarter."

No vocational plans or special abilities. No athletic interests. The AMI is really based on the low t (earthiness) and on obvious need. The boy looks as if he needed a lot. His Irish pug-face is so ugly that it is attractive, especially when the watery blue eyes fix steadily on you.

Medical: Early history unknown. No serious illnesses or injuries of record. Enuretic to age 15 and intermittently at least to 20. PX reveals no significant pathology except poor teeth and flat feet.

Running Record: At first he made a good impression and seemed adaptive. After a time it developed that he had been associating almost every night with one of the most troublesome of Boston's youthful gangs. This was a loose organization of youths specializing in automobile stealing, breaking and entering, jackrolling, robbery of drunks. While the boy was with us the gang manhandled a couple of policemen severely enough to precipitate a general "clean-up" of the gang. It developed that our boy had been a fringer, or persistent hanger-on, for more than a year. Shortly after this episode he began to appear at the Inn in alcoholized condition and we gave up on him, returning him to the referring agency.

During the succeeding half-dozen years he has had a bad time of it. Exempted from military service because of his record, he became more alcoholic and was more frequently involved in robberies. He has spent four of the past five years under detention, is now serving a sentence which will probably extend beyond the publication date of this volume.

Summary: Asthenic mesomorphy with good energy but with enough gynandroid or asthenic interference to incapacitate him for fighting and athletics. Good health except for history of enuresis; dull normal mentality. Persistent delinquency of appropriation.

ID 2-2-3 (7)
Insufficiencies:
    IQ 1
    Mop 1
Psychiatric:
    1st order ....
    2nd order 1
        C-penia (3-2-1)
    C-phobic 1
    G-phrenic ....
Residual D:
    Primary crim. 3

Comment: Outlook considered poor by local authorities. He has grown more alcoholic and with advancing maturity has lost the youthful winsomeness which served him so well in earlier years. He now seems more like a weak and broken-down character. The important point is that he has always been essentially a weak character, perhaps closer to the CPI borderline than to anything that could be called dangerous criminality. With his asthenic and gynandroid complication he had no more business aspiring to make the grade as a tough criminal than he would have trying to make a professional football team. His supply of energy was remarkable but was perhaps also his undoing, for if he had not had it he would perhaps have been more inclined to compromise and adapt, as most of us have to do. In a sense this is a singularly unfortunate youth. Really a weakling and fairly close to the borderline both mentally and physically he yet is considered "normal" by conventional standards. He has therefore been given rather stiff sentences and will in future be treated by the law with comparatively little mercy. If he commits a major crime it will be difficult to make out a case that he was the victim of a psychiatric disorder. Yet he is a victim of constitutional inadequacy as surely as anybody is.

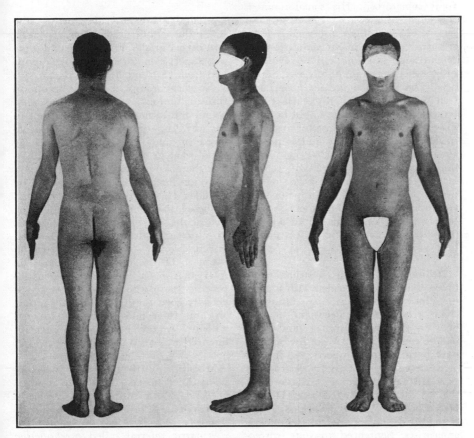

Description: Somatotype 3½-5-2. A 20-year-old slightly asthenic meso-morph of average stature. Arms a little asthenic or underdeveloped, and there is an appearance of general inadequacy which belies the rather hard facial expression. Narrow, scoliotic trunk and flaccid abdominal muscles. Yet this is *almost* a tough physique and it is closer to the golf-ball than to the tennis-ball *habitus*. Primary *g*+1; secondary *g*, no trace. Primary *t* 2, secondary *t* 2. Features pudgy, knobby. He is said to have a "Shanty Irish" look. Nose like a radish. Hands and feet crude and heavy. General strength 3, hand strength 2. Coordination only fair. He walks with a surly lurch. Not good at any kind of athletics or at fighting.

Temperament: This youth is smooth. He is highly somatotonic and full of latent energy but appears relaxed. He is alert and competent. There are no somatorotic energy leaks. He makes no false movements, wastes no energy in vocal somatorosis. His somatotonia is concealed, as are the claws of the cat family. He is ruthless, courageous, loves risk and gambling. No indications of cerebrotonic restraint and no evidence of "conflict" or strain of any sort. Superficially he seems to present a perfectly well-integrated and highly efficient pattern of temperament. It would be most difficult to make out a case for any kind of manifest psychopathy, unless persistent criminality is *in itself* a manifestation of pathological aggression. It may be. The pathology in such a case as this would then be both cerebropenic and visceropenic, but at a rather abstract level. ψ 3–2–1, and quite frankly a guess. (Possibly the psychiatric index should be 1–1–1.)

Delinquency: Persistent truancy between 6 and 10. Associated with a gang in minor stealing at 10. "Stubborn child" record at 12. Persistent stealing between 12 and 15. Robbery and automobile stealing at 16. All of his offenses have been against property. No history of violence or of wanton destructiveness. His has been gentle predation like that of the silent-winged owls. He has always been an insider with a gang, has been called "the brains" of delinquent enterprises. Sentenced to state correctional school at 14 and 16.

Origins and Family: Eighth of eleven, urban family, Scotch-Irish on both sides. Father a ne'er-do-well, alcoholic, with a long history of minor delinquency. Several paternal relatives delinquent and at least three are mentally defective. Mother a heavy woman of Scotch-Irish stock and described as "of good intent but ineffectual." She held the family together with much agency help until she weakened in her early forties and died of cancer, when our boy was 14. The father then drifted away from the family. Boy transferred to foster homes. Six of the siblings have records of delinquency. None is known to be feebleminded.

Mental History, Achievement: Finished the eighth grade after repeating two earlier grades. Frequently under police supervision for truancy. IQ reports run from 78 to 99, here called 90.

No vocational plan. He has an opportunistic outlook, expects to take what comes and to make the best of it but in *his* way. He regards himself as a privileged predator, not as a criminal. He takes what he wants where he finds it, and thereby receives the plaudits of possibly the majority of those in whom he confides. He is proud of clever stealing, of being the brains behind the scene, and of the fact that he has been caught only a comparatively few times. To steal is praiseworthy—all business is stealing—but to be caught is regrettable. The AMI that of a poised, competent-appearing youth who makes almost a universally good impression. Official report on him from one of the correctional schools: "A good boy who has been influenced by bad companions."

Medical: Birth and early development called normal. No serious illnesses or injuries. An entirely negative medical history. PX reveals no significant pathology. This is a healthy youth. On psychiatric referral called *psychopathic personality, with criminal trend,* which is possibly misleading.

Running Record: During a short stay at the Inn he demonstrated an urbane sophistication and a kind of friendly alertness. In the House he was inscrutable, quiet, and elusive. There were no complaints against him. Most of the staff agreed that he would be a good risk for the school program. However, two are needed to make a bargain and he had the same love of school that a cat has of water. In the end we had a complimentary opinion of his capacities and abilities but also felt a frustrating sense of lack of equipment with which to reach him.

Too young for military service during the war, he has now spent another three years in his gentlemanly predatory pattern. Within a year after leaving us he was arrested for breaking and entering and for larceny, was returned to a state correctional school. During the following year he married but was soon in court again on charges of stealing. A number of starts at jobs were abortive. A few months prior to the present writing he was inducted into military service. Many who know him regret that this experiment was not tried earlier.

Summary: Well-poised mesomorphy with high-grade athletic ability and excellent health. Mentality within the normal range. No indications of first-order psychopathy. Persistent good-natured stealing.

ID o–o–4 (4)
Insufficiencies:
  IQ ....
  Mop ....

Psychiatric:
  1st order ....
  2nd order .... (?)
  (3–2–1)
  C-phobic ....
  G-phrenic ....
Residual D:
  Primary crim. 4

Comment: The outlook is likely to be good. The military institution may succeed where others have seemed to fail. Although this youth has been more or less surrounded by defective and delinquent people, in both the hereditary and the environmental sense, he himself *appears* to present a pattern of essential strength and competence. Several social workers from different agencies have indicated that he is the star of his family. He is at any rate not grossly defective, or in any overt sense insufficient, and he presents no signs of serious psychopathy. If his identification with delinquency should prove persistent in adult life, so that he becomes a "hardened criminal," this may have to be called "idiopathic" criminality. Idiopathic is a term sometimes used by the medical profession in tacit apology for ignorance concerning the nature of a malady.

189. COMPANY B, PLATOON 2
Primary Criminality: Nos. 185–200

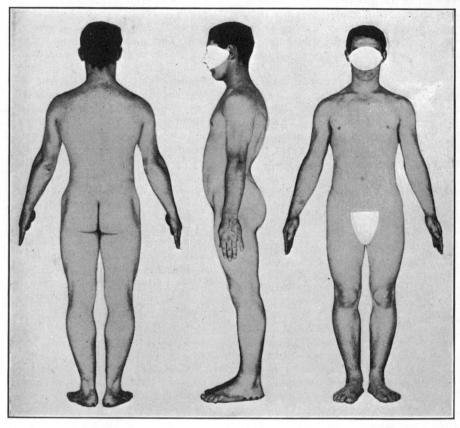

Description: Somatotype 3–6½–1. A 16-year-old extreme mesomorph an inch above average stature. Powerful, well-knit physique with no gross dysplasias or weaknesses. A slightly lordotic posture. Full mesomorphic development throughout, with a generous endowment of latent endomorphy. Legs especially powerful. A fighter's physique. Primary and secondary g±. Primary t 4, secondary t 3. Features strongly and evenly developed but coarsely shaped. He has an alert, brilliant eye. General strength 5, hand strength 4. Coordination superb. With a panther-like smoothness of movement he is fast and efficient. Good at athletic games and a terrific fighter.

Temperament: He is somatotonic but it is well-sustained and unhurried somatotonia. There are no indications of psychopathy, other than persistent criminality. He is always up to something but has a bland smile, is smoothly if not delightfully mendacious; lies purposefully and to the point. He is strongly identified with a delinquent outlook and with a program of unrestrained sexual expression. He is direct and ruthless, but rather graciously and relaxedly so; gives no indication of inner conflict; no signs of strain. He does not agglutinate with any group. There is just a trace of gynandrophrenic unctuousness in his speech and behavior, but he is not essentially gynandroid and is well removed from the *DAMP RAT* syndrome. ψ 3–2–1. Same comment as for No. 189.

Delinquency: Truancy began at 7. Sent to correctional school because of truancy at 11. Larceny and breaking and entering at 12, and intermittently until 20. Sent or returned to correctional schools fifteen times between 14 and 18 for larceny, breaking and entering, and automobile stealing. Armed robbery at 17. Between 14 and 20 about thirty instances of known larceny, breaking and entering, or robbery. Finally sent to state prison at 20. Never guilty of violence against a person or of wanton destructiveness. Merely a persistent thief with secondary police attention growing out of sexual offenses—too vigorous a wooing of young girls.

Origins and Family: Third of six, urban family, both parents immigrant Poles. Father of average physique, described as "hard drinking, cunning and sly with social agencies." He has several court appearances for drunkenness. Mother short and heavy, called "emotional, greedy, exploitative." She has no delinquency record. Boy reared in the home until transferred to correctional schools. Two of the other siblings have court records.

Mental History, Achievement: Finished the eighth grade after some failures which resulted from truancy. The last three grades were achieved at correctional schools. He failed badly at mathematics. IQ reports range from 88 to 106, here called 95. He gives the impression of a certain alertness and practicality of mind without the elements of intellectuality. He is well oriented to reality and has a good eye to the main chance.

No vocational plan and no special abilities. The AMI that of a well-spoken youth with good social address and a steady "honest" eye. He looks a little as if he ought to be a seminary student, and there is just the faintest fragrance of gynandrophrenia about him.

Medical: Infancy history not available. No record of serious illnesses or injuries. PX reveals no significant pathology except carious teeth.

Running Record: At the Inn he was something of a "smoothy" and was regarded as an enigma. Numerous efforts were made to break through his well-polished defense but none was very successful. We felt in the end that he knew us better than we did him. A psychiatrist to whom he was referred wrote, "I cannot quite make out this boy." That he carried on delinquent activities while with us we and the police strongly suspected but he was not caught. Two psychiatric referrals brought the diagnoses: *primary behavior disorder,* and *psychoneurosis, paranoid trend.* We saw little that was paranoid or psychoneurotic in him. On the work program in the House he was efficient and on rare occasions cooperative but generally was able to meet the situation by some smooth evasion. We did not try him on outside jobs or on a training program. Indeed we had the feeling that we never did quite catch up with him at all in any fundamental sense. He was an elusive character. Shortly following his sojourn with us he was inducted into military service.

He stayed in for about three years, was finally given a medical discharge after a good deal of hospitalization. Meanwhile he got married and started a family. In civilian life for more than a year now he remains vague about any general plans but has kept out of serious trouble and has worked for several months. In some quarters he is more darkly suspect than ever.

Summary: Endomorphic mesomorphy with asthenic chest and arms. Mentality about average. Excellent health. Somewhat gynandroid but no indications of psychoneurotic difficulties. Vigorous stealing to which the military experience *may* have brought an abrupt end.

ID 0–1–4 (5)
  Insufficiencies:
    IQ . . . .
    Mop . . . .
  Psychiatric:
    1st order . . . .
    2nd order . . . .   (?)
      (3–2–1)
    C-phobic . . . .
    G-phrenic   1
  Residual D:
    Primary crim. . . . .   4(?)

Comment: Outlook probably good but this is a puzzling youth and any predictions concerning him need still to be guarded. From a constitutional point of view he seems to have almost a clean slate. Perhaps the asthenic weakness of the chest and arms could be regarded as a physiological insufficiency and as contributive to some kind of internal conflict or frustration but if we start out on that road any physical characteristic short of a perfect 1–7–1 physique might be so regarded (during a period when mesomorphic values and objectives are in the ascendancy). To fall short of mesomorphic perfection does not yet entitle one to a license to steal even in a New Deal democracy. The gynandroid problem may be associated with the boy's criminalistic motivation but to use such a concept as an "explanation" is too simple and too easy. Probably twelve million American males carry around that degree of gynandromorphy without accumulating charges of larceny on their records. In some way which I do not pretend to understand, the youth is "slippery." He plays a double hand and carries more cards in it than "poor unfortunate boys" are generally supposed to carry. Maybe this is feminine circumvention arising from gynandrophrenia in just this particular pattern of personality. But I still have an uneasy sense of ignorance of the motivation of criminality. This problem seems to be about as complex as that of personality in general and I am afraid that in order to define *a criminal* it will first be necessary to standardize and to master a descriptive psychology—and then to use it for a few generations until it works as smoothly as, let us say, the language of automobile mechanics now works. This is going to be an arduous undertaking, for many psychologists will for a long time prefer to ride their horses.

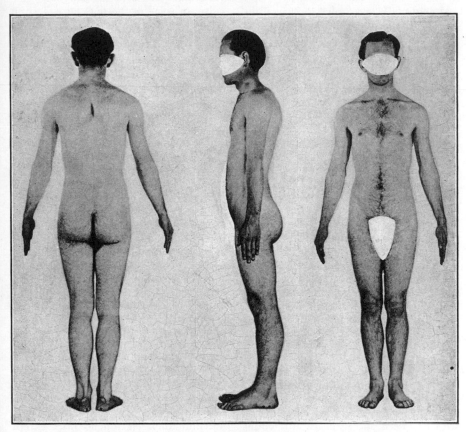

Description: Somatotype 4–4½–3. A 20-year-old endomorphic mesomorph two inches above average stature. Asthenic chest and arms; peculiarly long, narrow trunk; heavy legs; massive head, with dysplastically
mesomorphic neck and facial structure. If the head and neck can be taken
as developmentally comparable to the keel of a ship it would seem that the
Potter started this one with valiant mesomorphy in mind. Primary $g+1$, secondary $g\pm$. Primary t 2, secondary t 3. Features a little coarse but well
formed and symmetrical. Wide, level eyes; broad forehead. Fine hands. The
boy has been called handsome. General strength 3, hand strength 3. He is
not quite well coordinated; might be called ungraceful without being
clumsy. He lacks both the feminine lightness of the well-coordinated gynandromorphs, and the feline or equine bodily sureness of the mesomorphic
athletes. Yet he is no weakling. Unable to fight effectively and not good at
games, he is a good runner; has led police on many a merry chase.

Temperament: Somatotonia predominates manifestly and constantly. He is extraordinarily aggressive, occupies the center of attention wherever he may be; is noisy, extraverted, unrestrained. The extraversion is both viscerotonic and somatotonic. His broad grin is contagious and his indiscriminate amiability tends to break whatever ice other people's cerebrotonia may have frozen into the social picture. He has good orientation to people, appears to know "by instinct" who are the easy ones from whom he can get what he wants. The temperamental pattern is Italian-Dionysian with a paranoid undercurrent, but there are no indications of any first-order psychopathy. ψ 4–2–1.

Delinquency: Early and continued history of persistent stealing. Chronic runaway and truant. Sentenced to state correctional school at 13 as a "stubborn child." Returned many times; an enterprising runaway from correctional schools. Twice arrested for carrying a dangerous weapon although never known to use it.

Origins and Family: Born extramaritally of immigrant Italian parents who later married and produced six more. Father a large, vigorous mesomorph who has been successful in this country; now moderately prosperous and violent-tempered. Mother of short, heavy physique, long in close contact with social agencies and regarded as mendacious or tricky but not legally delinquent. The boy was born when his mother was 14, was sent to Italy at 4 to live with relatives, remained there until 12, and then returned to the family in this country.

Mental History, Achievement: The only schooling here has been in ungraded classes. He has a language difficulty although he spoke English before being sent to Italy and now speaks it fairly well. IQ reports vary from 60 to 102 and this is perhaps a legitimate variation because of the language difficulty. In some of the tests he was given credit for what he "would have known" under normal conditions. Here we put his IQ at 90.

No vocational plan. Outlook one of sustained Dionysian incorrigibility. The AMI that of impish or vigorous mischievousness. He will take nothing seriously, has been babied and overcaseworked, is a great favorite with social workers. When we first knew him he was in contact with five different agencies, playing off one against another.

Medical: Early medical history not known. Between 12 and 16 he was referred to medical clinics about thirty times for many sorts of complaints, principally eye trouble (congenitally defective vision), infections, refusal to eat American food, and abdominal and many somatic pains. No significant pathology was found other than visual. Several psychiatric referrals yielded the usual echolalial diagnoses. PX reveals only flat feet and hyperhidrosis.

Running Record: Here he behaved liked a growing but unbroken puppy. Consistently good natured, unrestrainedly Dionysian, mendacious, a smart and watchful thief. He did no work except when forced to do so, promptly abandoned each job undertaken. Two attempts at a school program were merely wasted time. With the passage of a year he seemed to grow harder and sharper, more mercenary, or more calculatively exploitative. Also he grew heavier and healthier in appearance. Somatic complaints were endless. Because of the history of "interrupted childhood" social workers buzzed around him like bluebottle flies. Possibly he was a little spoiled.

Exempt from military service on psychiatric grounds, he has continued for another half-dozen years in the pattern of good-natured irresponsibility with frequent episodes of stealing. He has now grown much larger and heavier, seems physically prosperous, but still prefers "rackets" to any sort of secure or legalized way of living. A few months before the present writing he visited his parents, stayed a couple of weeks, then "cleaned them out—stole everything movable," and disappeared. A month later he joined the Merchant Marine but got lost or deserted at the first port.

Summary: Heavy, gnarled mesomorphy with good strength but poor coordination. Normal subaverage mentality. Visual insufficiency. He is Dionysian but seemingly free from serious psychopathy. A persistently delinquent or exploitative outlook.

ID 1–0–4 (5)
Insufficiencies:
   IQ . . . .
   Mop 1
Psychiatric:
   1st order . . . .
   2nd order . . . . (?)
    (4–2–1)
   C-phobic . . . .
   G-phrenic . . . .

Residual D:
   Primary crim. 4

Comment: Prognosis good and bad. For the boy, perhaps good; for society, probably bad. An essentially healthy and vigorous youth who seems to be having a good time, he is long accustomed to irresponsible exploitation as a way of life. He would like to have a large family of children and to have them reared by Boston social agencies. At least so he says and from the present perspective that looks like a fairly likely outcome. To blame him would be to blame a puppy for eating frankfurters off the floor.

He has been referred to many psychiatric clinics and has been given numerous diagnoses. Yet from what I have seen of him there is no indication of attentional or psychotic disorder. A military draft board rejected him on the ground of *psychopathic personality* but the boy put on an act for that. He perhaps does have some physiological insufficiency in addition to the defective vision but possibly no more of such insufficiency than we all carry around.

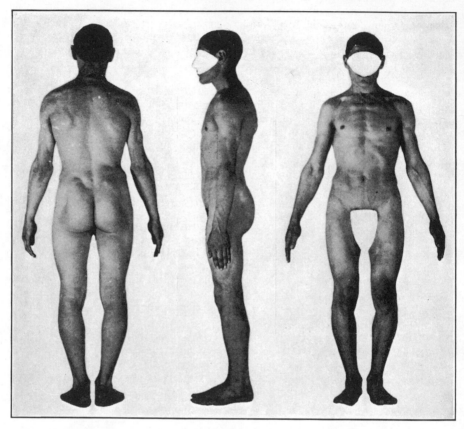

Description: Somatotype 2½–5½–2. A 16-year-old Italian mesomorph of average stature. Heavy bones, gnarled or scruboak mesomorphy—a kind of physique which in later life becomes very heavy. Short thick neck, bunchy muscles, and a certain hard lumpiness throughout the body. Legs strong and well developed, as is the trunk. Arms imperfectly developed with a trace of the "arrested" characteristic. Primary and secondary $g\pm$. Primary and secondary t 2. Features coarse, irregularly shaped, hands and feet crude. General strength 4, hand strength 3. Coordination poor. He moves with a peasant-like heaviness, seems incapable of delicate muscular adjustment. Incompetent at all games and unable to fight although strong and vigorously energetic.

Temperament: He is viscerotonically somatotonic, and well sustained in the pattern. Aggressive, pushy, he is always in the forefront of what is going on and is well oriented to people. No discernible cerebrotonic interference. He is sociable; happiest where the crowd is thickest and noisiest. Immediate adaptation: usually good. Long-run picture: apparently both Dionysian and paranoid. He has the gambler's *persona*. ψ 4–2–1.

Delinquency: Early truancy and unmanageability in school and at home. Persistent minor stealing between 8 and 14. Involved in gambling of one sort or another since early childhood. Sent to state correctional school at 12 and at 14 as incorrigible.

Origins and Family: Sixth of eight, urban Jewish family, both parents immigrant from eastern Europe. The father has a long history of agency contacts and is considered of borderline mentality but not actively delinquent. Called a "low grade exploiter." Mother short and very heavy. She has a history of violence, quarreling with neighbors, fighting with her children, "flying into rages during court sessions," and so on. Arrested several times on morals charges. Boy lived at home until 12, then sent to correctional school. At least two of the siblings are mentally defective.

Mental History, Achievement: Completed the fourth grade, then became uncontrollable in school and quit. IQ reports cluster between 72 and 82, here called 80. He was several times considered for commitment at one of the schools for the mentally retarded but was never sent. He gives an impression of better mental alertness than is indicated by the IQ, thinks school is impractical, has never learned to write but is good at arithmetic and at keeping track of sums. As one watches and interviews this boy the impression grows that the recorded IQ does not quite fairly tap his mental resources. He is cunning, energetic, and in a sense smart and competent.

His interests are centered on gambling and he has a definite vocational plan to live by what he calls rackets, particularly the "slot machine, juke box, and taxicab rackets." The AMI that of a bright, alert youth who knows how to "pour it on" to the social workers about his rejections, sibling rivalries, and intrafamilial warfare.

Medical: Apparently a healthy and vigorous infant, very active from infancy but with a long history of minor complaints having to do principally with upper respiratory infections. PX reveals no significant pathology except poor teeth. He has a remarkable hyperflexibility of all joints—a gynandroid characteristic commonly encountered in Jewish males.

Running Record: In and out of the Inn intermittently for two years, he showed social intelligence in his ability to sell himself to members of the staff and also a certain business acumen or acquisitive intelligence in his relations to other boys. Of more sustained physical energy than perhaps anyone else at the Inn, he always had irons in the fire and something going on. He had a passion for gambling tricks, for trading, for employing other boys at shoe-shining and so on. We of the staff liked him, in a way, and I do not altogether know the reason why. Possibly it was because of his enormous energy combined with a total absence of physical combativeness. While he was aggressive in the highest degree there was in him no threat of physical danger. He couldn't fight; he and everyone else knew that and even the most vicious of our bullies seemed therefore to respect his physical "neutrality." He would walk among tough Irish fighters capable of tearing him to pieces as wolves can tear a pig, and would shout them down with sheer vocal somatorosis without a blow being struck on either side although the rafters might shiver with reverberations from the encounter. He could openly cheat these same toughs at gambling and could somehow seem to make them take it. We twice started him on a school program, both times abortively, also got him several outside jobs but he never held a job for more than a week or so. At the end of our contact with him he seemed fairly prosperous. He had several rackets going but we knew we had not converted him to anything.

During the succeeding several years this youth has continued in essentially the same pattern. Three times he came to police attention through gambling charges, once on a dangerous weapon charge. Recently he was caught by federal authorities in a kidnapping enterprise which went awry. He has risen at least to noncom status in the professional criminal ranks of the city.

Summary: Vigorous endomorphic mesomorph with no fighting ability. Mentality above borderline; good health. No indication of first-order psychopathy. Persistent primary criminality.

ID 1–1–4 (6)
  Insufficiencies:
    IQ 1
    Mop ....
  Psychiatric:
    1st order ....
    2nd order .... (?)
      (4–2–1)
    C-phobic ....
    G-phrenic 1
  Residual D:
    Primary crim. 4

Comment: The outlook is regarded as dubious. In official circles he is beginning to be looked upon as a confirmed criminal. At the Inn he gave an impression of really having himself better in hand than the record would indicate. This is a kind of case where the Freudian system of explanation of misbehavior seems plausible, and may be sound. One generalization concerning Jews seems to be safe. They are as a rule highly energized people, overly somatotonic but not good at physical combat. They tend to get into the most astonishing intrafamilial entanglements and the resultant wrangling often results in prolonged warfare. Lacking physical combativity they lack effective means for settling or *ending* disputes. So jealousies smoulder and emotional attachments and aversions tend to develop into chronic mental abscesses. Among Jews both sexes are more gynandroid than in any other breed with which I am familiar. The two sexes are closer together, physically and temperamentally, and therefore sexuality may tend to be forgotten at times and then rediscovered anew—with attendant religious excitement.

In a case like this boy's it is entirely possible that the usual Freudian explanation makes sense. Early bad conditioning and hate associated with (the usual) familial mess may offer "a primary reason" for the later criminality—this of course in association with the ψ 4–1–1 temperament. At any rate the history as we have it does not seem to offer a simpler or more plausible explanation unless you care to fall back on the even lazier idea of an "instinct of criminality."

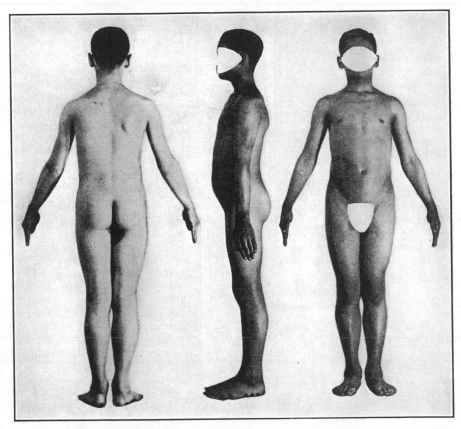

Description: Somatotype 4–5–1½. A 15-year-old immature endomorphic mesomorph two inches under average stature. A compact, vigorous, highly energized physique which in a few years will be hefty and barrel-bodied. No noticeable dysplasia. The arm segments are not yet fully developed. Primary *g*+1, secondary *g*+1. Primary *t* 3, secondary *t* 2. Features coarse, prominent. General strength 3, hand strength 2. Coordination excellent. A well-poised, self-sufficient physical personality. Movement is smooth and integrated. He shows a generalized feminoid softness. Inept at athletics. A good swimmer but unable to fight.

Temperament: Well-sustained hostile somatotonia evenly expressed, with no trace of epileptoid variation in temper. No straining in the somatotonic role. He is relaxed, poised. The body is always effectively alert, erect in posture, ready for action. He has great energy, requires little sleep—never sleeps more than six hours a night. He loves physical adventure and dangerous risk above all things, says he gets more kick out of a "job" when cops are in the neighborhood. He is direct, bland, well met and usually well dressed. No sign of cerebrotonic restraint or of somatorotic straining. Excellent example of extraversional (first psychiatric component) aggression. ψ 3–2–1.

Delinquency: Almost constant early truancy, a frequent runaway before 10. Persistent early stealing. Many charges of larceny between 8 and 12. Sent to state correctional school at 11 and during the succeeding eight years made his home intermittently at these institutions. Between 15 and 19. numerous arrests for larceny, gang association, unnatural sex practices. Long-standing general identification with criminality. At 19, armed robbery.

Origins and Family: Fourth of five, urban family. Father of English descent and a wiry, muscular millworker who has always been moderately alcoholic but is considered reputable. He has ulcers. Mother Portuguese. She was a delinquent before marriage, deserted when this boy was about 5. Boy reared in the home until 11, thereafter almost entirely in correctional schools. Three of the siblings have been involved in some kind of delinquency of record.

Mental History, Achievement: Quit school in the fourth grade but credited with finishing that grade at correctional schools. IQ reports fall between 70 and 80, here put at 73. Because of mesomorphic poise he gives a first impression of

better intelligence but the good impression is not sustained.

No vocational plan. He is an accomplished athlete. From early childhood he has been a fighter of note and at 18 and 19 did some professional boxing, but he lacks the legs for first-flight competition. The AMI that of a sturdy youth who is parsimonious of speech but with proper encouragement can recite enough of the catechism to get a hearing at the average agency.

Medical: Large baby, apparently normal early development. No serious illnesses or injuries and no history of temper tantrums. An entirely negative medical background. PX reveals no significant pathology except high blood pressure.

Running Record: At the Inn he was a moronophile, surrounding himself with the more mesomorphic of the feebleminded and agglutinating with the most delinquent group. In his relations with the staff he was smooth. He always spoke calmly and deliberately, gave the impression of sophistication. He took none of us into his confidence but managed to give some the impression that he was a reformed youth and something of an envoy for the side of the angels in the other camp. However, within two or three months it developed that he had meanwhile been engaged in a series of well-planned robberies and had influenced other youngsters to participate. He was apprehended in an armed holdup and was returned to one of the correctional schools after having rather adroitly led a double life while with us.

Exempt from military service because of the record, he has for another six years continued in essentially the same pattern as before. He was employed at several defense jobs during the war but always quit after a few months. On at least two occasions was in trouble with police because of rackets associated with labor agitation. Meanwhile he has repeatedly been detained for short periods in consequence of persistent automobile stealing.

Summary: A powerful mesomorphic physique with nearly first-rate athletic ability. Borderline mentality; excellent health. No indications of first-order psychopathy. Persistent criminality.

ID 2–0–4 (6)
  Insufficiencies:
    IQ 2
    Mop . . . .
  Psychiatric:
    1st order . . . .
    2nd order . . . . (?)
      (3–2–1)
    C-phobic . . . .
    G-phrenic . . . .
  Residual D:
    Primary crim. 4

Comment: The outlook ought to be good on constitutional grounds but probably is not. We can unearth no evidence of psychopathy that would "explain" the delinquency. But delinquent he is and to a fairly high degree. I have an idea that he represents the sort of personality which, with a higher IQ, often develops into a first-rate and successful criminal. I have met and interviewed a few such men. They often had his manner and they tended to look like him. Unfortunately this class is but poorly represented in the present series and the boys who do give promise of first-rate criminal attainment are still too young to have arrived at their full professional stature. To complete a proper study of delinquency a couple of hundred top-flight criminals who are *not* easily apprehended and have *not* been babied or overcaseworked ought to be included. But that will be another book for somebody to write.

Our category of primary criminality leaves much to be desired. To give this youth a weight of 4 in that category is merely to say, (1) that he is far more delinquent than could be predicted from manifest insufficiency or psychopathy, and (2) that the delinquency has not been a transitory episode but has been persistent and seems to stem from some persistent *desire* to be delinquent. We here run into the problems of will and moral responsibility, but the aim of the present study is only to accomplish a clearer delineation or definition of these problems.

Too bad the army rejected this boy. That might have been a good experiment and he might have made a first-rate soldier. Compare this case with No. 187.

193. COMPANY B, PLATOON 2
Primary Criminality: Nos. 185–200

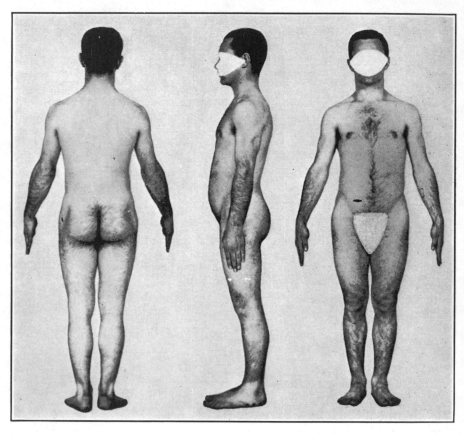

Description: Somatotype 4–5½–1½. A 19-year-old endomorphic meso-morph an inch under average stature. Solid, compact athletic physique ex-cept for a slight failure of full mesomorphic development in the distal seg-ments of arms and legs. Primary $g+1$; secondary g, no trace. Primary t 3, secondary t 3. Features a little coarse but strong and evenly formed. General strength 4, hand strength 3. Excellent athletic coordination. The entire body seems to function as a single muscle. He moves with a catlike grace sugges-tive of reserve power. A good boxer and basketball player, he loves the gym-nasium.

Temperament: He has a gunpowder-like touchiness, violently explosive temper. Somatotonic, loud and aggressive, he walks about like a schoolboy with a chip on his shoulder; seems insatiable in his thirst for violent altercation, yet manifests no gratitude to the altercator. This is not the epileptoid pattern. There is nothing rhythmic about his explosions and the latter seem to be natural expressions of his personality, not periodic tantrums. He is physically relaxed but in a poised, athletic sense—not in the armchair sense. Relaxed like a cat on the prowl, not like one sleeping in the noonday shade. He has three passions —for gambling, for white girls, and for suppressing the "arrogant white race." Psychiatrists have called him paranoid but the aggression is more overt than covert. ψ 4–3–1.

Delinquency: Under police surveillance at the age of 5 for destructiveness and window smashing. General uncontrollability between 6 and 12. At state correctional schools about half the time between 12 and 18 for stealing, breaking and entering, lewdness, destruction of property, jackrolling, possession of dangerous weapons, assault and battery, burglary.

Origins and Family: Fifth of eight in a highly delinquent urban family. Father in and out of correctional and penal institutions most of his life; killed in a brawl when this boy was 4. He was a powerful full-blooded Negro. Mother a mulatto, considered feebleminded and easily led; long record of delinquency and disorderly conduct. She died in her thirties of an unnamed "central nervous system infection" when the boy was 12. All other siblings mentally retarded; five have delinquent records.

Mental History, Achievement: Finished no grades in public school but completed about the equivalent of a fifth-grade education at correctional schools. IQ reports range from 76 to 90, here put at 85. He is not feebleminded but is alert, opportunistic, in some respects competent at seeking what he wants. Particularly efficacious in his pursuit of girls. Very popular with a coterie of semidelinquent teen-age white girls.

No vocational plans; gifted in music. He has what is known as hot rhythm. Considered one of the best young drummers around the city, a tireless piano player and an unofficial champion at hot or somatorotic dancing. The AMI that of superabundant energy, competent pugnacity, and healthy mesomorphy.

Medical: No early data. No record of serious illnesses or injuries. Childhood rickets probably accounts for the leg bowing and possibly for the narrowing of the lower part of the thoracic cage. He seems to have enjoyed almost perfect health. On psychiatric referral called *psychopathic personality, paranoid trend.*

Running Record: Through two years the Inn maintained an interest in this boy and tried him on virtually every program that was offered. Meanwhile a nearly continuous effort was made by other agencies to cajole or decoy him into the pleasant pastures of middle class morality. He proved more than equal to all these efforts. In the House he was a vicious influence, strove to organize gang warfare, roamed at night with a predatory and destructive Negro gang. They preyed on drunks, had a joyous trick of decoying, and beating and robbing sexually intoxicated whites who were seeking sexual adventure or education in the Negro quarter. School programs, conferences, participation in activities, camp, and attempts at vocational training all seemed equally ineffective in reaching this youngster. He merely made use of such facilities as the Inn offered and it was he who seemed really to possess the upper hand in the situation. He said: "Nobody's ever going to punish me. All they can do is lock me up and feed me good."

For another half-dozen years he has continued in about the same pattern. Exempt from military service because of his record, he has spent about half of the intervening time under detention, usually for robbery or holdup, once for "assault with intent to kill." When not in jail he still lives mainly off social agencies but does so with a kind of friendly assurance which so often renders vigorous mesomorphs immune to resentment.

Summary: Highly energized mesomorphy with good athletic and fighting ability. High health; dull normal mentality; somatorotic temperament. Long history of violence and of the delinquency of predatory appropriation.

ID 1–2–4 (7)
Insufficiencies:
  IQ 1
  Mop ....
Psychiatric:
  1st order ....
  2nd order 2
    Somatorotic (4–3–1)
  C-phobic ....
  G-phrenic ....
Residual D:
  Primary crim. 4

Comment: Outlook generally considered dubious. For more than a decade now he has spent a good half of his time under detention and is just about as loyal to the predatory outlook as some other youths have been to their *alma mater*. Such a case challenges the conventional mental stereotype of delinquency as an expression of weakness. Mentally and physically competent, he seems to be strong enough—constitutionally rugged enough—to absorb such punishment as the environment offers and to continue resolutely on his delinquent course. From his point of view the outlook may be good. He remains true to his ideals in quite a one-minded way, enjoys himself, has a fairly large following of female admirers both white and black, gets plenty to eat. He is something of a hero in his circle, as fighting mesomorphs usually are, and he may find it possible to carry on his way of life without radical change for some time to come. Almost certainly he will be involved in further delinquency. Already a score or so of social agencies have spent hundreds of casework hours and many thousands of dollars on him and on his immediate family. None of this ammunition seems to reach him. His fortifications appear to be impenetrable. One of our staff calls him a case of *le grand paranoia*.

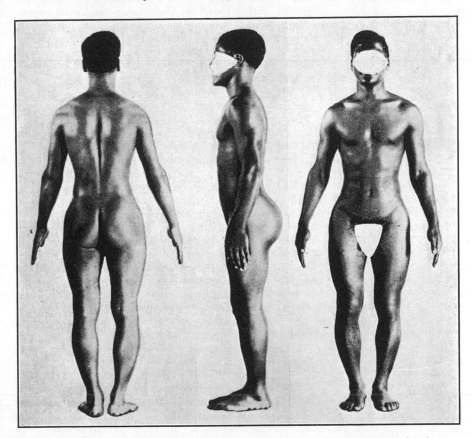

Description: Somatotype 2½–5½–2. An 18-year-old Negro youth of average stature and of almost extreme mesomorphy. Compact, muscular, with long trunk and short powerful legs. He has an odd narrowing of the central trunk with a high waist. The common Negroid (Nilotic) brittleness or ectomorphic interference in the arms and legs is absent. He stems from the heavier West Coast Negro stock. Hips peculiarly wide although not gynandroid —he is hard like black walnut. Shoulders and chest broad. Primary g±, secondary g, no trace. Primary t 3, secondary t 2. Features broad and sprawling. General and hand strength 4—a very powerful boy. Coordination excellent. He moves with tiger-like suppleness, is an adroit wrestler, can jump five or six feet sideways without effort. He is a good sprinter but has had little interest in organized athletics.

Temperament: He gives somewhat the impression of a lazy or endomorphic tomcat in the sun. A smooth personality without somatorosis. He seems overly relaxed until he moves or speaks. Self possession and balance are then conspicuous. The voice is richly resonant. He is predominantly somatotonic with no straining in the role and no waste motion. Readiness for action lurks immediately beneath a placidly disarming exterior. No overt trace of cerebrotonic or paranoid tension. He seems years older than he is. In the lobby or on the athletic floor he was often taken for the Director. ψ 3-2-1.

Delinquency: Early history of persistent stealing, between 10 and 14. No record of early school history available (alias difficulties and origins in a distant state). Numerous charges of stealing at 14 and 15, when he was "disowned" by his parents as incorrigible. Sent to correctional school at 15, promptly ran away, and was then more or less of a tramp or drifter for the succeeding four years. Numerous difficulties with police during this period on account of vagrancy and minor stealing. Meanwhile he developed high-grade symbiotic parasitism with social agencies.

Origins and Family: First of two, rural family. Father called Irish-German, said to have been a respectable average citizen of marginal economic status who had "many medical problems." Mother not described but said to have been of the same stock. The parents separated and disappeared after this boy left. No trace of them can be found. The other sibling has a delinquent history. On this family we have only indirect and scanty information.

Mental History, Achievement: Quit in the first year of high school with a poor record. IQ reports fall between 86 and 95, here put at 90. Like most well-poised mesomorphs he at first seems more intelligent than the IQ indicates, and perhaps he is.

No vocational plan or ambition except that of avoiding work. The AMI is based on remarkable candor of expression and objective directness of address. His gift is that of natural salesmanship. His whole personality gives off sincerity as a ripe cheese gives off fragrance.

Medical: No early data. As a child he had many infections, was three times hospitalized with pneumonia between 2 and 6. Two operations for hernial repair. Much trouble with teeth—caries and abscesses. PX reveals extremely flat feet, moderately high blood pressure, and an edematous puffiness about the eyes which might indicate renal or cardiac pathology.

Running Record The enduring memory this boy left at the Inn was that of the smooth mendacity with which he presented his case and took us in. His unquestionable sincerity quickly won him a room here and a place on the school program. He had wonderful viscerotonic extraversion. His words were resonant with earnestness. He transfixed the listener with a steady stare which could not be evaded, and with the hard consonants he tended to vaporize the latter a little, as if to keep his attention pointed. These are sure signs of sincerity and trustworthiness, as you will find on consulting any first-rate treatise on business psychology.

He told such a convincing story of an urge for better things that he was started successively on programs of high school education, vocational training, job placement, and development of athletic ability. In each instance he dropped out within a week or was caught at some kind of theft. The Inn was stubbornly persistent in its effort to find something good in this youth, for we thought we saw at least potential "business ability" in him, but after a year we were convinced that he had the best of us. He had developed a sort of *persona* of professional leg pulling, seemed to think of himself as a sleek tomcat and of the social agencies as his own private mousoria. One thing about him pleased us. His superb relaxation was misleading to more than one of the bullying mesomorphs who made up our company. To the unobservant or unwary he seemed an easygoing youth with whom all sorts of liberties could be taken. But when he went into pugilistic action he did so with an initial and usually terminal ferocity which was most educational.

Caught several times at thievery during the year following his stay with us, he was finally inducted into military service. There he was in frequent difficulty and within a few months after psychiatric discharge was in jail again for stealing. We have no direct report on his military career but an agency reports that he was repeatedly AWOL and spent much of his military time under penal detention. He is beginning to be regarded as a confirmed delinquent.

Summary: Beautifully poised feloid or catlike mesomorphy with good athletic and fighting ability. Mentality normal; several traces of physiological insufficiency. No indications of a disturbing psychopathy. Persistent appropriative delinquency.

ID 2-0-5 (7)
Insufficiencies:
IQ ....

Mop 2
Psychiatric:
1st order ....
2nd order .... (?)
(3-2-1)
C-phobic ....
G-phrenic ....
Residual D:
Primary crim. 5

Comment: Prognosis dubious. For ten years he has lived an essentially delinquent pattern of life. Yet there are some things in his favor. So far as we know his delinquency has been confined to stealing and to failure to live up to responsibilities and expectations. There is no record of violence or destructiveness and none of alcoholism. He does not seem to have deteriorated in any measurable way and he seems to maintain good control of himself. There is really no indication of psychopathy unless the criminality is *ipse facto* a psychopathic indication—in which case criminology and possibly business and politics are merely minor psychiatric subheadings. Such a person might conceivably "change his mind" about stealing and exploiting, just as Southern Democrats have been known even in midlife to begin suddenly to vote Republican. The best point in his favor may be his health. With high blood pressure and with a faint early indication of cardiorenal insufficiency he may presently find himself in a position where getting religion will be easy.

195. COMPANY B, PLATOON 2
Primary Criminality: Nos. 185–200

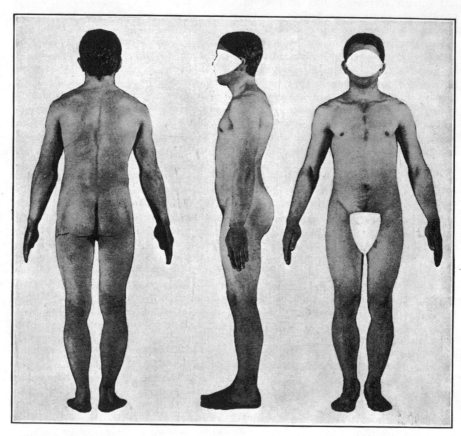

Description: Somatotype 4–5½–1. A 19-year-old endomorphic meso-morph an inch under average stature. Very compact physique, well buffered with endomorphy and showing virtually no trace of ectomorphy. No gross dysplasias. Chest a little less developed than other segments. Head round and heavy. Primary and secondary $g\pm$. Primary t 3, secondary t 3. Features regular and even but broad and coarse. Mouth excessively large, overly re-laxed. Hands comparatively soft and inadequate. Feet flat, poorly formed. General strength 4, hand strength 2. Coordination first rate. He moves with relaxed poise, yet has the fighter's quickness and precision of movement. Good swimmer. Fairly good at basketball. He is a terrific hitter but lacks the heart, or the "killer instinct," for championship fighting.

Temperament: No somatorotic signs. He is well relaxed, never seems to strain. Well poised and apparently self-sufficient. He is smooth in social manner, makes good contact with people. When pressure is brought to bear on him, though, he becomes surly and hostile and there are temper explosions. For the most part he is as poised as an elevator starter in a department store but under stress he lacks the *ultimate* poise of secure mesomorphy. If he has an outstanding temperamental characteristic it is that of cerebropenia. ψ 4–2–1.

Delinquency: At 6 called destructive, willful, uncontrollable. At 10 called stubborn, contrary, mendacious. Much minor stealing between 10 and 15. At 14 called a clever thief and liar. At 15 in trouble because of throwing knives in fights and because of persistent sexual aggression. Strongly identified with a delinquent gang at this age and later. Many episodes of larceny between 15 and 17. Possession of gun at 17. In trouble at 16 because of organizing and running an alleged harem as an adjunct to the gang.

Origins and Family: Offspring of a brief urban marriage, the parents having separated before the boy was born. Father thickset and Irish, called incorrigible, hypomanic, and subject to depressions. In his late thirties, long after his contact with this boy's mother, he was committed for a time to a state mental hospital where he was labeled *alcoholic, unstable,* with a *manic tendency.* He has high blood pressure. Mother Old American, from a delinquent family and with a history of minor delinquency before marriage. Called in social agency records "an utterly irresponsible person." Boy reared with the father and stepmother until 19, then in foster homes under agency management.

Mental History, Achievement: Finished the seventh grade, quit in the eighth after several repetitions. IQ reports range between 82 and 96, here called 90. At first he seems competent and mentally poised. As acquaintanceship progresses it soon grows clear that the mental fabric is of the thinnest quality.

No vocational plans or special gifts. The AMI that of a seemingly competent youth who is known to be a mendacious smoothy and thereby presents quite a challenge.

Medical: Early history not known. Numerous hospital referrals for minor complaints but no serious illnessess. He has long suffered from sinusitis, has had other chronic infections, and is doubtless a near relative of the infectious syndrome. Persistent enuresis at least to 17 and probably to the present. Several psychiatric referrals because of being a "behavior problem"; no diagnoses except echolalial reiterations of that complaint. PX reveals no significant pathology other than dental caries and evidences of sinusitis.

Running Record: At the Inn he was superficially well behaved so long as allowed to roam at will. When an effort was made to persuade him to work he was smoothly evasive. When the matter was pushed further and an attempt was made to *force* him to work, he blew up like a powder magazine, became momentarily hypomanic. He was a corruptive influence in the House without seeming to be somatorotic. Without scruple or inhibition, he had a smooth way of influencing other boys to execute his will. His viscerotonic extraversion was irresistible. For a time he was generally known among the boys as The Boss. He had a way of looking directly into your face and you knew you were up against something implacable. He gave the impression of ultimate ruthlessness. At the end of his stay we had the feeling that he had all the marbles and that we had got nothing but experience.

He left for a government works project, stayed there a few weeks, broke parole, stole and deserted. Six months later he reappeared in another part of the country as a vagrant. Late in the war his draft board or federal agents caught up with him and he was inducted into military service. After a few months he was listed as a deserter, was later heard from in a western state but was not apprehended and as of the present writing is still at large.

Summary: Extreme mesomorphy with just enough primary *g* to wreck him as a fighter. Good poise. Mentality in the lower range; enuresis and history of many infections. A persistent delinquent without grossly apparent serious psychopathy.

ID 2–0–5 (7)
Insufficiencies:
  IQ ....
  Mop 2
Psychiatric:
  1st order .... (?)
    (4–2–1)
  2nd order ....
  C-phobic ....
  G-phrenic ....
Residual D:
  Primary crim. 5

Comment: Outlook regarded by local authorities as poor. "He is of the criminal stamp," says one of his former parole officers. Another officer who knew him six years ago predicts that he may become a killer. He certainly has a ruthless outlook, is dangerously explosive, and likes to use weapons. He may have a psychotic component. If so it is of the Dionysian-somatotonic or hard-manic variety. The father, of apparently similar pattern although not seen by us, did not require hospitalization until his late thirties. In dealing with this youth one had the feeling that it was a pity he was not a drinker. Alcohol affects some personalities badly but with others it is unquestionably a useful drug. There was a sense of lurking menace about this boy which is rarely felt in the presence of an alcoholic. In some respects the effect of alcohol is like that of a loud bark in a dog. Barking dogs may be a nuisance but are rarely a menace.

The hard-manic psychosis usually manifests itself late and in my experience it is the most difficult of the psychotic patterns to detect and predict from early behavior. This youth is probably close to the borderline of first-order psychopathy. I have the impression that he will stay on the right side of that more or less indeterminate line, but within a narrow belt on that same right side of the line it is very likely that many of our "true criminals" and dangerous personalities dwell.

COMPANY B, PLATOON 2
Primary Criminality: Nos. 185–200

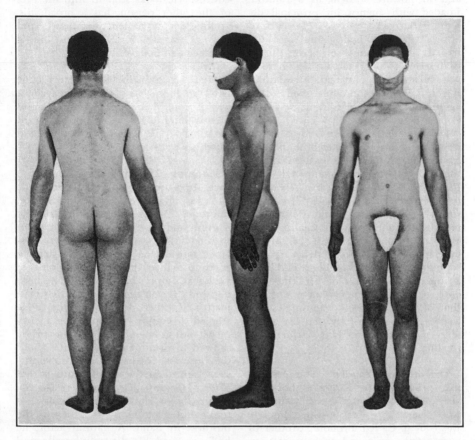

Description: Somatotype $3\frac{1}{2}$–$5\frac{1}{2}$–$1\frac{1}{2}$. A 17-year-old endomorphic meso-morph an inch under average stature. First region: extreme mesomorphy. Note the predominance of the transverse neck diameter over the anteropos-terior diameter (VHP, p. 40). Except for the unexpectedly gynandroid high waist and for just a trace of asthenic failure in the arms and legs he presents a good example of extreme mesomorphy throughout. Primary $g+1$; second-ary g, no trace. Primary t 3, secondary t 3. Pug face. Features even and sym-metrical but coarse. He is good looking at a little distance. Short, heavy hands. General strength 4, hand strength 4. Coordination good in the sense that he moves with a feline silent economy of effort but there is a fatal gynic softness. He is not a fighter and is not very good at games; has been called "deadly with a knife."

BIOGRAPHIES

Temperament: A good picture of predominant somatotonia well buffered with viscerotonia. He is poised, relaxed, and in posture straight as a ramrod. Loaded with energy, his principal delight is derived from risk. He loves to "crash" theaters, ball games, and the like. It is the danger of being caught that seems to offer the thrill. There is no somatorosis, no maladaptive straining in the somatotonic role. The hostile aggression is overt and frank. ψ 3–2–1.

Delinquency: He ran with a delinquent gang as a youngster of 6 and had continued in the same pattern up to the time when we encountered him. Early truancy or disregard of school altogether. Petty stealing and pilfering of stores between 6 and 10, bicycle stealing from 10 to 12, automobile stealing from 14 to 17. He had done some jackrolling, some panhandling, some decoying and robbing of homosexuals. There had been a number of charges of breaking and entering. Delinquency almost entirely that of theft, none of wanton destructiveness. Between 13 and 17, five times sent to state correctional school for stealing.

Origins and Family: Youngest of five, urban family. Father a short but very powerfully built French-Canadian who deserted the family when this boy was 8 or 9. Called alcoholic. Mother of average physique and Irish extraction, regarded as ineffectual although not as an active delinquent. Boy reared at home until 12 after which he had lived mainly in correctional institutions.

Mental History, Achievement: Finished grade school at one of the correctional institutions. IQ reports fall between 75 and 80, here put at 77 although he gives the impression of a higher IQ, as forthright mesomorphs often do.

No vocational plan other than that of professional stealing, which he regards as the only worth-while career. No special abilities except stealing. The AMI is based on a sprightly eagerness of manner and a disarmingly forthright address. He looks straight into the eyes of the other person, has a broad, disarming smile; a generous, level, and "honest" mouth. In talking with him it is difficult to believe ill of him.

Medical: Said to have been a large baby and to have enjoyed excellent health from birth. No record of illnesses of any kind. PX reveals no significant pathology. He seems as sound and tough as a butternut.

Running Record: His response to such opportunities as were offered at the Inn was that a healthy flea to a nice, juicy dog. There was a not unfriendly warmth and a certain viscerotonic grace in him but it was as impossible to convince him of the wrongness of stealing as to convince the flea. His point of view was simply that here is a fine tasty dog but "If you don't like me there are plenty of other dogs in Boston." He seemed to enjoy working the agency racket just as he enjoyed stealing and he showed a certain healthy candor about the business. He had a team of youngsters trained in the art of stealing from stores. His own act was to engage the proprietor or clerk in candid conversation while accomplices achieved the business in hand. A natural actor, he had practiced his disarming smile and his forthright address until he had become something in the way of an amateur hypnotist. Of this art he was proud.

We gave up on him after a few months. During the intervening years he appears to have made progress in his profession. Exempt from military service because of his record, he has spent possibly a third of the time under detention and there are half a dozen new entries on his record, all of them associated with robbery. He is classed locally as a confirmed and moderately competent thief.

Summary: Extreme mesomorphy, short stature, excellent health and strength. Mentality near borderline; no indications of serious psychopathy. Persistent identification with stealing as a profession.

ID 2–0–5 (7)
  Insufficiencies:
    IQ 2
    Mop ....
  Psychiatric:
    1st order ....
    2nd order .... (?)
    (3–2–1)
    C-phobic ....
    G-phrenic ....
  Residual D:
    Primary crim. 5

Comment: In the light of the history the outlook must be called dubious. He is so deeply identified with what society calls crime that any radical shift in motivation seems doubtful. His role in life as he sees it is that of minor and immediate predation. He wants to live as a hawk does, from talon to mouth. He thinks of himself as a hawk and he looks upon the human scene as his to plunder if he can. When he is caught he is a good sportsman about it, or claims he is. Says he holds no grievance against police—they took that trick, maybe he'll take the next. This is objectivity or twentieth-century mental hygiene at its best and objectivity is a characteristic of the second component. He is as objective as a duck hawk harrying a flock of teal.

From this boy's point of view his "delinquency" is a perfectly normal adaptation. There is no cornering him on moral, ethical, or exhortative grounds, or on psychological or psychiatric grounds. All this has been tried by experts with no effect whatever and his generation has seen an orgy of that kind of exertion the like of which was perhaps never known on this earth before. There still remains the argument that "What you are doing does not pay." This is a point of view he can understand but believes is mistaken, and his life possibly for decades to come will offer an interesting testing ground for the argument.

197. COMPANY B, PLATOON 2
Primary Criminality: Nos. 185–200

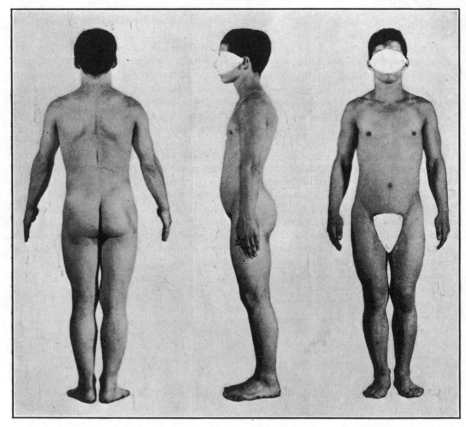

Description: Somatotype 3–6½–1. A 17-year-old gristly mesomorph five inches under average stature. No dysplasias, uniform segmental development. This physique is about as tough and unbreakable as the human organism gets. Primary $g\pm$; secondary g, no trace. Primary t 3 despite dumpiness or squatness. Secondary t 2. Features plain and heavy although balanced or symmetrical. Hands and feet stubby, excessively coarse. General strength 5, hand strength 3. Coordination good. The body functions as an integrated unit and he is a terrific close-in fighter although too compact and bunchy for most kinds of athletics.

Temperament: The outstanding characteristics are maladaptive ruthlessness and hard tenacity of purpose. He is considered harsh or hostile—a tough character—and he has a somatotonic love of danger and risk. He is restless, with the somatorotic "stamp of psychoneurosis." He is known as a ruthless youth and is much feared as an enemy. Has been called paranoid by psychiatrists but the aggression is clearly extraversional, not introversional. It is the first psychiatric component, not the second, that predominates. He is feared because he is a hitter, not because he "thinks too much." ψ 4–2–1.

Delinquency: Early truancy and the typical early delinquency of the street gang; minor stealing, precocious sophistication, school difficulties, staying out all night and the like. At 15 he was one of the ringleaders of a South End gang which perpetrated a long series of holdups and robberies. In this gang he was closely associated with another tough youngster who later became a murderer. He himself was at least once apprehended with a revolver. At 19 he could be described as *primarily* identified with major delinquency of both kinds—stealing and violence.

Origins and Family: Third of seven, urban Irish family. Both parents described as healthy but paranoid and difficult to get along with. Father only intermittently employed but without a court record and he has stuck to his family. Mother described as patriotically loyal to her family and clan. At least three of the seven children have been involved in major delinquency.

Mental History, Achievement: Completed two years of high school with a mediocre but passing record. IQ reports fall between 90 and 108, here called 100. He gives the impression of being cagey, or cunning and hard. He always seems to know what he wants and is ready to go about getting it.

No vocational plan. Talented in music. He can play a number of instruments—through this ability was prominent and popular in high school. His chief interest is in fighting. Every year he enters various boxing tournaments, seems unwilling or unable to accept the fact of his physical limitation in this direction. The AMI that of stalwart mesomorphic directness. He has wide level eyes, an open honest face, and a direct mesomorphic stare.

Medical: Normal birth and development. No known illnesses or injuries of a serious nature. PX reveals no significant pathology. He is a powerful, rugged youth with a very slight elevation in blood pressure and flat, South Irish feet.

Running Record: At the Inn it was clear within a very few weeks that his identifications with delinquency were too well established to be affected by such influences as we could bring to bear. His response to the situation here was like that of a wild dog willing to accept fodder during an emergency but with no intention of submitting to domestication. He scarcely took the trouble even to laugh at the work program or at our job placement efforts, frequently appeared drunk, was known to bring a revolver into the House, and soon became a source of tension within the community. Within a month he held up a local lunchroom and the Inn felt it advisable to release him to police custody.

Following his contacts with us he continued in a career of robbery and holdup, was several times caught, and was exempted from military service because of his record. During the ensuing half-dozen years he has spent about three quarters of the time under detention and has begun to be regarded locally as a "hardened criminal."

Summary: Powerfully built endomorphic mesomorph with a trace of weakness in the arms and upper chest. Robust health and average mentality. Somatorotic. Stubbornly persistent iden-tification with delinquency both of stealing and of violence.

ID 0–3–5 (8)
  Insufficiencies:
    IQ ....
    Mop ....
  Psychiatric:
    1st order ....
    2nd order 3
    (4–2–1)
    C-phobic ....
    G-phrenic ....
  Residual D:
    Primary crim. 5

Comment: Outlook regarded by lo-cal authorities as poor. The boy is con-sidered an established criminal and he has so looked upon himself since early childhood. One of the most unequivocal delinquents in the series although the economic status of his family and the general integrity and continuity of it *as a family* would perhaps fall within the upper third of our group of families. The youth is more powerful than his fa-ther or than any of his known immedi-ate relatives, so his motivation cannot well be explained in terms of the *disap-pointed mesomorphic expectancy* syn-drome (see p. 524) unless perchance his disappointment arises from a sense of physical inferiority to John L. Sullivan —in which case a few more of us ought to suffer with similar symptoms.

The environment in which he has lived may be called bad. But he himself has been one of the elements that par-ticularly made it bad and to explain his delinquency in terms of "environmen-tal influence" would to some extent in-volve an *argumentum ad hominem.* If there is such a thing as a "born crimi-nal" this youth is probably an example of the phenomenon, but I for one do not know how to make the diagnosis. One man who has known the boy from infancy says, "He has it (criminality) in his eye, and he has had it in his eye all his life."

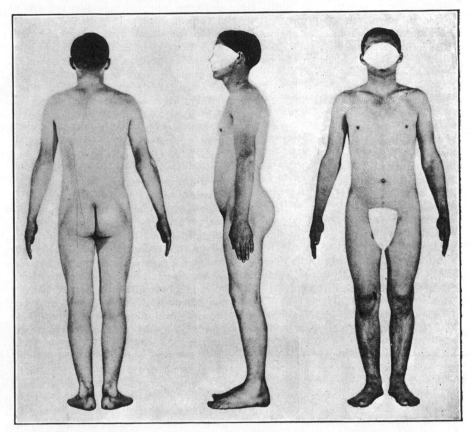

Description: Somatotype 4–5–2. A 19-year-old endomorphic mesomorph of average stature. Legs, trunk, and neck sturdy. Arms and upper chest show a trace of asthenic failure or underdevelopment—enough to interfere seriously with his fighting ability. From the point of view of professional athletics or pugilism a fatal weakness exists. Primary and secondary $g\pm$. Primary t 3, secondary t 2. Coarse, bland features with a wide pug nose. The eyes have a hard steady stare. General strength 4, hand strength 3. Coordination excellent. He is a fairly good athlete and a respected fighter although unsuccessful at professional boxing.

Temperament: The hallmark is a persistent and almost unvaryingly hostile stubbornness. He is somatorotic only when pressed or when someone attempts to discipline him or to make him work. The reaction is then *violently* somatorotic, like that of a trapped wild animal. He may be said to be latently, rather than manifestly somatorotic. He is not conspicuously aggressive or noisy but is surly, resistant, uncooperative. The voice becomes sharp and rasping when he is angry. No indications of cerebrotonic interference. This is the kind of boy who would rarely be called "neurotic." ψ 3–2–1.

Delinquency: Excessive truancy beginning during the first year of school. Minor stealing of so persistent a nature that he came to police attention before 10. Between 10 and 15, continued stealing, larceny, at least six episodes of breaking and entering. Between 15 and 17, close identification with a gang of major delinquents, jackrolling, breaking and entering, robbery, possession of a gun. At 16, sent to state correctional school for robbery. At 17, dishonorable discharge from CCC for larceny.

Origins and Family: Youngest of four, urban family. Both parents Polish immigrants and both of husky physique. The father has a long delinquent history, including more than thirty court appearances, mainly for drunkenness and crimes associated with liquor; also assault and battery, brawling, stabbing, use of aliases. He deserted or disappeared when the boy was 15. Mother called "assaultive, violent, quarrelsome." She has a court record with several appearances for alcoholism, was uncooperative in accepting treatment for venereal disease, and was institutionalized permanently with central-nervous system complications when the boy was 12. Boy reared for the most part in foster homes under agency control. Of the three siblings two have delinquent records.

Mental History, Achievement: Finished the first year of high school, quit in the second year with failing grades. IQ reports cluster at 90 with very slight variation. He gives the impression of dullnesss and slow mentality but also of a certain stolid watchfulness.

No vocational plan; no special gifts. The AMI is based on the underlying ruggedness or manliness. This boy is no complainer. At 12 he was called by one social worker "a self-reliant little man."

Medical: Infancy history not known. No serious illnesses or injuries. PX reveals no significant pathology except badly carious teeth and flat feet.

Running Record: At the Inn he adapted just far enough to insure a day-to-day security but never cooperated beyond that point. He was a poisonous influence in the House and in outlook was one of the most delinquent boys we had. Independent, surly, and uncooperative, he manifested about the attitude of the average department store clerk during the late war. When in danger of being dropped from the program he would accept an outside job but always would quit the job within a few days.

After we gave up on him he roamed about or drifted for another year, then was inducted into military service and at this point we have lost his direct trail. We know only that within a few months he was AWOL, that six months later he was out of the service, delinquent and in serious trouble in another part of the country. Shortly after this he disappeared. During the succeeding four years he has not been heard from either by his relatives or by police. A close acquaintance believes he is dead but another thinks he is serving a long prison sentence under an alias. At the moment this youth is one of our mystery boys.

Summary: Scrub-oak mesomorphy with only fair athletic ability but with good health. Mentality normal or dull normal. Long and dead-in-earnest identification with delinquency.

ID 0–1–6 (7)
  Insufficiencies:
    IQ ....
    Mop ....
  Psychiatric:
    1st order ....
    2nd order   1
      C-penia (3–2–1)
    C-phobic ....
    G-phrenic ....
  Residual D:
    Primary crim.   6

Comment: Outlook probably poor. He seems to be headed toward criminality as a career and since he has good health and is not particularly alcoholic it may be that he will be able to keep at it for a long time. But with dull mentality his chances for conspicuous success at so hard a game are slight. He probably will not be President, at any rate not a Republican president.

People of this sort of mental endowment usually accept their humble lot and derive what vicarious thrill they can from life. They become clerks, bartenders, psychiatrists or sociologists, and on Saturday evenings play bridge or read detective stories. Meanwhile the high-grade or gifted criminal personality rides high in the romantic imagination of nearly everybody. Many of us would rather be Robin Hood than any other character ever imagined. But a story like this present one is disillusioning. It takes some of the romance out of one of the most romantic corners of the mind. This youth "should never be allowed" to aspire to lofty criminality. He ought to be locked up.

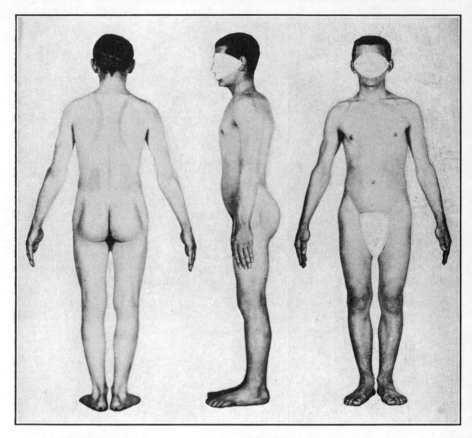

Description: Somatotype 2½–5½–2. A 17-year-old mesomorph an inch under average stature and showing the gnarled characteristic of timberline or scrub-oak mesomorphy. All segments of the body very heavy boned but the arms in particular seem comparatively weak in muscle. They are, however, powerful arms and this youth is no weakling in any sense. Primary g±; secondary g, no trace. Primary t 2, secondary t 2. Features coarse, heavy, asymmetrical. Hands and feet big and crude. General strength 4, hand strength 3. Coordination rather poor. His walk is described by one member of the staff as a peasant shuffle—but is a "peasant shuffle" actually the normal gait of scrub-oak mesomorphy? The boy walks a little like a bear. He has a predilection for athletics but does not adapt well to social games. We tried him in the gymnasium on nearly everything from basketball to boxing. Reactions are a little slow. He is quite a fighter when it is "for keeps" but he was not an effectual boxer.

Temperament: A picture of relaxed, resourceful, and aggressive somatotonia *without a smile.* A menacing youth with a foreboding face and manner. Behind the menace lies both physical power and a violent, destructive temper. There is a remarkable absence of that quality sometimes called "sweet reasonableness." He looks upon life through the eyes of a predator. There is little barking or other waste of energy but destructive violence lurks close to the surface. No sign of cerebrotonic interference. Often called paranoid but the aggression is more extraversional than introversional. His one passion is for gambling and the higher the stakes the better. His pattern of a lethally quick temper is very different from that of an epileptoid personality. This youth is like a gun with a hair trigger. He is not subject to periodic tantrums. ψ 3–2–1.

Delinquency: Destructive and uncontrollable during his first years of school. "Stubborn child" complaint at 9. Stealing, breaking and entering, systematic looting between 10 and 15. Three times sent to correctional schools between 13 and 16. Robbery, possession of dangerous weapons, racketeering between 15 and 18. Armed robbery at 18, repeated instances of larceny between 18 and 20. Close identification with delinquency from early childhood to the present.

Origins and Family: Eighth of eleven, urban family. Father immigrant from Ireland and a burly, powerful man who served a number of sentences for larceny, robbery, drunkenness. Mother Irish, called "a large vigorous woman." She has had contact with social agencies through most of her life. Boy reared in the home until 10, then because of court record and uncontrollability removed and placed in foster homes under agency management. Four of the siblings died in childhood. At least three have court records. This boy and his brothers long regarded as leaders of a tough gang. They are husky youths and have always been known as honest fighters who preferred fists to weapons.

Mental History, Achievement: Finished the eighth grade. IQ reports fall between 80 and 90, here called 85. He makes a first impression of better intelligence than this. He has a watchful tenacity and a mesomorphic objectivity which give an interviewer the sense of being confronted by one who is master of the situation. Responses in the man-to-man situation are effective; those in the paper-and-pencil situation are inadequate. Perhaps our IQ records rest too heavily on the latter.

No vocational plan except the frankly expressed one of living by his wits and by exploitation of social agencies. His achievement is in the field of fighting. Few young men can stand up to him in a fist fight although he has not quite the stamina for top-flight competition. The AMI is a potent one with his direct, objective address, stalwart manliness and vigorous, ruddy health.

Medical: No early data. A "behavior problem" at least as early as 4. A vigorous, violent, and destructive child. Smoked at 6, a window smasher and neighborhood tough at 7. No history of illness of any kind. PX reveals no pathology except carious teeth, flat feet, and an active tic.

Running Record: Throughout several months of interrupted contact with the Inn he made use of the facilities offered only as a falcon might use a temporary resting place and observation perch. He yielded no hostages to the future, neither sought nor accepted advice, entered upon no educational or vocational program. However, without actually hitting anybody he established a healthy respect or fear in the minds of boys and staff alike. We were all glad enough to let him alone. I recall feeling toward him about as I used to feel toward the larger and more silent dogs in the front yards I had to invade as a Wear Ever aluminum salesman during summer vacations. In conferences with me he was watchful, self-sufficient, and I think he rather got the better of those interviews. Anyhow he was not entrapped by any persuasions and we knew in the end that we had no equipment that could reach him. I think that a mesomorphic priest after thoroughly outboxing him might have won him. But despite the movies and romantic fiction there are not many such priests.

For another half-decade this youth has lived out his role of appropriative predation. Exempt from military service because of his record, he has continued in the pattern of larceny and robbery, spending more than half the intervening time under detention. As yet there has been no indication that anybody has reached him. In the late twenties he still gives promise of retaining a criminal outlook.

Summary: Vigorous mesomorphy with high-grade athletic ability and excellent health. Mentality well above borderline. No indications of first-order psychopathy and none of the second order unless the predatory aggression is *ipse facto* psychopathy.

ID 1–0–6 (7)
Insufficiencies:

IQ	1
Mop	
Psychiatric:	
1st order	
2nd order	(?)
(3–2–1)	
C-phobic	
G-phrenic	
Residual D:	
Primary crim.	6

Comment: Outlook regarded by police and penal authorities as poor. He comes about as close as any in the series to what might be called "willful" criminality. Physically, mentally, and temperamentally he is essentially normal or gifted. In strength and health he is endowed far above the usual lot of our species. He regards society as delinquent and therefore as his oyster. The first premise of this argument is difficult to refute and if the first is granted the second can be met only by the more or less dangerous argument that society has the greater force. That is about the way matters stand with this young man. He believes that he has the advantage of the argument and he has the courage of his convictions. *Subtle* argument based on abstracted intellectual grounds will no more reach him than it would reach the falcon. Perhaps muscular Christianity with Joe Louis as priest could accomplish a conversional reform. But who is going to convert Joe to the cloth?

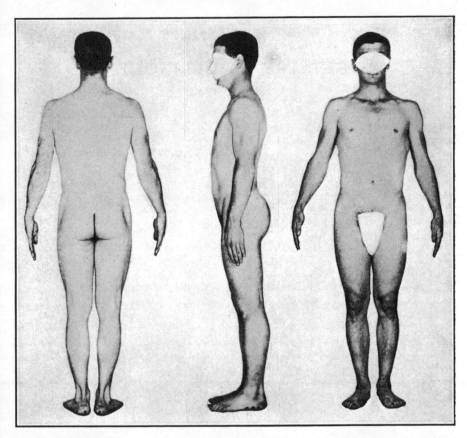

Description: Somatotype 4–5½–2. A 21-year-old mesomorph two inches above average stature. A large, powerfully built youth with no apparent physical weaknesses. Not quite *extreme* mesomorphy and therefore not quite in the professional athlete or professional fighter class but very close to this territory. There is strength and a mastiff-like menace in the face and throughout the body. No dysplasias. Primary and secondary $g\pm$. Primary t 4, secondary t 3. Features large and coarsely molded but regular and level. A fighter's face. General and hand strength 4. Coordination excellent. He moves with firm, elastic step. All muscles of the body behave like a well-drilled unit. He suggests a slightly fattened or softened mastiff.

Part Three

PSYCHIATRY OF DELINQUENCY

CHAPTER 4

STATISTICAL REVIEW

1. Tabulation

Among the many ways of losing or covering up the trail of an idea perhaps the easiest is to clothe it in too many statistics, and the principal concern of the present study is not with statistical prestidigitation but with an experimental demonstration of a biographical method. Yet now and then to array in the sun, as if on a clothesline, the more elemental of the statistical undergarments of an idea is probably not unhealthful to the idea. It is in that washday spirit that we turn to the business of reviewing the distributions and of contemplating the more apparent relational implications of those variables which have been constantly recurrent through the 200 biographies.

Table 11 presents the entire battalion of 200, arrayed in marching order. Table 12 presents the means for each of 19 variables within the different units of the battalion.

TABLE 11
THE PRINCIPAL VARIABLES*

No.	Total D	IQ	Mop	1st order	2nd order	C-phobic	G-phrenic	Primary crim.	Somatotype	Psychiatric index	Stature	Primary g	Secondary g	Primary t	Secondary t	Gen'l strength	Hand strength	Gen'l ath. ability	Paternal extraction	Maternal extraction	IQ score	Military service	Value to the service
COMPANY A, PLATOON 1: 36 WITH MENTAL INSUFFICIENCY PREDOMINANT																							
Section 1																							
1	2	1	0	0	1	0	0	0	5½-4½-1	3 1 1	68	2	2	2	1	4	2	2	It.	It.	80	Yes	±
2	3	1	0	0	1	1	0	0	4½-4 -3½	2 1 1	63	3	2	3	4	2	3	2	O.N.E.	O.N.E.	85	Yes	±
3	5	2	1	0	2	0	0	0	3 -5½-2½	2 1 1	67	1	1	3	3	4	3	4	Scand.	It.-I.	80	No	
4	6	2	2	0	2	0	0	0	3½-3½-4½	1 2 3	68	3	3	2	2	2	2	2	F.-Can.	I.	77	No	
5	6	2	2	0	2	0	0	0	2 -3½-4½	1 3 2	72	2	3	3	3	3	3	1	I.-O.N.E.	E.	77	Yes	—
6	6	2	2	0	2	0	0	0	4½-4½-2½	3 2 2	68	3	1	2	2	3	2	2	X.	I.	75	Yes	—
7	6	2	2	0	0	0	0	2	3½-5 -1½	2 1 1	65	2	2	1	1	4	2	2	It.	It.	77	Yes	—
8	7	2	1	0	2	0	2	0	3 -4½-3	2 2 1	67	2	3	2	2	2	2	1	Gr.	I.	75	Yes	—
9	7	2	2	0	1	1	0	1	2 -4½-3½	2 2 1	67	1	1	2	2	2	2	1	Sla.	F.	75	Yes	—
10	7	2	2	2	0	0	0	1	4 -3 -4	2 1 3	73	2	2	2	2	2	2	1	Scand.	E.-I.	75	Yes	—
11	7	2	2	0	1	0	0	0	3 -5½-2½	4 2 1	68	2	1	2	1	4	4	3	Gr.	Gr.	72	No	
12	8	2	0	0	1	2	1	2	4½-5 -1½	3 1 1	67	4	2	2	2	3	3	2	F.-Can.	I.	75	No	
13	8	2	2	0	2	1	0	1	4 -5½-1½	4 1 1	68	2	2	3	1	4	3	4	G.	G.-I.	72	No	
Section 2																							
14	6	3	3	0	0	0	0	0	4 -3½-3	2 1 2	71	5	2	2	3	2	2	1	O.N.E.	O.N.E.	70	No	
15	7	3	0	0	1	1	1	1	4 -4 -2½	4 1 1	68	3	2	3	3	3	2	2	E.-I.	X.	71	Yes	—

TABLE 11

THE PRINCIPAL VARIABLES* (Continued)

No.	Total D	IQ	Mop	1st order	2nd order	C-phobic	G-phrenic	Primary crim.	Somatotype	Psychiatric index	Stature	Primary g	Secondary g	Primary t	Secondary t	Gen'l strength	Hand strength	Gen'l ath. ability	Paternal extraction	Maternal extraction	IQ score	Military service	Value to the service
16	7	3	0	0	3	0	0	1	2½-5 -2½	2 2 1	71	2	1	3	3	4	3	5	Gr.	F.-Can.	67	Yes	±
17	7	3	1	0	3	0	0	0	3 -5½-2	3 2 1	68	3	1	3	2	4	4	4	N.	N.	70	No	
18	7	3	3	0	0	1	0	0	4½-5 -1½	2 1 1	69	3	2	2	1	3	1	2	X.	O.N.E.	65	No	
19	7	3	3	0	1	0	0	0	5½-3 -2	2 1 1	68	4	3	2	2	2	1	1	O.N.E.	I.	70	Yes	±
20	7	3	3	0	0	0	0	1	2½-5 -3	1 1 1	65	3	2	1	2	2	2	2	I.	I.	67	No	
21	8	3	2	2	0	1	0	0	3½-5 -2	3 2 2	65	3	2	2	2	3	2	1	Li.	Li.	67	No	
22	8	3	2	0	2	1	0	0	4 -4½-3	4 2 1	70	3	3	3	3	3	2	3	F.	G.	67	Yes	−
23	8	3	2	3	0	0	0	0	4 -52−	4 3 1	72	3	3	3	2	3	3	2	O.N.E.	E.	70	No	
24	9	3	2	2	0	1	1	0	3 -4½-3	3 4 2	69	4	4	3	3	3	3	1	I.	I.	70	Yes	−
25	9	3	2	3	0	0	1	0	4 -4½-3	4 3 3	68	4	3	3	3	2	1	1	I.	I.	65	No	
26	9	3	3	0	2	1	0	0	4 -4 -4	3 2 2	71	3	4	2	3	2	2	1	E.	I.	67	No	

Section 3

No.	Total D	IQ	Mop	1st order	2nd order	C-phobic	G-phrenic	Primary crim.	Somatotype	Psychiatric index	Stature	Primary g	Secondary g	Primary t	Secondary t	Gen'l strength	Hand strength	Gen'l ath. ability	Paternal extraction	Maternal extraction	IQ score	Military service	Value to the service
27	6	4	0	0	1	1	0	0	2½-6 -1½	3 2 1	67	2	1	2	2	5	4	5	Po.	Li.	56	Yes	±
28	6	4	1	0	1	0	0	0	4½-4½-1½	3 1 1	68	2	2	2	1	2	2	2	F.-Can.	I.	63	Yes	−
29	7	4	0	0	2	0	0	1	3½-4½-2	4 1 1	70	3	2	2	1	3	3	2	I.	I.	64	Yes	±
30	7	4	1	0	2	0	0	0	4½-4½-2½	2 1 1	70	3	2	2	3	3	2	2	I.	I.	60	Yes	−
31	7	4	1	0	1	0	0	1	2 -3 -5½	1 3 2	70	2	1	3	2	3	5	3	Scand.	I.-F.-Can.	63	No	
32	8	4	0	0	1	3	0	0	4 -4½-1½	3 1 1	66	3	2	2	2	3	2	2	I.	I.	63	No	
33	8	4	0	0	3	0	0	1	4 -4 -4	2 2 2	72	4	2	1	1	2	2	1	F.-Can.	I.	60	No	
34	6	5	0	0	1	0	0	0	2 -6 -1½	3 3 1	67	1	1	3	1	4	3	5	It.	I.	56	Yes	±
35	8	5	0	0	2	1	0	0	2 -6 -1½	3 2 1	69	1	1	3	2	4	5	5	N.	N.	50	No	
36	9	5	1	3	0	0	0	0	5 -3½-1½	5 1 2	65	2	3	2	2	2	1	2	It.	It.	55	No	

COMPANY A, PLATOON 2: 46 WITH MEDICAL INSUFFICIENCY PREDOMINANT

Section 1

No.	Total D	IQ	Mop	1st order	2nd order	C-phobic	G-phrenic	Primary crim.	Somatotype	Psychiatric index	Stature	Primary g	Secondary g	Primary t	Secondary t	Gen'l strength	Hand strength	Gen'l ath. ability	Paternal extraction	Maternal extraction	IQ score	Military service	Value to the service
37	2	0	1	0	1	0	0	0	3½-5 -2	3 1 1	67	2	3	2	3	3	2	2	O.N.E.	E.-I.	90	Yes	+
38	3	0	1	0	1	0	1	0	3 -4 -3	2 2 1	67	3	2	3	3	4	4	3	Scand.	E.	95	No	
39	2	0	2	0	0	0	0	0	3 -4½-3	1 1 1	71	3	2	3	3	3	3	3	E.-F.	I.	115	Yes	±
40	3	1	2	0	0	0	0	0	3 -3½-4	1 2 1	72	3	2	1	2	2	2	1	O.N.E.	O.N.E.	85	Yes	+
41	3	1	2	0	0	0	0	0	3 -4 -3½	1 2 1	68	2	2	2	3	2	2	2	N.	N.	85	Yes	±
42	4	0	2	0	1	0	1	0	3 -4½-2½	2 1 1	68	3	2	2	3	2	2	2	E.	E.	100	No	
43	5	0	2	0	2	0	1	0	4 -4½-2½	3 2 1	68	3	3	2	3	2	2	1	R.-J.	R.-J.	89	Yes	±
44	5	0	2	0	1	0	2	0	3 -4 -4	2 3 2	70	3	4	3	2	2	2	1	F.-Can.	O.N.E.	95	Yes	±
45	5	0	2	0	1	0	2	0	4 -4 -4	3 2 2	72	4	4	2	2	1	2	1	F.-Can.	I.	95	Yes	±
46	6	0	2	0	2	1	1	0	3½-4½-4	2 3 1	73	3	3	4	2	3	2	2	F.	E.-I.	110	Yes	−
47	6	0	2	0	2	0	2	0	4½-5 -2	5 2 1	72	3	2	3	3	3	3	2	I.	I.	90	No	
48	6	1	2	0	2	1	0	0	4 -5½-1½	4 2 1	70	2	2	3	1	4	3	1	X.	X.	85	Yes	±
49	6	1	2	0	2	1	0	0	4 -5 -1½	4 2 1	69	3	3	2	3	4	3	4	I.	I.	85	Yes	−
50	6	1	2	0	1	1	1	0	6 -2½-2	3 1 2	68	4	2	3	3	2	2	2	F.-Can.	F.-Can.-I.	85	No	
51	6	1	2	0	1	0	2	0	3 -4 -3	2 1 1	69	4	2	2	3	2	3	2	I.	I.	85	Yes	±
52	6	1	2	0	1	0	2	0	4 -4½-2½	3 2 1	71	3	4	3	3	2	2	2	O.N.E.	O.N.E.	80	Yes	±
53	6	1	2	0	2	0	0	1	2 -5½-2	2 2 1	67	1	1	4	2	4	3	4	F.-Can.-I.	O.N.E.-I.	83	Yes	±
54	7	0	2	2	0	1	2	0	5½-3 -2½	5 1 3	71	4	3	3	3	2	1	1	I.	I.	90	Yes	−
55	7	0	2	0	2	2	0	1	2 -4½-3½	2 3 1	68	2	2	2	3	2	2	2	I.	I.	95	Yes	−

Section 2

No.	Total D	IQ	Mop	1st order	2nd order	C-phobic	G-phrenic	Primary crim.	Somatotype	Psychiatric index	Stature	Primary g	Secondary g	Primary t	Secondary t	Gen'l strength	Hand strength	Gen'l ath. ability	Paternal extraction	Maternal extraction	IQ score	Military service	Value to the service
56	5	0	3	0	2	0	0	0	2 -4 -4	1 3 1	66	1	2	3	3	2	2	2	It.	E.-I.	105	No	
57	6	0	3	0	3	0	0	0	2½-5 -3	2 2 1	68	2	2	1	2	3	3	2	I.	G.-I.	90	Yes	±
58	6	2	3	0	1	0	0	0	4 -5½-1½	2 1 1	71	3	1	3	1	3	3	2	O.N.E.	I.	77	Yes	±
59	7	1	3	2	0	0	1	0	3 -4 -3½	2 3 2	66	3	2	1	2	2	3	1	O.N.E.	I.	80	Yes	−
60	7	1	3	0	2	0	0	1	3 -5 -2	3 2 1	66	2	2	1	1	2	1	1	X.	I.	80	Yes	−
61	7	2	3	0	2	0	0	0	3½-5 -2½	2 1 1	67	2	2	1	1	2	2	1	Po.	Po.	75	Yes	−
62	7	2	3	0	2	0	0	0	3 -5½-1½	2 1 1	67	4	2	2	1	3	2	2	It.-I.	I.	78	No	
63	8	2	3	0	2	1	0	0	2½-5 -2	2 2 1	67	3	2	2	2	3	3	1	F.-Can.	I.	73	No	
64	8	2	3	0	3	0	0	0	2½-4½-3½	2 2 2	69	2	2	3	3	3	2	1	E.-I.	I.	77	No	
65	8	2	3	0	1	1	0	1	3 -5 -2½	3 2 1	70	3	2	2	3	2	2	2	I.	I.	77	Yes	−
66	6	0	4	0	2	0	0	0	3½-5 -1½	3 2 1	65	2	2	3	2	3	1	2	F.-Can.	F.-Can.	93	No	
67	7	2	4	0	1	0	0	0	3½-4½-3	3 2 1	66	2	2	1	2	3	2	1	It.	It.	75	Yes	−
68	8	1	4	0	2	0	1	0	4 -4 -4	3 2 2	73	3	2	4	3	3	3	2	O.N.E.	O.N.E.	85	Yes	−
69	8	3	4	0	0	1	0	0	3½-5 -2½	- - -	70	3	2	2	2	3	3	1	P.	P.	70	Yes	−
70	9	3	4	0	2	0	0	0	3½-5 -2	4 2 1	68	3	2	4	3	4	3	4	I.	I.	70	No	

TABLE 11

THE PRINCIPAL VARIABLES* (*Continued*)

No.	*Total D*	*IQ*	*Mop*	*1st order*	*2nd order*	*C-phobic*	*G-phrenic*	*Primary crim.*	*Somatotype*	*Psychiatric index*	*Stature*	*Primary g*	*Secondary g*	*Primary t*	*Secondary t*	*Gen'l strength*	*Hand strength*	*Gen'l ath. ability*	*Paternal extraction*	*Maternal extraction*	*IQ score*	*Military service*	*Value to the service*
Section 3																							
71	5	0	5	0	0	0	0	0	3 -5 -2½	– – –	68	2	2	2	3	1	1	1	La.	Li.	93	No	
72	5	0	5	0	0	0	0	0	2½-5 -3	– – –	67	2	2	3	3	3	2	2	N.	N.	95	No	
73	6	0	5	0	1	0	0	0	2 -4½-3½	1 2 1	66	2	2	3	2	3	3	3	E.-I.	E.-I.	95	Yes	±
74	6	1	5	0	0	0	0	0	3 -5 -2½	– – –	68	2	2	3	2	2	2	2	O.N.E.	Scand.	85	Yes	±
75	7	1	5	0	1	0	0	0	3 -3½-4½	1 3 1	71	2	2	3	3	3	3	2	O.N.E.	I.	85	No	
76	8	2	5	0	0	1	0	0	3½-5 -1½	– – –	64	4	3	1	1	3	2	1	I.	I.	77	Yes	–
77	8	3	5	0	0	0	0	0	4 -4½-1½	– – –	66	4	3	1	2	2	1	1	Scand.	G.	67	Yes	–
78	9	1	5	2	0	0	1	0	3½-4½-2	– – –	67	4	2	1	2	1	1	1	Sy.	Sy.	83	No	
79	9	1	5	0	0	0	2	1	4½-3 -4½	2 1 3	71	6	5	3	4	1	2	2	I.	I.	80	No	
80	9	1	5	0	1	0	0	2	3 -5 -2½	2 1 1	66	3	2	1	1	2	2	1	I.	I.	85	No	
81	9	4	5	0	0	0	0	0	4 -4 -4	– – –	71	4	3	1	2	1	1	1	Sy.	Sy.	60	No	
82	7	0	6	0	1	1	0	0	3 -4½-3½	– – –	70	2	2	2	2	1	3	1	I.	I.	90	Yes	–
COMPANY A, PLATOON 3: 18 WITH FIRST-ORDER PSYCHOPATHY PREDOMINANT																							
83	4	1	1	2	0	0	0	0	4 -5 -3	3 2 2	72	3	3	3	4	4	4	4	F.-O.N.E.	G.	80	No	
84	6	0	0	3	0	0	3	0	4 -5 -3	4 2 2	71	3	3	3	3	2	3	3	F.-Can.	F.-Can.-I.	110	No	
85	6	0	0	3	0	0	2	1	4 -5 -3	4 3 2	72	3	2	3	3	4	3	4	I.	I.	115	Yes	±
86	8	0	2	3	0	3	0	0	4 -4½-3	3 2 2	68	3	2	2	2	2	1	1	X.	O.N.E.	95	Yes	–
87	6	0	0	4	0	0	2	0	3½-5 -2½	4 2 1	67	3	3	3	3	3	4	2	O.N.E.	O.N.E.	90	Yes	±
88	7	0	0	4	0	1	1	1	2½-4 -4	2 3 3	70	2	3	2	3	3	2	1	I.-G.	G.	95	No	
89	8	1	0	4	0	2	1	0	4 -4½-3	5 2 1	69	3	3	2	3	2	2	1	X.	Po.	80	Yes	–
90	8	0	0	4	0	0	0	4	4 -5½-1½	4 3 2	67	2	2	3	3	4	2	2	E.-I.	I.	90	No	
91	9	2	2	4	0	1	0	0	3 -5 -3	3 3 3	69	2	1	3	3	3	2	2	P.-Li.	P.-Li.	77	Yes	–
92	7	0	2	5	0	0	0	0	5 -4 -2	5 2 2	68	4	2	2	2	2	1	1	It.	It.	100	No	
93	7	1	1	5	0	0	0	0	3 -5½-2	4 3 1	68	3	2	3	3	4	2	3	I.	I.	85	Yes	–
94	8	0	2	5	0	1	0	0	2 -4 -4	1 5 3	68	2	2	2	2	2	1	1	I.	I.	90	No	
95	8	0	1	5	0	0	2	0	2 -4 -4	1 2 5	68	2	3	2	2	1	2	1	I.	O.N.E.	115	No	
96	9	1	3	5	0	0	1	0	5 -4 -2	5 2 2	68	5	5	3	4	2	1	1	X.	I.	85	No	
97	9	1	0	7	0	0	1	0	5 -4 -3	4 3 3	73	3	4	2	2	2	1	1	Scand.	Scand	85	No	
98	8	0	0	8	0	0	0	0	2½-5 -3	3 4 2	69	3	2	3	3	3	2	1	F.-Can.	I.	90	No	
99	8	0	0	8	0	0	0	0	5½-4 -1½	5 2 3	70	3	2	3	3	3	1	1	O.N.E.	F.-Can.	90	No	
100	9	1	0	8	0	0	0	0	7 -3½-1	6 1 1	68	2	2	2	2	3	3	4	It.	It.	85	No	
COMPANY B, THE CHAPLAIN'S UNIT: 5 WITH ID ZERO																							
101	0	0	0	0	0	0	0	0	5 -3½-3½	1 1 1	70	5	2	3	4	2	2	3	Scand.	Scand.	115	Yes	+
102	0	0	0	0	0	0	0	0	1 -6 -2	1 1 1	66	2	1	2	2	5	4	5	Sy.	Sy.	105	Yes	±
103	0	0	0	0	0	0	0	0	4 -6 -1	1 1 1	69	2	2	3	3	5	4	4	R.	P.	100	Yes	+
104	0	0	0	0	0	0	0	0	2½-4½-3½	1 1 1	72	2	2	4	4	3	4	3	Scand.	Scand.	120	No	
105	0	0	0	0	0	0	0	0	2½-4½-4	1 1 1	70	2	2	4	4	3	4	4	O.N.E.	O.N.E.	118	Yes	+
COMPANY B, PLATOON 1, SECOND-ORDER PSYCHOPATHY: 9 BORDERING ON FIRST-ORDER PSYCHOPATHY																							
Section 1																							
106	2	0	0	0	2	0	0	0	7 -3 -1½	4 1 1	72	3	2	3	2	3	1	3	Scand.	Scand.	120	No	
107	4	0	0	0	3	0	1	0	4 -4½-3	2 2 1	67	3	3	3	3	3	2	2	N.	N.	90	Yes	–
108	6	0	2	0	3	0	1	0	5 -4½-2	5 1 1	70	4	3	3	3	3	2	2	O.N.E.	O.N.E.	110	Yes	–
109	7	0	0	0	3	2	2	0	4 -3½-4½	3 2 3	72	3	4	3	3	2	2	2	F.-Can.	I.	90	No	
110	7	0	0	0	3	2	0	2	6 -3 -1½	6 1 1	70	3	1	3	3	3	3	3	O.N.E.-I.	O.N.E.	110	Yes	–
111	6	0	2	0	4	0	0	0	5 -4 -2	4 3 2	69	3	2	2	2	3	2	2	O.N.E.	F.-I.	90	Yes	–
112	6	1	1	0	4	0	0	0	5 -4 -2½	2 2 3	69	3	2	2	2	2	1	1	I.	I.	85	Yes	–
113	6	1	0	0	4	0	1	0	3½-6½-1	4 2 1	70	3	2	3	1	5	3	3	N.	N.	80	No	
114	6	0	0	0	5	0	1	0	3½-4½-3	4 2 2	71	3	2	3	3	3	3	2	I.	I.	90	Yes	±
18 WITH MINOR SOMATOROSES																							
Section 2																							
115	1	0	0	0	1	0	0	0	2 -2½-6½	1 2 1	72	2	1	3	4	4	4	4	O.N.E.	I.	95	Yes	+
116	1	0	0	0	1	0	0	0	3 -4½-4	2 2 1	73	2	1	3	3	3	3	2	O.N.E.	I.	95	Yes	+
117	1	0	0	0	1	0	0	0	5 -4½-1½	3 2 1	68	3	2	3	2	3	2	3	Ass.-J.	Ass.-J.	115	No	
118	2	0	1	0	1	0	0	0	4 -5½-1½	2 2 1	64	2	2	3	3	4	1	3	X.	P.-Au.	115	Yes	–
119	2	0	0	0	1	1	0	0	3 -7 -1	3 1 1	67	2	1	4	2	5	3	5	P.	P.	95	No	
120	2	0	0	0	1	0	1	0	4½-5 -2½	2 1 1	72	3	2	4	3	3	3	3	I.	O.N.E.	100	No	
121	3	0	0	0	1	1	0	1	2½-7 -1	2 1 1	69	2	2	5	3	5	4	5	I.-O.N.E.	I.-O.N.E.	95	Yes	+

TABLE 11

THE PRINCIPAL VARIABLES* (Continued)

No.	Total D	IQ	Mob	1st order	2nd order	C-phobic	G-phrenic	Primary crim.	Somatotype	Psychiatric index	Stature	Primary g	Secondary g	Primary t	Secondary t	Gen'l strength	Hand strength	Gen'l ath. ability	Paternal extraction	Maternal extraction	IQ score	Military service	Value to the service
122	2	0	0	0	2	0	0	0	3½-5½-1½	2 1 1	66	2	2	3	2	4	3	3	O.N.E.	E.-I.	90	Yes	+
123	2	0	0	0	2	0	0	0	4 -4½-3½	2 1 1	75	2	3	3	4	2	3	2	E.-I.	E.-I.	100	Yes	
124	3	0	1	0	2	0	0	0	3 -5½-2	2 1 1	68	2	1	3	3	3	3	3	X.	I.	105	Yes	±
125	3	0	0	0	2	0	1	0	4 -4 -4	2 2 2	69	3	4	3	4	2	2	3	N.	N.	110	Yes	±
126	3	0	0	0	2	0	0	1	2½-4½-4	2 2 1	73	3	2	3	4	4	4	4	O.N.E.	O.N.E.	115	Yes	+
127	3	0	0	0	2	0	0	1	5½-4½-1	2 1 1	67	2	2	2	2	4	3	4	Po.-I.	I.	90	Yes	±
128	4	0	1	0	2	1	0	0	4 -4 -4	3 2 1	72	3	2	3	2	3	3	3	X.	I.	100	Yes	±
129	4	0	0	0	2	0	2	0	2½-4½-3½	2 3 2	68	2	3	3	4	3	3	3	E.	O.N.E.	115	Yes	−
130	5	1	1	0	2	1	0	0	3 -5 -3	3 2 1	68	2	2	1	2	3	4	3	F.-Can.	I.-F.	83	Yes	−
131	5	1	1	0	2	0	1	0	2½-4 -4	2 2 1	70	2	2	4	3	3	3	3	N.	N.	85	Yes	−
132	6	1	1	0	2	1	1	0	3½-5 -2½	3 1 1	68	2	3	1	2	3	3	2	F.-I.	I.	83	Yes	−
Section 3																		**11 COMPARATIVELY UNCOMPLICATED CASES**					
133	1	0	0	0	1	0	0	0	7 -2 -1½	2 1 1	73	4	2	2	2	2	2	3	Ru.-J.	Ru.-J.	100	No	
134	3	1	0	0	1	0	0	1	3½-5½-2	3 1 1	73	2	2	4	4	4	4	4	E.-I.	E.-I.	83	No	
135	3	0	0	0	3	0	0	0	1½-2½-6½	1 3 1	73	2	2	3	4	2	4	4	O.N.E.	F.-E.	105	No	
136	3	0	0	0	3	0	0	0	4 -4½-2	3 1 1	68	3	2	2	2	4	3	4	O.N.E.	Scand.	125	Yes	±
137	3	0	0	0	3	0	0	0	5 -3½-2½	5 2 1	72	3	3	3	2	3	2	2	P.-J.	P.-J.	110	No	
138	4	0	0	0	3	1	0	0	5 -5 -1	4 1 1	67	3	2	3	3	3	2	3	X.	F.-Can.	100	No	
139	4	0	1	0	3	0	0	0	1½-2½-6½	1 3 1	70	2	1	1	2	4	4	2	E.	F.-Can.	95	No	
140	4	0	1	0	3	0	0	0	1½-5 -3½	2 4 1	68	2	1	3	2	4	3	2	It.	It.	110	No	
141	4	0	1	0	3	0	0	0	2 -7 -1	4 2 1	68	1	1	4	3	5	4	5	F.-Can.	I.	105	No	
142	4	0	0	0	4	0	0	0	3 -5½-1½	4 2 1	69	3	1	3	2	4	4	4	Scand.	Scand.	115	Yes	±
143	5	0	0	0	4	0	0	1	3 -4½-4	2 3 2	72	3	2	3	4	3	3	3	O.N.E.	O.N.E.	120	Yes	−
Section 4																		**21 WITH MULTIPLE COMPLICATIONS**					
144	5	0	1	0	2	0	1	1	3 -4 -4½	2 4 2	71	2	2	4	3	4	4	3	I.	Li.-P.	90	Yes	±
145	5	0	0	0	2	1	0	2	2 -7 -1	5 2 1	64	2	2	3	2	5	3	5	Po.	Po.-It.	100	Yes	−
146	6	1	1	0	2	1	1	0	3 -4½-3	2 2 2	69	2	2	3	3	3	3	3	I.	I.-E.	85	Yes	−
147	6	0	2	0	2	1	1	0	4 -4 -3½	4 3 2	69	3	1	3	3	3	3	3	I.	I.	90	Yes	−
148	7	1	1	0	2	1	1	1	4 -4 -4	2 2 2	69	2	1	4	4	2	2	3	X.	F.-Can.	85	Yes	−
149	5	1	1	0	3	0	0	1	3½-5½-1½	4 2 1	64	2	1	4	3	4	2	3	R.-J.	I.	80	Yes	±
150	5	0	1	0	3	0	0	1	2 -5 -3½	2 3 1	68	2	1	3	3	3	3	3	It.	It.	100	Yes	±
151	6	0	0	0	3	1	1	1	5 -5 -1½	5 2 1	69	3	3	3	4	4	3	3	Po.	Po.	95	No	
152	6	0	1	0	3	0	1	1	4 -3½-4½	2 2 3	73	3	2	2	2	2	2	1	E.-I.	E.-I.	90	No	
153	6	0	2	0	3	0	0	1	3 -5 -2½	3 2 1	65	2	1	2	2	4	3	3	P.	P.	95	No	
154	6	1	1	0	3	0	0	1	2½-4 -5	1 3 2	70	2	1	2	2	3	3	2	F.-Can.	I.	83	Yes	±
155	6	1	1	0	3	0	0	1	3 -5 -2	3 2 1	64	2	2	3	3	3	2	3	E.-I.	F.-Can.	83	No	
156	6	1	1	0	3	0	0	1	2 -5½-1½	4 2 1	65	2	1	2	2	4	4	2	Li.	Li.	85	No	
157	7	0	2	0	3	1	0	1	3 -4½-4	2 2 2	72	2	1	3	4	3	4	4	I.	I.	118	No	
158	7	0	1	0	3	1	0	0	4½-4½-2½	5 1 1	74	4	2	3	2	4	3	3	I.	I.	93	Yes	−
159	7	1	2	0	3	1	0	0	3½-4½-3½	2 2 1	69	2	1	1	3	2	2	1	O.N.E.	O.N.E.	80	Yes	−
160	7	2	0	0	3	1	0	1	3 -4 -4	2 4 2	70	2	1	2	3	3	3	3	I.	I.	77	Yes	−
161	7	1	0	0	4	2	0	0	1½-4½-4½	2 4 2	71	2	1	4	3	3	3	3	N.	N.-W.	80	No	
162	7	1	0	0	4	0	0	0	3 -5 -2½	5 3 1	66	3	1	3	2	3	2	2	R.-J.	G.-J.	85	Yes	−
163	7	1	0	0	4	0	0	2	3 -5½-1½	5 3 1	67	2	1	4	3	5	3	5	I.	I.	80	No	
164	8	0	0	0	4	2	0	0	4 -5½-1½	5 2 1	68	2	1	3	3	5	4	5	F.-Can.	F.-Can.-I.	90	No	
Section 5																		**3 ALCOHOLICS**					
165	7	0	0	0	0	4	1	2	4 -4 -2	3 1 1	68	3	1	3	2	3	3	3	I.	I.	95	No	
166	8	0	2	0	2	4	0	0	5 -4 -1½	3 1 1	68	4	3	3	2	3	2	2	O.N.E.	Po.	100	Yes	−
167	8	0	0	0	2	4	2	0	3½-5½-2	3 2 2	70	3	3	3	3	3	2	3	I.	Da.-F.	100	Yes	−
Section 6									THE PSYCHIATRIC REAR GUARD: 17 GYNANDROPHRENES														
168	1	0	0	0	0	0	1	0	4 -3½-4	2 1 1	69	3	3	3	3	2	3	3	I.	O.N.E.	100	Yes	±
169	2	0	0	0	1	0	1	0	5 -2½-4	2 1 2	68	5	4	2	3	1	1	1	G.	G.-O.N.E.	115	Yes	±
170	3	0	0	0	1	0	2	0	2½-4 -4	1 2 1	71	3	3	3	3	3	4	3	X.	E.-I.	100	Yes	±
171	3	0	0	0	1	0	2	0	3½-4½-3	2 2 1	71	3	3	3	4	3	3	3	O.N.E.	F.-Can.-I.	125	Yes	±
172	3	0	0	0	1	0	2	0	4½-5 -2	3 2 1	73	4	3	3	2	3	2	2	N.-W.	N.-W.	115	No	

TABLE 11

THE PRINCIPAL VARIABLES* (Continued)

No.	Total D	IQ / Mop	1st order / 2nd order / C-phobic / G-phrenic	Primary crim.	Somatotype	Psychiatric index	Stature	Primary g / Secondary g / Primary t / Secondary t / Gen'l strength / Hand strength / Gen'l ath. ability	Paternal extraction	Maternal extraction	IQ score	Military service	Value to the service
173	4	0 0	0 2 0 2	0	2 -5 -3	1 5 2	74	2 3 3 3 3 3 2	O.N.E.	O.N.E.	120	Yes	—
174	4	0 0	0 2 0 2	0	3 -4 -3	3 3 1	68	2 4 3 3 3 3 3	P.	P.	95	No	
175	4	0 1	0 1 0 2	0	2½-4½-3	2 2 2	69	2 4 3 3 2 3 1	I.	I.	110	No	
176	5	0 0	0 2 1 2	0	4 -3 -4½	3 2 4	72	4 4 3 3 2 2 2	X.	R.-J.	115	Yes	—
177	6	0 1	0 2 1 2	0	3 -5½-2½	4 2 1	70	2 3 4 3 4 4 3	W.-N.	W.-N.	120	Yes	
178	6	0 1	0 2 1 2	0	2½-3½-4½	2 3 2	69	2 3 3 3 2 3 3	I.	R.-J.	115	No	
179	6	0 1	0 1 2 2	0	4½-4 -2	5 1 1	67	3 4 3 3 2 2 2	X.	O.N.E.	120	No	
180	3	0 0	0 0 0 3	0	3½-4 -3	2 1 2	70	4 2 1 2 1 3 1	O.N.E.	O.N.E.	110	No	
181	5	0 0	0 2 0 3	0	4 -4 -4	4 2 2	75	4 4 3 3 2 2 2	N.-W.	N.-W.	100	Yes	—
182	5	0 1	0 1 0 3	0	4 -4 -3	4 1 1	70	2 4 2 3 2 2 2	G.-I.	F.-Can.-I.	100	Yes	—
183	5	1 0	0 0 1 3	0	4 -4½-3½	2 1 1	72	2 4 3 2 2 2 2	Li.	G.	85	No	
184	7	0 0	0 1 2 4	0	5 -4 -3	3 1 2	72	3 3 3 3 2 2 2	I.-O.N.E.	I.	115	Yes	—
COMPANY B, PLATOON 2: 16 WITH CRIMINALITY THE PREDOMINANT FACTOR													
185	5	1 1	0 1 0 0	2	3 -5½-1½	2 2 1	65	2 1 2 2 4 2 3	E.-I.	I.	85	Yes	±
186	6	1 1	0 0 2 0	2	4 -4½-2½	2 2 1	70	2 2 2 2 3 3 3	G.-Scand.	Scand.	83	Yes	—
187	5	2 0	0 0 0 0	3	3 -5½-2½	3 2 1	71	2 1 4 2 4 4 5	O.N.E.	I.	75	Yes	+
188	7	1 1	0 1 1 0	3	3½-5 -2	3 2 1	68	3 1 2 2 3 2 3	I.	I.	85	No	
189	4	0 0	0 0 0 0	4	3 -6½-1	3 2 1	69	2 2 4 3 5 4 5	E.-I.	E.-I.	90	Yes	±
190	5	0 0	0 0 0 1	4	4 -4½-3	3 2 1	70	3 2 2 3 3 3 3	P.	P.	95	Yes	—
191	5	0 1	0 0 0 0	4	2½-5½-2	4 2 1	68	2 2 2 2 4 3 3	It.	It.	90	No	
192	6	1 0	0 0 0 1	4	4 -5 -1½	4 2 1	66	3 3 3 2 3 2 3	Ru.-J.	Ru.-J.	80	No	
193	6	2 0	0 0 0 0	4	4 -5½-1½	3 2 1	67	3 1 3 3 4 3 5	O.N.E.	Po.	73	No	
194	7	1 0	0 2 0 0	4	2½-5½-2	4 3 1	68	2 1 3 2 4 4 5	N.	N.	85	No	
195	7	0 2	0 0 0 0	5	4 -5½-1	3 2 1	67	2 2 3 3 4 2 4	I.-G.	I.-G.	90	Yes	—
196	7	0 2	0 0 0 0	5	3½-5½-1½	4 2 1	67	3 1 3 3 4 4 3	I.	O.N.E.	90	Yes	—
197	7	2 0	0 0 0 0	5	3 -6½-1	3 2 1	63	2 1 3 2 5 3 5	F.-Can.	I.	77	No	
198	8	0 0	0 3 0 0	5	4 -5 -2	4 2 1	68	2 2 3 2 4 3 4	I.	I.	100	No	
199	7	0 0	0 1 0 0	5	2½-5½-2	3 2 1	67	2 1 2 2 4 3 4	P.	P.	90	Yes	—
200	7	1 0	0 0 0 0	6	4 -5½-2	3 2 1	70	2 2 4 3 4 4 5	I.	I.	85	No	

* 1. *Paternal and Maternal Extraction.* An indication of the predominant national or racial stock in the immediate ancestry of the father and mother. Abbreviations:

Ass.	Assyrian	*I.*	Irish	*P.*	Polish
Au.	Austrian	*It.*	Italian	*Po.*	Portuguese
Da.	Danish	*J.*	Jewish	*R.*	Russian
E.	English	*La.*	Latvian	*Ru.*	Rumanian
F.	French	*Li.*	Lithuanian	*Scand.*	Scandinavian
F.-Can.	French-Canadian	*N.*	Negro	*Sla.*	Slavic
G.	German	*N.-W.*	(or *W.-N.*) Mixture of	*Sy.*	Syrian
Gr.	Greek		Negro and white	*X.*	Unknown
		O. N. E.	Old American, of North		
			European origin		

2. *Military Service.* A *Yes* or *No* indication as to whether or not the youth served in one of the armed forces—Army, Navy, or Marines—during the period of the study.

3. *Value to the Service.* The application of a 3-point rating scale to an estimate of the outcome of the military careers of the 115 who were in the service. The symbol *plus* (+) indicates that after all the available information—much of it confidential—has been reviewed, the boy appears to have more than earned his way. He seems to have been of value to the military effort. The symbol *minus* (−) indicates that from a strictly military point of view his presence was probably more costly than it was worth; that his induction turned out to be a poor bargain for the government. Most of the "minuses" are boys who spent a large part of their time under medical, psychiatric, or disciplinary care, or were

2. The Somatotype

All but two of the variables represented in Table 12 can be plotted as simple one dimensional functions. Consequently they can be considered more or less illuminatively in terms of means or averages, but first the two polydimensional variables, somatotype and psychiatric index, need to be considered within the frame of their own polydimensional structure.

Figures 19 and 20 present a two-dimensional comparison of the somatotype distribution for 4,000 college students with the distribution for the 200 of the present study. The population of 4,000 contributing to Figure 19 was drawn mainly from Harvard, the University of Chicago, and Oberlin, with smaller groups from three other colleges. This is the same statistical population as that presented in Table 23 A on page 268 of *Varieties of Human Physique*. In the figure each of the 200 black dots represents an approximate somatotype average for 20 cases.

To try to represent in two dimensions what occurs in three is never perfectly satisfactory. Yet these two figures do reveal some singular differences, even on a flat graph. Figure 19 represents a crossing and intermingling of three distributions, each of which approximates (in its own dimension) the familiar bell-shaped curve often called "biologically normal." In the colleges there appear to be nearly as many ectomorphs as mesomorphs, and although there are appreciably fewer endomorphs, the distribution of the endomorphy follows almost the same symmetrical pattern that is seen in the vicinity of the other two poles. In the everyday parlance of the Constitution Laboratory there is in the college normal distribution a degree of lightening in the southwest, with massing in the southeast and a slightly heavier massing in the north. It should be noted that in the college population there is no appreciable massing in the northwest, as compared with the east and northeast; and also that in this population there is a fairly good representation from the extreme south (the mesopenes).

The population of 200 for the Hayden Goodwill Inn (Figure 20) departs quite sharply from the college distribution, with a distinct and rather heavy

---

deserters. Those who were given medical discharges for cause other than actional injury also are rated minus. The symbol *plus or minus* (±) means either that our information is too incomplete to justify a guess, or that the balance between plus and minus seems to be about an even one.

It should be emphasized that the estimates of *value to the service* are in no sense official military ratings; also that these are not estimates of value in general, or of value in any sense other than specifically military. In no instance are the ratings to be interpreted as reflecting personal discredit on the boy, except possibly in those few cases where primary criminality is regarded as the predominant factor in the difficulty. Even in those cases I am not sure that the "primary criminality" is to be blamed particularly on the boy. I have written the biographies as a reporter, and reporters get to have sympathies. These are in nearly all cases with the boy as an individual already born. They are not always with the social system that lacked the wisdom or the courage to advise the boy on whether to be born or not; and, having been born, on what to do with himself.

TABLE 12

SUMMARY OF MEANS WITHIN THE DIFFERENT UNITS OF THE BATTALION

Predominant weakness	Company	Platoon	Section	Nos.	Total D	IQ	Mop	Psychiatric, 1st order	Psychiatric, 2nd order	C-phobic	G-phrenic	Primary criminality	Somatotype	Psychiatric index	Stature	Primary B	Secondary B	Primary τ	Secondary τ	General strength	Hand strength	General athletic ability	IQ score
Mental insufficiency	A	1	1 (ones, twos)	1–13	6.0	1.8	1.4	0.2	1.3	0.4	0.2	0.7	3.6-4.5-2.8	2.4-1.5-1.5	67.8	2.2	1.9	2.2	2.0	3.0	2.5	2.1	76.6
			2 (threes)	14–26	7.6	3.0	2.0	0.8	0.9	0.5	0.2	0.2	3.7-4.5-2.6	2.8-1.9-1.5	68.8	3.3	2.5	2.5	2.4	2.8	2.1	2.0	68.1
			3 (fours, fives)	27–36	7.2	4.3	0.4	0.3	1.4	0.5	0.2	0.3	3.4-4.7-2.3	2.9-1.7-1.3	68.4	2.3	1.6	2.3	1.7	3.1	2.7	2.9	59.0
			Means for the platoon		6.9	2.9	1.3	0.4	1.2	0.4	0.2	0.4	3.6-4.5-2.5	2.7-1.7-1.4	68.3	2.6	2.0	2.3	2.1	3.0	2.4	2.3	68.7
Medical insufficiency	A	2	1 (ones, twos)	37–55	4.9	0.4	1.9	0.1	1.2	0.4	1.9	0.1	3.6-4.3-2.8	2.6-1.8-1.3	69.5	2.9	2.5	2.6	2.6	2.6	2.4	1.9	91.4
			2 (threes, fours)	56–70	7.2	1.5	3.3	0.1	1.7	0.2	0.1	0.1	3.1-4.8-2.6	2.4-1.9-1.2	67.9	1.9	1.9	2.3	1.9	2.8	2.3	1.7	80.3
			3 (fives, six)	71–82	7.3	1.2	5.1	0.2	0.3	0.2	0.3	0.3	3.3-4.5-3.0	1.5-1.8-1.5	67.9	3.1	1.5	2.0	2.3	1.9	1.9	1.5	82.9
			Means for the platoon		6.3	1.0	3.2	0.1	1.1	0.2	0.5	0.2	3.3-4.5-2.8	2.4-1.9-1.3	68.6	2.8	2.3	2.3	2.3	2.5	2.2	1.7	85.6
First-order psychopathy	A	3	Means for the platoon	83–100	7.5	0.4	0.8	4.8	0	0.4	0.7	0.3	3.9-4.5-2.7	3.7-2.6-2.2	69.2	2.8	2.6	2.6	2.8	2.7	2.1	1.9	92.1
None; chaplain's unit	B		Means for the unit	101–105	0	0	0	0	0	0	0	0	3.0-4.9-2.8	1-1-1	69.4	2.6	1.8	3.2	3.4	3.6	3.6	3.8	111.6
Second-order psychopathy	B	1	1 (Bordering on first order)	106–114	5.6	0.2	0.6	0	3.4	0.4	0.7	0.2	4.8-4.2-2.3	3.8-1.8-1.7	70.0	3.1	2.3	2.8	2.4	3.0	2.1	2.2	96.1
			2 (Minor somatoroses)	115–132	2.9	0.2	0.3	0	1.6	0.3	0.3	0.2	3.4-4.8-2.3	2.2-1.6-1.1	69.4	2.3	2.1	3.0	2.9	3.4	3.0	3.2	99.2
			3 (Uncomplicated)	133–143	3.5	0.1	0.3	0	2.8	0.1	0	0.2	3.4-4.3-2.9	2.8-2.1-1.1	70.3	2.5	1.7	2.8	2.7	3.5	3.2	3.3	106.2
			4 (Multiple complications)	144–164	6.3	0.6	0.9	0	3.0	0.6	0.3	1.0	3.2-4.8-2.9	3.1-2.5-1.5	68.4	2.3	1.4	3.2	3.0	3.4	2.9	3.0	88.7
			5 (Alcoholics)	165–167	7.7	0	0.7	0	4.0	0	0	0.7	4.2-4.5-1.8	3.0-1.3-1.6	68.7	3.3	2.3	3.0	2.7	3.0	2.7	3.0	98.3
			6 (Gynandrophrenes)	168–184	4.2	0.1	0.3	0	1.2	0.5	2.2	0	3.6-4.1-3.3	2.6-1.9-1.6	70.6	2.9	3.4	2.8	2.9	2.3	2.6	2.2	109.4
			Means for the platoon		4.6	0.2	0.5	0	2.3	0.5	0.7	0.4	3.6-4.5-2.9	2.8-2.0-1.4	69.6	2.6	2.2	2.9	2.7	3.1	2.8	2.8	99.2
Primary criminality	B	2	Means for the platoon	185–200	6.2	0.8	0.5	0	0.5	0.2	0.1	4.1	3.4-5.4-1.8	3.2-2.1-1.0	67.7	2.3	1.6	2.8	2.4	3.9	3.1	3.9	85.8
			Means for the battalion		5.7	0.9	1.3	0.5	1.4	0.4	0.5	0.6	3.5-4.6-2.7	2.8-1.9-1.4	69.0	2.7	2.2	2.6	2.5	3.0	2.7	2.5	89.2

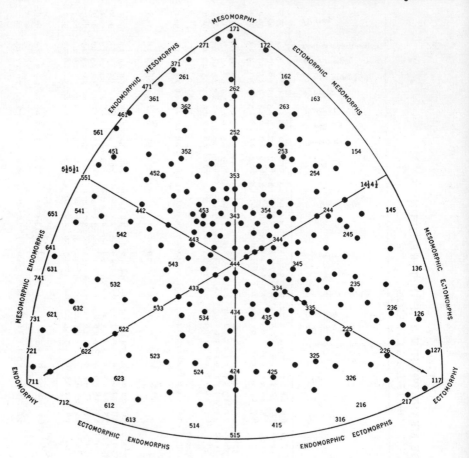

FIGURE 19.   The Distribution of Somatotypes for a Male College Population of 4000. Each Black Dot Represents 20 Cases.

massing in the northwest; also with a falling away in the east, northeast, and southeast, and with dramatic absence of the contingency from the south. Mesopenes appear to be a great rarity in the HGI population. Ectomorphs are rare, and oddly, ectomorphic mesomorphs are rare in comparison with the preponderance of endomorphic mesomorphs. Mesomorphic endomorphs are of just about the same frequency of occurrence at the HGI as in the college population, but ectomorphic endomorphs—the western half of the southern or mesopenic population—are almost unknown at HGI. There is only one clear-cut example of this group among the 200. This is No. 169, a harmless gynandrophrene who is a 5-2½-4 in somatotype. From the eastern half of the southern population there is not a single example that departs from the territory of the midrange somatotypes.

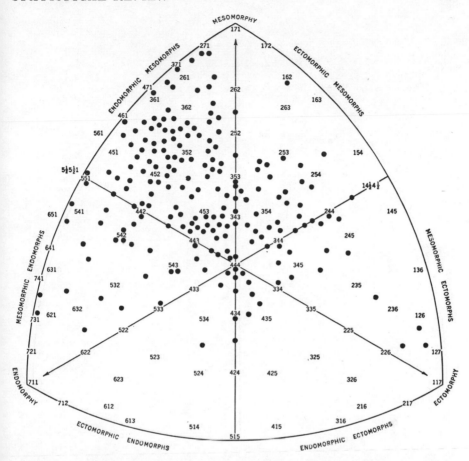

FIGURE 20.   Distribution of Somatotypes for 200 Delinquent Boys. Boston Study.

If a straight line be drawn horizontally across the HGI distribution so as to pass through the point 4–4–4, only 32 cases will be found to fall below the line, or on the mesopenic side. We may call such a line the divider for mesomorphy. It would be parallel to a straight line connecting the point 7–1–1 with the point 1–1–7. If now the divider for ectomorphy be also drawn, likewise through the point 4–4–4 but parallel to a line connecting the point 7–1–1 with the point 1–7–1, it will be found that 153 of the cases fall on the ectopenic side. Similarly, 107 of the cases will be found on the endopenic side of the divider for endomorphy.

As a generalization, then, the 200 delinquent youths are decidedly mesomorphic. They are also decidedly ectopenic. There seems to be no strongly defined tendency either way with respect to endomorphy. It would appear that the level of delinquency we have sampled in this study is one which on

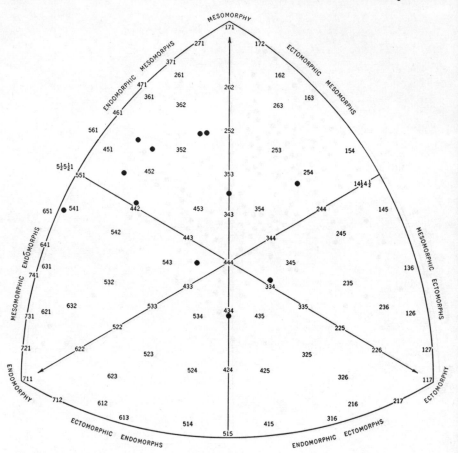

FIGURE 21. Somatotype Distribution for Company A. Platoon 1. Section 1. Mental Insufficiency, Mild. Nos. 1–13.

the whole calls for—or appeals to—a somewhat higher degree of elemental physical vigor than is represented in the college population. This is true, at any rate, in so far as elemental vigor is expressed by the second component. So far as the somatotype is concerned our sample of delinquents, far from being weaklings, are a little on the hefty and meaty side.

Figures 21 through 35 show the somatotype distributions for each of the fifteen sections constituting the whole battalion of 200. The means for the primary components in these fractional somatotype distributions are given in Table 12.

Figure 21. Company A, Platoon 1, Section 1. Mental Insufficiency, Mild: Cases 1–13. This distribution looks like a random sampling from Figure

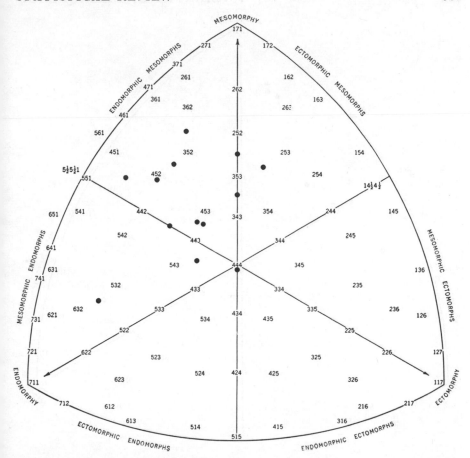

FIGURE 22. Somatotype Distribution for Company A. Platoon 1. Section 2. Mental Insufficiency, Moderate. Nos. 14–26.

20, the distribution for the whole 200. There seems to be no particular "tendency" here in any direction.

Figure 22. Company A, Platoon 1, Section 2. Mental Insufficiency, Moderate: Cases 14–26. Here the distribution of somatotypes appears to have begun to draw just slightly toward the northwest. There are no cases southeast of 4–4–4, and only 1 case is east of that point.

Figure 23. Company A, Platoon 1, Section 3. Mental Insufficiency, Severe: Cases 27–36. There seems to be some accentuation of the migration to the northwest, although with one dramatic exception. The exception is No. 31, who is a feebleminded Scandinavian-Irish 2–3–5½ with a tremendous soma-

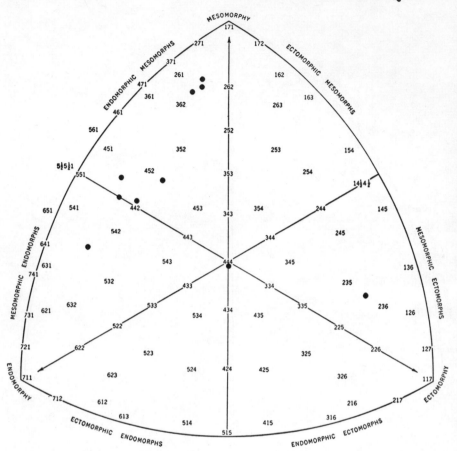

FIGURE 23. Somatotype Distribution for Company A. Platoon 1. Section 3. Mental Insufficiency, Severe. Nos. 27–36.

torosis and one sound or nondelinquent parent (in itself a rare circumstance in Company A).

The mean somatotype for the whole platoon of mental insufficiency is 3.6–4.5–2.5 (Table 12), as compared with 3.5–4.6–2.7 for the battalion as a whole. There is no significant correlation within the delinquent population as we have sampled it, between somatotype and mental insufficiency. There is a slight tendency for the distribution to retreat into the northwest as the gravity of the mental insufficiency advances.

Figures 24, 25, and 26. Company A, Platoon 2, Sections 1, 2, and 3. Medical Insufficiency Mild, Moderate, and Severe: Cases 37–55, 56–70, and 71–82. These three distributions as a whole might very well represent a random sampling from Figure 20. The "moderate" group (Figure 25) seems to con-

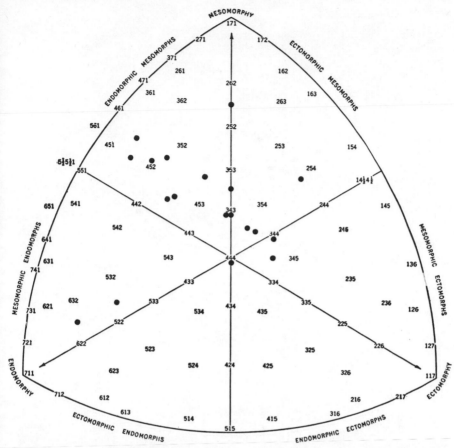

FIGURE 24. Somatotype Distribution for Company A. Platoon 2. Section 1. Medical Insufficiency, Mild. Nos. 37–55.

centrate a little to the northwest but such a tendency is not reflected in either the mild group or the severe group. The mean somatotype for the whole platoon of medical insufficiency is 3.3–4.5–2.8, which also agrees very well with the mean somatotype 3.5–4.6–2.7 for the entire battalion. Certainly there is no significant correlation between degree of medical insufficiency and somatotype within the population of 200.

Figure 27. Company A, Platoon 3. First-Order Psychopathy: Cases 83–100. The striking thing about this distribution is the sharp contrast with the distribution of somatotypes ordinarily found in mental hospitals. Compare Figure 27 with Figure 7 (see p. 70) which represents, so far as I know, a good sample of the psychotic population in general. The two distributions are very different. However, if Figures 8 and 10 (see p. 71 and 73) are also

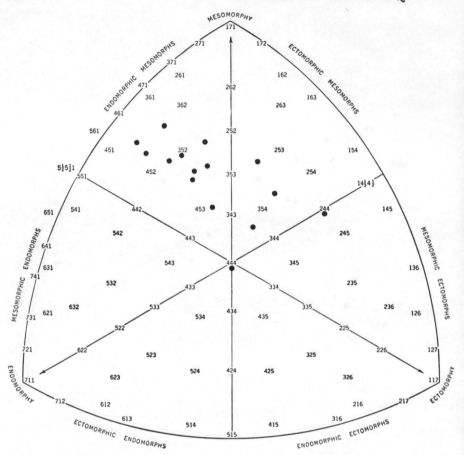

FIGURE 25. Somatotype Distribution for Company A. Platoon 2. Section 2. Medical Insufficiency, Moderate. Nos. 56–70.

examined, a possible answer to that perplexity will present itself. In most mental hospital populations the third psychiatric component is predominant, with a corresponding preponderance of ectomorphy. But among the psychotics and semipsychotics at the HGI the third psychiatric component is conspicuously weak in comparison with the first (see p. 750).

For what so small a sample as 200 is worth the logical inference would seem to be that hebephrenia is not a major problem in civil delinquency, or at any rate not among delinquent youths who have enough persistence and self-assertiveness to reach reasonably decent stature in juvenile troublemaking. At the HGI the predominant *psychiatric* component is the first, with the second falling between the first and third. This order exactly reverses the typical mental hospital order, where the third is overwhelmingly predomi-

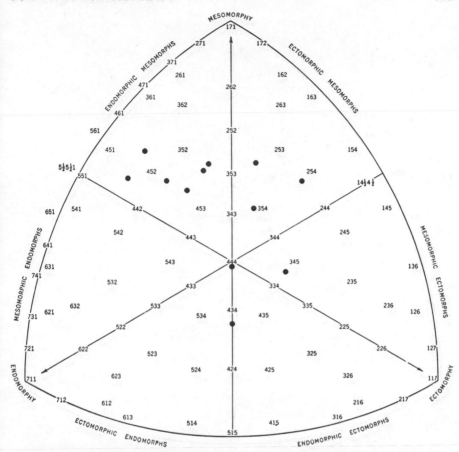

FIGURE 26. Somatotype Distribution for Company A. Platoon 2. Section 3. Medical Insufficiency, Severe. Nos. 71–82.

nant and the first is the rarest. In the mental hospital systems of New York, Massachusetts, and Illinois, taken as an average, only about 8 per cent of psychotics get labeled manic-depressive, or predominantly first psychiatric component. But if the 18 psychotics and semipsychotics from the HGI series were to be given the Kraepelinian typological labels, 13 of them, or 72 per cent, would be predominantly first psychiatric component.

The somatotype distribution for this 18 is so concentrated in the (ecto-penic) west that only 4 cases fall east of the midpoint. The mean somatotype for the platoon is 3.9–4.5–2.7, and this agrees closely with the mean somatotype for the whole 200 except for an elevation of about half a standard deviation in endomorphy.

Figure 28. Company B, Chaplain's Unit. No Delinquency: Cases 101–105. These 5 are well distributed on the somatotype chart, unless it is worthy of

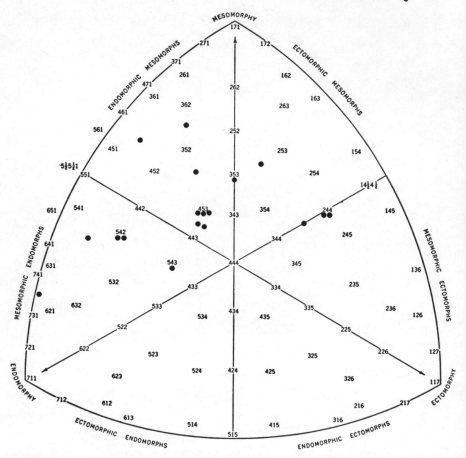

FIGURE 27. Somatotype Distribution for Company A. Platoon 3. First-Order Psychopathy. Nos. 83–100.

note that among the 5 are to be found 3 of the most northeastern half-dozen of the whole 200.

Figure 29. Company B, Platoon 1, Section 1. Second-Order Psychopathy, Bordering on First Order: Cases 106–114. These are the near-psychotics, a very small group which seems to reflect just about the same somatotype distribution as that seen in Figure 27—the psychotics. Only a single case among the 9 falls east of the center point. In this study the psychotics and the near-psychotics are morphologically ectopenic; psychiatrically Dionysian. Mean somatotype: 4.8–4.2–2.3; mean psychiatric index: 3.8–1.8–1.7.

Figure 30. Company B, Platoon 1, Section 2. Second-Order Psychopathy, Minor Somatoroses: Cases 115–132. The somatotype distribution looks very

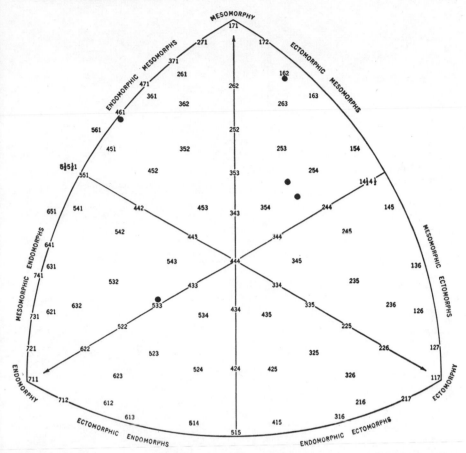

FIGURE 28. Somatotype Distribution for Company B. The Chaplain's Unit. Nos. 101–105.

much like a skeletal outline of that for the whole 200. Here is found one of the 3 extreme ectomorphs of the series—No. 115, a 2–2½–6½—who discovered in time that he *is* an ectomorph and, having given up trying to be what he is not, seems now to be a success. Two of the most extreme mesomorphs of the series are also found here—Nos. 119 and 121. Both of these seem to have discovered that they *are* extreme mesomorphs, and since therefore there is no reason for them to "protest," both have relaxed and have become in their own way successes. Mean somatotype: 3.4–4.8–2.8.

Figure 31. Company B, Platoon 1, Section 3. Second-Order Psychopathy, Comparatively Uncomplicated: Cases 133–143. These 11 cases present a singularly wide spread in their somatotype distribution, including as they do the most extreme endomorph (No. 133), 1 of the most extreme meso-

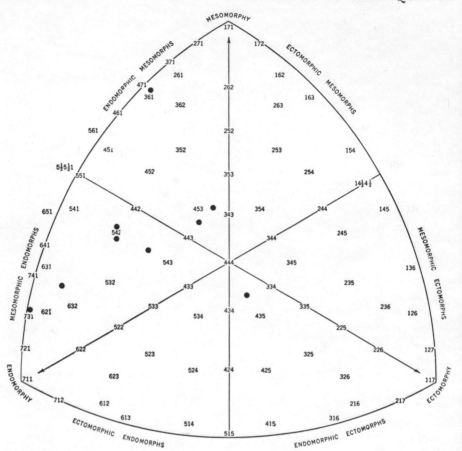

FIGURE 29. Somatotype Distribution for Company B. Platoon 1. Section 1.
Second-Order Psychopathy. Nos. 106–114.

morphs (No. 141), and 2 of the 3 extreme ectomorphs of the series (Nos. 135
and 139). The endomorph is a curiosity in a delinquency series, for he presents what seems to be a perfectly clear case of simple viscerosis—a condition
which rarely gets anybody into trouble (see page 515). The mesomorph was
an extremely somatorotic youth who now seems to have made peace with
his dysplasia and to have "settled down." No. 135 is the only extreme ectomorph in the series who is free of the asthenic characteristic, and his history
is one that might be interpreted as a case of "pure" environmental delinquency. No. 139 is an excellent example of ectomorphy with markedly asthenic structure. Mean somatotype for the section: 3.4–4.3–2.9. This is a
good example of how unenlightening averages may be (by failing to reflect
the spread) when you are dealing with biological distributions.

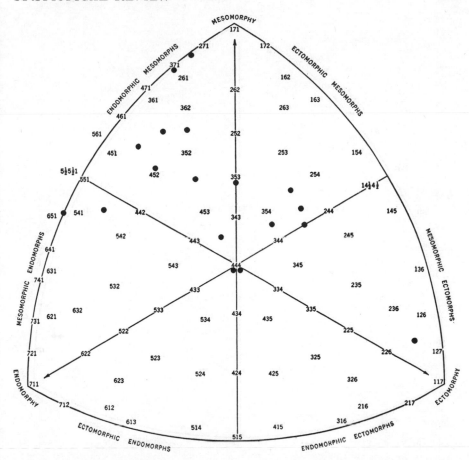

FIGURE 30. Somatotype Distribution for Company B. Platoon 1. Section 2. Second-Order Psychopathy, with Minor Somatorosis. Nos. 115–132.

Figure 32. Company B, Platoon 1, Section 4. Second-Order Psychopathy, with Multiple Complications: Cases 144–164. This distribution has about the same proportions as that for the whole series but lacks the extreme somatotypes. There are no endomorphs, no pronounced ectomorphs, and only 1 extreme mesomorph. The distribution suggests that of catatonic schizophrenia (Figure 11, page 75), which might perhaps better be called "schizophrenia with multiple complications." Or perhaps this group illustrates an entity that should be called "catatonic delinquency." The extreme mesomorph in the group is No. 145, who offers a fine study in Adlerian psychology. Mean somatotype for the section: 3.2–4.8–2.9.

Figure 33. Company B, Platoon 1, Section 5. Second-Order Psychopathy, Cerebrophobes or Alcoholics: Cases 165–167. It would be a little difficult

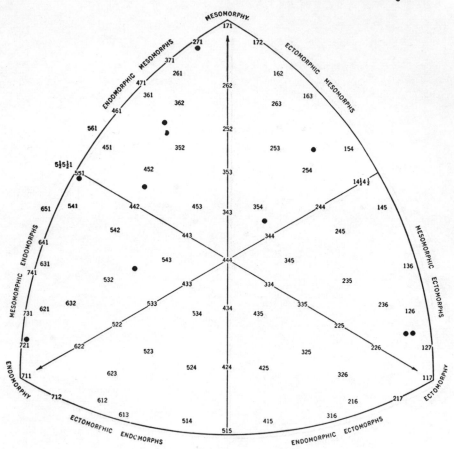

FIGURE 31. Somatotype Distribution for Company B. Platoon 1. Section 3. Second-Order Psychopathy; Comparatively Uncomplicated Cases. Nos. 133–143.

to establish a biological generalization on 3 cases. Among the 200 there appear to be only 3 in whom alcoholism can be called the primary difficulty. Morphologically these are 3 ectopenes—mean somatotype: 4.2–4.5–1.8. Psychiatrically they are well over toward the Dionysian side, mean psychiatric index: 3.0–1.3–1.3. For what such slight evidence is worth, alcoholism might seem to be more associated with *lack* of the third component than with conflict between that component and the second. In earlier studies, however, I have often had the feeling that alcoholism is more of a problem in the "conflict" personalities—the 4–4–4's and related overloaded somatotypes—than in the ectopenes. Possibly the *delinquent* alcoholics will turn out to be morphologically and temperamentally more faithful to Dionysus (who also has been known as Bacchus).

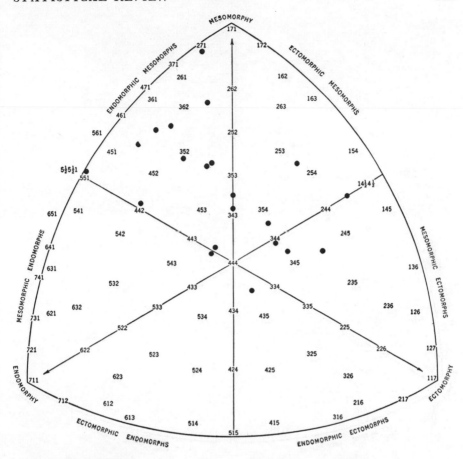

FIGURE 32. Somatotype Distribution for Company B. Platoon 1. Section 4. Second-Order Psychopathy; Cases with Multiple Complications. Nos. 144–164.

Figure 34. Company B, Platoon 1, Section 6. Second-Order Psychopathy, Gynandrophrenes: Cases 168–184. This group which includes the homosexuals, near homosexuals, and psychiatrically gynandrophrenic men, shows one striking morphological characteristic—absence of pronounced strength or weakness in any of the primary components. There is quite a remarkable avoidance of the whole periphery of the somatotype distribution, and this is one delinquent population among whom the somatotypes in the west and northwest do not conspicuously predominate. The problem of homosexuality is one about which we know little. So far as I am aware there has never been even a good morphological study of homosexuals of either sex, and I have long been puzzled to find a clue to the identity of that population. Here may possibly be a clue. Perhaps the males, at any rate, are usually of

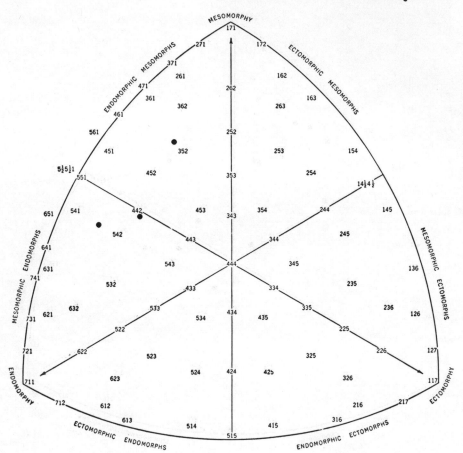

FIGURE 33. Somatotype Distribution for Company B. Platoon 1. Section 5. Alcoholics. Nos. 165–167.

midrange and often of overloaded somatotype, i.e., with somatotypes total-ing 12 or nearly 12 in the three primary components. Among the 17 in this group 7 show somatotypes with total strength of 11½ or more. Such a clue may be rather a remote one, but I think it will hold good that homosexual males are rarely pronounced endomorphs, mesomorphs, or ectomorphs and that they rarely show a pronounced lack of any of these components. It is also worth noting that in the gross sense they are not conspicuously gynan-dromorphic. Study a group of known homosexual males either in a mental hospital or at some recognized homosexual hangout, and you will find that primary gynandromorphy is not one of the conspicuous signs.[1] Mean soma-

[1] For primary gynandromorphy in the male go to a School of Music. I once somatotyped 90 male students in one of the well-known schools of music, and found the mean primary

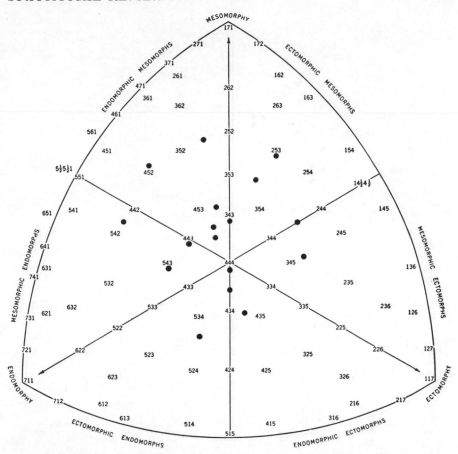

FIGURE 34. Somatotype Distribution for Company B. Platoon 1. Section 6. Gynandrophrenes. Nos. 168–184.

totype for the gynandrophrenes: 3.6–4.1–3.3. This is the lowest mesomorphy and the highest ectomorphy found in any of the delinquent groups, but mesomorphy is still predominant. A very interesting study, in the light of this finding, would be that of a civilly nondelinquent or nontroublesome group of homosexuals. My guess is that the three primary components would tend still further to converge.

Figure 35. Company B, Platoon 2, Primary Criminality: Cases 185–200. This distribution of somatotypes is sufficiently dramatic. The "criminals"

---

g to be 3.2 (mean for the college population, 2.2; standard deviation .8; for the general population the mean is probably a little lower). Among these students of music there were undoubtedly some homosexuals, for many of them were extreme *DAMP RATs*; but if I can recognize the homosexual brand of *DAMP RAT,* it was not common among the extreme gynandromorphs in that particular group.

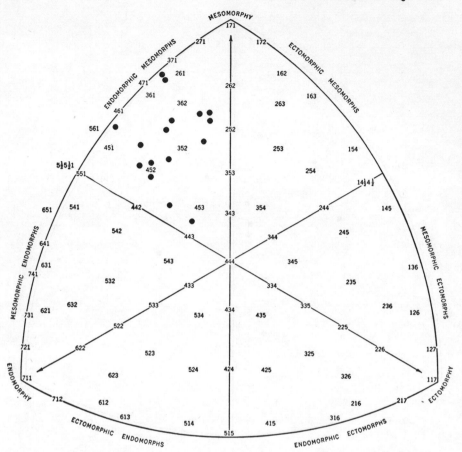

FIGURE 35. Somatotype Distribution for Company B. Platoon B. Platoon 2. "Criminals." Nos. 185–200.

are so remarkably concentrated in the northwest that the entire 16 of them are contained within an area that embraces only about one-eighth of the somatotypes. It is of interest that there are no 7's in mesomorphy among the group but that all except one show a 5 or a 6 in that component. The one exception is a 4½ in mesomorphy, which is still nearly a standard deviation above the general average. Mean somatotype: 3.4–5.4–1.8.

Before drawing any conclusions about the "high correlation" between criminality and a home in the northwest it might be well to ponder some obvious further considerations. Suppose, for example, we were to consider the somatotypes of the 16 most famous generals in history. Where would these somatotypes fall on the distribution? Almost certainly, I think, in just about the same area as the 16 criminals here presented. Very much the same thing will be found, too, if instead of generals we somatotype the most vigorously successful businessmen or the leading politicians. To study the pictures of celebrities of all sorts in *Time* magazine from week to week is an instructive exercise. Take a hundred of them in sequence and jot down what you think the somatotypes are, then plot these on the somatotype chart. If they do not fall mostly in the northwest, you are not a very good somatotyper.

The structural northwest means energetic vitality and freedom from inhibition, two cardinal factors in success at most of the things men undertake. It follows, I suppose, that the great majority of successful men are from the structural northwest; that is to say, men who successfully follow occupations in which success is largely conditioned upon energetic vitality and lack of inhibition. Two professions which I hope are otherwise unrelated appear especially to call for these qualities. They are professional criminality and the writing of fiction. Many dilettantes enter both of these fields or flit about the edges but I have never heard of anybody really "arriving" at either calling who was not structurally well into the northwest. It may be impossible for a person with much cerebrotonia to write good fiction. Consider how hard it must be for the stuff to flow when for every step of the way there are almost an infinity of alternative directions of flow. To be cerebrotonic means to be caught in a maze of alternatives and perhaps that is why cerebrotonic people are forever trying or wanting to write fiction but cannot do it.

The writer of fiction needs to be a bright, buoyant northwesterner. Excellent candidates for the prototype would be H. G. Wells (about 4½–5–1½), Conan Doyle (about 3½–6–1½), Alexander Dumas (probably 5–5–1½), or Erle Stanley Gardner, a currently successful writer of whodunits and (according to one of his friends) about a 3½–5½–1½. From such men, *it flows*. Sometimes cerebrotonics or others, envious of the way it flows, name it vulgarly. But it is often the cerebrotonics who love to drown therein their overly painful awareness.

Figure 35 is not altogether to be explained away. It may be that most—or nearly all—of the persistent criminals who are not demonstrably mental, medical, or psychiatric delinquents do come from the northwest. This would not mean that a northwest somatotype predisposes toward criminality, but it might mean that to make a go of being a criminal requires a certain kind and amount of guts that is usually found only in the northwest.

It should be clear that the somatotype alone has virtually no predictive value. To try and predict such a thing as criminality from the somatotype would be like trying to predict where a bullet will strike by describing only the gun and the bullet and powder charge. You still have to deal with such variables as how the gun is aimed. But to know the latter variable without knowing the former, which are the "constitution" of the weapon itself, leaves you equally without predictive knowledge.

PSYCHIATRY OF DELINQUENCY

If it were to be established that a very large proportion of primary criminals find their biological origins in somatotypes from the northwest, the fact would attach no stigma of criminality to those somatotypes in general but would offer a valuable clue to an understanding of criminality, and hence to its control. Until we know *who* the criminals are, talk of *why* and *how* is premature. Meanwhile Figure 35 may have a practical vocational guidance value. The fact that from the northwest come *all* of those residual criminals among 200 who for a decade have been able resolutely to stay with the profession of criminality may indicate a special northwestern adaptation to the profession. If you are of some other structural pattern it might be well to reconsider any vocational ambition toward professional criminality, or toward professions requiring similar attributes.

3. The Psychiatric Index

The mean psychiatric index for the whole 200 is 2.8–1.9–1.4 (Table 12), or roughly 3–2–1½. To me this was an astonishing finding. I had supposed that the predominant psychiatric component in delinquency would be the third, since most contemporaries have centered their sociological reflections on such an assumption. The psychiatric index 3–2–1½ would place the HGI boys, as an average, in the lower bracket or milder degree of psychoneurotic involvement, with most of the difficulty coming from the northwest, some from the northeast, and comparatively little from the south. Table 13 gives the correlations between the components of the psychiatric index and the primary morphological components.

TABLE 13

CORRELATIONS BETWEEN THE COMPONENTS OF THE
PSYCHIATRIC INDEX AND THE MORPHOLOGICAL
COMPONENTS: HGI SERIES
(N=200)

	1	2	3
Endomorphy	+.45	−.46	+.08
Mesomorphy	+.20	+.001	−.37
Ectomorphy	−.52	+.39	+.34

These correlations lend a degree of further support to the hypothesis advanced in Chapter 2 that the primary psychiatric components may be meaningfully interpretable in relation to poles rotated clockwise 60 degrees ahead of the poles of the morphological distribution. The first psychiatric component, showing a negative correlation with ectomorphy and positive correlations with both endomorphy and mesomorphy, seems as it did in the Elgin study to be oriented to a pole lying somewhere in the direction of the 7–7–1

746

peak. That is to say, the first psychiatric component appears to indicate a recognizable viscerotic-somatorotic cerebropenia even in a population which is not in general psychotic. Such a finding seems greatly to strengthen the likelihood that what we have been calling psychiatric components are far more generalized patterns for the expression of temperament than would be implied by a "disease entity" approach to psychiatric classification. It begins to look as if a Dionysian psychosis or psychoneurosis may be no more a disease than being a 5–5–1 is a disease. The thesis that psychotic and psychoneurotic involvements are levels in a continuum rather than *different things* seems also to grow more tenable.

The second psychiatric component shows a more sharply defined negative correlation with endomorphy than it did in the Elgin Study, and a positive correlation with ectomorphy, but no correlation in this instance with mesomorphy. A good "reason for" this absence of a positive correlation where one would be expected is however easily found by looking at the distribution for mesomorphy. The HGI series is heavily mesomorphic and the distribution is unbalanced toward the upper ranges of the 7-point scale. But with respect to all three of the psychiatric components the distribution is unbalanced in the other direction. On the 7-point scale most of the cases, not being psychotic, pile up at the low end. For these correlations we are thus using only a very narrow range of the scale for one of the variables, in about 80 per cent of the cases, and that tends to mask or lower the correlations. In the case of the correlations with mesomorphy any positive correlation is further masked by the fact that the distributions are skewed in opposite directions. Thus although the positive correlation of the first psychiatric component with mesomorphy is disproportionately lower than that with endomorphy, it does not follow that the Dionysian personality actually derives its pattern disproportionately from an endomorphic influence in this series of cases. And although the second psychiatric component fails here to show the positive correlation with mesomorphy that it does show with ectomorphy, it does not follow that the paranoid personality here derives its pattern independently of the mesomorphic influence.

In this series the third psychiatric component is correlated negatively with mesomorphy and positively with ectomorphy, as in other studies, but the positive correlation with endomorphy is insignificantly low. The fact is that in this series there are very few cases showing any particular strength in the third psychiatric component, and the absence of the hebephrenic mesopenes is one of the most surprising findings of the study.

The most remarkable thing about the psychiatric index is its constancy throughout the battalion. Except for the Chaplain's Unit in Company B (Figure 28), which seems to be made up of temperamentally "normal" individuals (psychiatric index 1–1–1), there is no platoon which fails to reflect the same order of strength in the components that is shown by the battalion as a whole. Only Section 3 in Platoon 2 of Company A—those youths presenting the severest medical insufficiency—reverses the predominance of the first psychiatric component over the second (the *really* sick ones seems to be less Dionysian); and no section in the battalion reverses either the predominance of the second component over the third or of the first over the third.

This homogeneity of expression of the psychiatric components, with the Dionysian factor almost uniformly dominant, is indeed the most conspicuous common bond found in the HGI series. Perhaps that will turn out to be the long-sought highest common factor needed for framing a definition of delinquency. Possibly we shall someday define civil delinquency in terms of the Dionysian and paranoid manifestations of cerebropenia, thus establishing in fact as well as in theory the continuum of psychiatric and criminological practice. A second dimension of the continuum, expressing the continuity of psychiatric and medical practice, has been healthfully emphasized in recent medical education, and this may constitute a parallel medical advance of great importance.

Table 12 gives the means for the components of the psychiatric index within each platoon section of the battalion. The first platoon of Company A—the platoon of mental insufficiency—reflects almost exactly the same psychiatric pattern as does the battalion as a whole. Platoon mean: 2.7–1.7–1.4; battalion mean: 2.8–1.9–1.4. This platoon is feebleminded-Dionysian (mean IQ: 68.7), with a dash of paranoia and only a trace of hebephrenia. How wonderful a pattern that is! Some of the happiest personalities of my acquaintance are to be found among those 36 boys. Free, with delicious resentments, gloriously uninhibited. How tragic that they are so seldom told how happy they are. It brings to mind the legendary stereotype of the beautiful princess reared by jealous guardians to believe that she is ugly. We did what we could at the Inn to correct such an injustice, but in that philanthropy we did not always have cooperation from other agencies.

Platoon 2 of Company A is the platoon of medical insufficiency, and here too the same pattern is found. Platoon mean: 2.4–1.9–1.3. The Dionysian ebullience is perhaps dampened just a little by the medical insufficiency but this appears statistically only in Section 3, where the latter is severe enough to reverse the dominance between the Dionysian and paranoid components. Considering the insufficiencies as a whole—both mental and medical—neither the somatotypes nor the psychiatric indices show any particular departure from those for the battalion as a whole. In other words there is no evidence here that the factor of insufficiency per se is exerting any causative effect on the delinquency. The indication would be, rather, that where delinquency occurs particular patterns of somatotype and of psychiatric index are more likely to be found as constants than are the insufficiencies.

Platoon 3 of Company A—the psychotic platoon—presents another of the interesting findings of the study. The mean psychiatric index (3.7–2.6–2.2) not only exceeds that for the battalion as a whole (2.8–1.9–1.4) in all three components, but exceeds it about equally in all three components. For what so small a number of cases are worth it does not seem to be psychosis, or the psychotic level of involvement, that bears a relationship to getting-into-trouble delinquency, but it seems rather to be a particular pattern or ratio of predominance among the psychiatric components. The psychotics who have a flair for civil delinquency appear to be first of all Dionysian, secondarily paranoid, and only a little hebephrenic.

Turning to Company B, the Chaplain's Unit appears to be innocent of any psychiatric achievement at all, but Section 1 of the first platoon—the 9 boys who border on psychotic territory—present the mean psychiatric index 3.8–1.8–1.7. This is the high-water mark in Dionysianism for the battalion but the paranoid component has fallen back not only far below the mark for the psychotics but a little below the mean for the battalion. In this series of 200 the near-psychotics are jolly extraverts, fully as Dionysian as the psychotics, but they are far less paranoid and also they are markedly less hebephrenic. For what it is worth the indication is that so far as delinquent youths are concerned the difference between a psychotic and a near-psychotic level lies largely in the second and third psychiatric components, that both levels are predominantly and about equally Dionysian.

Section 2 of this first platoon of Company B is made up of 18 youths who present only minor somatoroses. The mean psychiatric index is 2.2–1.6–1.1, which is well below the means for the battalion in all three psychiatric components and may be not far above the means for the general population. The nearly complete absence of the hebephrenic component in these delinquent youngsters who are neither insufficient nor psychotic is one of the most striking findings of the study.

Section 3 has the mean psychiatric index 2.8–2.1–1.1. This is the group of 11 youngsters who show comparatively uncomplicated second-order psychopathy, although somewhat graver psychopathy on the whole than is encountered in Section 2. The first two psychiatric components rise noticeably but the third remains almost at a minimum. In Section 4, which has 21 youths presenting relatively rich complications, all three psychiatric components rise to achieve the mean index 3.1–2.5–1.5, or a total psychiatric involvement averaging 7.1. This places the boys of Section 4, according to the definition advanced on page 89, just about at the middle point of the "psychoneurotic" level of psychiatric involvement. The 21 biographies from No. 144 through No. 164 should constitute collectively an operational definition of the average young male psychoneurotic in our culture—that is to say, if Boston can be considered within the culture.

The 3 alcoholics who make up Section 5 of this first platoon of Company B scarcely constitute a quorum, but for what weight their voices carry they vote for Dionysus by 3.0 to 1.3 to 1.3. The 17 gynandrophrenes of Section 6 present the psychiatric index 2.6–1.9–1.6 and this was as surprising to me as any finding in the study. I had previously entertained what is probably a common mental stereotype concerning the gynandrophrenic personality, with its associated *DAMP RAT*-ism and homosexuality, and had regarded it as of a more furtive and cerebrotic than Dionysian pattern. I had thought of gynandrophrenes as lonely-heart "sissies" who would tend toward the third psychiatric component, rather than as viscerotonic "sharers" or Dionysian "Oxford Groupers." But our gynandrophrenes at the HGI were far from hebephrenic. Their psychiatric indices reflect almost perfectly the mean psychiatric index of the platoon of second-order psychopathy as a whole, and that of the battalion as a whole. Once more the psychiatric index reflecting Dionysian predominance, and paranoid secondary predominance over hebephrenia, seemed to be the most constant element in the delinquency picture at the HGI—constant enough to cut across such seemingly divergent variables as the insufficiencies, the psychoses and psychoneuroses, and the gynandrophrenias.

We come finally to the 16 residual delinquents, or primary criminals, who constitute the second platoon of Company B, and there find the psychiatric index 3.2–2.1–1.0. Dionysianism strongly predominates. The second psychiatric component flourishes moderately. The third is not seen, not even a trace. Among the "criminals" of the HGI series no introvertive oneirophrenia is encountered. None of these 16 could be called "schizzy" or schizoid, and in early life not one was of the shy-and-lonely-child pattern. The outstanding characteristic of the group is extraversional irresponsibility. This is sustained and supported by a degree of watchful hostility sufficient to prevent any yielding of the "inner soul" to the common blandishments of the palliative agencies of our social order, but not sufficient in any instance to raise a question of paranoid involvement at a psychotic level.

In summary, so far as the psychiatric index goes the 200 delinquent youngsters as an average are just barely within the psychoneurotic range arbitrarily set up on page 89 (total strength in the three psychiatric components, 6.1). Their affiliation is strongly northwestern with good support from the northeast and poor support from the south. This affiliative pattern is virtually constant throughout the whole series and is characteristic of the insufficiencies, the first- and second-order psychopathies, and primary criminality alike, the latter group showing almost a perfect 3–2–1 ratio of strength in the primary psychiatric components.

4. Some Other Variables

The long and dismal story of the attempt to correlate single-dimension variables—such as stature, IQ, and so on—with complex variables like delinquency and criminality has been often enough reviewed. Every generation partially forgets what the previous one learned and enthusiasts of our own day have sacrificed themselves to the enterprise of trying to overcome by statistical transmogrification an initial failure of wisdom in the selection of variables. Chapter 2 of the first volume in the series (VHP) briefly chronicles recent adventurings of the sort, and includes some of my own. When younger I paid liberal tribute to this common academic monkey trap, but if energetic correlating of apples with elephants, so to speak, once looked like the road to a psychology it does not look that way now. Variables like stature, strength, IQ, "mental traits," and so on are of the utmost importance in considering the history of any personality—so important, I should say, that to omit any of them from the story is to fail to come up with a psychology—but such variables do not yield useful product-moment correlations with complex criteria like delinquency unless the criteria are in the first place narrowly defined to fit just these variables.

Table 12 (see p. 727) gives the means, within each section of the battalion, for stature, primary and secondary g, primary and secondary t, general strength, hand strength, general athletic ability, and IQ score.

Stature does not appear to be very significantly related to any of the kinds of delinquency here described. The mean for the 200 is 69.0 inches, which is probably very close indeed to the present mean for the adult male population as a whole (see p. 818). The primary criminals, at 67.7, are about an inch and a quarter shorter and this might possibly indicate a significant difference although the platoon of primary criminality has an enrollment of only 16. It will be recalled that Hooton[2] found a large penitentiary population to be of shorter than average stature, and also that within that population he found significant structural and other differences among different kinds of criminals. In a study extending over twelve years Hooton and his assistants made extensive observations on "some 15,000 sub-adult and adult male incarcerated offenders in ten states" (page 371). The excerpts to follow are from the summary chapter at the end of the publication.[3]

Old American criminals, classified according to type of offense, differ profoundly from each other in groups. . . . Some—usually those convicted of crimes of violence against persons—are comparatively large and brutish, presumably equipped with a moderate to excessive amount of sheer animal vigor. . . . Sex offenders include among the rapists no few of full-bodied and probably over-sexed ruffians, but also, and especially in the (nonrapist) sex category, a majority of shrivelled runts. . . . Thieves and burglars tend to be sneaky little constitutional inferiors, either physically stunted or malnourished, or both. . . . Robbers lean to several variants of the wiry, narrow, hard-bitten tough. . . . Forgers and fraudulent criminals are somewhat above the general level of criminal physique although well below that of comparable civilians.

The putatively law-abiding citizen . . . is larger, superior in physique and in most anthropological characters . . . to the White criminal of comparable ethnic and racial origin and drawn from approximately similar occupational levels.

[2] *Crime and the Man* (Harvard University Press, 1939).
[3] Pp. 374–388.

The evidence that the criminals are derived from the baser biological stuff of their various ethnic stocks seems to me to be conclusive. . . .

As in the Old American Whites, [Negro and Negroid] murderers tend to be bigger and brawnier, thieves and burglars smaller and physically less well endowed, bootleggers bulky, square-jawed, thick-necked and broad-faced. . . . Some of the offense proclivities which are associated with various types of physique seem to cut right across racial lines and to manifest themselves in Negroes and Negroids, as in Whites.

So I think that inherently inferior organisms are, for the most part, those which succumb to the adversities or temptations of their social environment and fall into antisocial behavior, and that it is impossible to improve and correct environment to a point at which these flawed and degenerate human beings will be able to succeed. . . . The bad organism sullies a good environment and transforms it into one which is evil.

Hooton repeatedly emphasizes the *physical inadequacy* along with the sense of undersizedness which he almost constantly encountered. One gathers the impression that in ordinary criminals Hooton saw for the most part skinny runts, and there is no doubt that he had good grounds for such an impression. The book has been attacked with violence in certain quarters, but nobody who knows Hooton ever doubted the keenness of his observation or the integrity of his report.

Our series of 200 is much too small for detailed comparison with the Hooton classifications according to types of (current) offense. In his 15,000 cases Hooton sees what appears to be overwhelming evidence of a general breakdown or degeneration of the quality of the structure of the organism. It may be in itself a criminal thing that Hooton did not take standardized photographs of his series, for without such photographs posterity will never be able to reconstruct what these men were—even grossly. A million measurements and a ton of verbal description, however well done, would not perfectly restore even the gross outline of one human organism in three dimensions.

But Hooton is one of a small group of contemporaries who have resolutely persisted in the retention of a modicum of common sense in the formula for academic social science. He considers it a datum of common sense that there are structurally superior and inferior human organisms, and that a relationship must exist between structural and behavioral inferiority. Hooton has searchingly looked for, seen, and tried to objectify his report on such a relationship—this in a period of fanatical suppression of even the secret thought of human physical quality. His report is couched in a somewhat different frame of language from that used in the present project, but without question the general impression he gathered from his 15,000 criminals was similar to our impression from ten years of observation at the HGI. It can be summarized in a single sentence: *Where essential inadequacy is present the inadequacy is well reflected in the observable structure of the organism.*

On this main point the two studies agree. On the minor question of stature there seems to be a difference between the two findings. Our HGI boys were not shorter than the general population, as were Hooton's criminals, although the 8 per cent of "criminals" in the HGI series were shorter.

In connection with the Hooton findings some students have invoked the Adlerian hypothesis that criminal behavior (as well as outstanding achievement) is inclined to be compensatory to some "inferiority" such as short stature. If there is sense in the compensation idea—that the trouble is associated with a too vigorous struggling to overcome or live down a (statural) weakness, we may say that in the HGI series the conspicuous characteristic was not the weakness itself but the vigor and somatotonia with which the compensatory struggle was carried on. Our youngsters in the criminal platoon are of moderately short stature but as a group they are *immoderately* mesomorphic and vigorous. It does not follow, I hope, that mesomorphic vigor is a cause of criminality, but neither would it follow that short stature is in itself such a cause even if it were to be shown that criminals in general are short.

The insufficiency group at the HGI when taken as a whole, both mental and medical, are about half an inch shorter than the mean for the battalion and among this group are many weaklings of every sort. The weaklings seemed to give the whole population at the Inn a halo of pitiful inadequacy. Anyone "making a survey" of delinquency and therefore interviewing or measuring our 200 boys casually (along with thousands of others), and not bothering to take standardized photographs or to work up the biographies —anyone thus looking superficially at our delinquent youngsters would certainly have gathered the impression that they were a weak or degenerate lot. They were ill-dressed and looked "run down at the heel." Casually, they looked weaker and perhaps smaller than they were. I have noticed that inmates of jails and penitentiaries tend to give this same impression. There too a heavy sprinkling of both mental and medical insufficiency is almost always seen, along with psychiatric difficulties and "primary criminality."

The population that Hooton and his associates surveyed yielded data justifying an emphasis both on physical inadequacy and on shortness of stature. Yet I think there is a possibility that Hooton's population of penitentiary inmates did not vary appreciably in either of these respects from our HGI population. There are two good reasons for such a view.

First, no taxonomic attempt was made in the Hooton study to differentiate the sheep from the goats; that is to say, the insufficiency people and the psychopaths from the primary criminals. They were all mixed together and for Hooton's statistical purposes were classified according to the nature of the current charges against them. His classifications were sociological, not psychological. Some of the Hooton groupings may have been composed mainly of a population that in the HGI study would have fallen into the first two platoons—the insufficiency platoons. Other groupings may have had only a sprinkling of such a population. Now there is no doubt that the insufficiency people tend to be weak, flaccid, and undernourished (asthenic). They are often narrow chested, round shouldered, furtive, and bedraggled in appearance, and to get one of them to stand up straight is sometimes quite an undertaking. They are frequently light in weight. It is the spoor of this insufficiency group that you seem to be crossing and recrossing with Hooton, over and over again, as you read *Crime and the Man.* Almost any group of men if mixed generously enough with insufficiency cases would make a below par showing in anthropometric measurements of every sort. In a penitentiary population there is doubtless a larger proportion of insufficient and asthenic men than is to be found elsewhere outside the mental hospitals and the universities, but this does not prove a relationship between insufficiency and primary criminality. The murderers and criminals of violence are anything but insufficient. These are husky, powerful athletes both in the Hooton study and in the HGI series. Possibly it is the insufficient and therefore unwary weaklings of delinquent propensity who are caught oftenest in the police net.

Second, although Hooton's criminals were of shorter recorded stature than the HGI boys the reason for the reported difference might very well be technical. Hooton's assistants who did the measurements for his studies took stature with an instrument called an anthropometer. This is a portable vertical rod with a sliding horizontal bar at the top. The subject stands adjacent to this flexible rod without support and the sliding bar is adjusted to the level of the top of his head. With such a device it is impossible to measure what we call full stature (see p. 32) since the subject has nothing against which to stretch, and when an anthropometer is used diurnal variations in height for the same subjects often amount to an inch or even two inches. These are apparently not true variations in stature but result from differences in posture and in technique. People tend to slump somewhat in their posture late in the day, so that their stature when taken by anthropometer is less, but when full stature is taken properly against a wall scale this diurnal variation is apparently not found (see footnote, p. 32).

I once took stature with an anthropometer for a series of 96 psychiatric patients, using all the care possible to get full stature, and then remeasured the same series of patients against a wall scale. By the latter method the patients averaged 1.7 inches taller. Patients in a mental hospital tend to slump markedly in their postural habits and the differences in stature as revealed by the two techniques are probably greater in such an institution than in the general population, but that may be also true of prison populations. It is possible that if Hooton's criminals had been measured for stature in the way the HGI boys were measured, the mean stature for the entire Hooton series might have been an inch or an inch and a half greater. This would have been enough to vitiate the differences in stature between most of Hooton's subgroups and the HGI series.

Primary g, with the mean for the whole series at 2.7, shows an increment of nearly a standard deviation (0.6) over the primary *g* for a college series of 4,000 and an Army series of 2,500 (see p. 20). This increment in the gynic characteristic is well distributed throughout the battalion except in the last platoon. The criminals alone appear to be of normal or average *g*. In Company A the first platoon (mental insufficiency) shows a primary *g* of 2.6; the second platoon (medical insufficiency), 2.8; the third platoon (psychotics), 2.8. In Company B both the Chaplain's Unit and the first platoon (psychoneurotic) has an average primary *g* of 2.6. Within the first platoon the particularly gynic sections are the first, fifth, and sixth; that is, the section bordering on psychosis, the alcoholics, and the gynandrophrenes.

Secondary g, with the mean for the series at 2.2, fails conspicuously to reflect the increment in primary *g*. I have not recorded secondary *g* for an extensive college series, but in the Army secondary and primary *g* showed almost the same mean for 2,500 cases (see p. 20) and I have no reason to doubt that the same would be true in a typical college population. At the HGI secondary *g* lagged behind primary *g* in every platoon and in all but one of the platoon sections. The gynandrophrenes (Section 6, Platoon 1, Company B) were the sole exception, with a mean secondary *g* of 3.4 which is two standard deviations above the mean for the series. The relationship of gynandrophrenia with secondary *g* is thus seen to be a far closer one than that with primary *g*.

It is a curious thing that homosexuality, in the male at any rate, does not appear to be closely related to primary *g*, although I believe I have never seen a male homosexual without a conspicuous secondary *g*. I have several times tried to pick out the known male homosexuals from a series of somatotype photographs, always without success. If there is a way to detect the fact of male homosexuality from the somatotype photograph alone I have not yet found it. I would expect, however, to achieve a nearly perfect score at recognizing the male homosexuals (as well as other psychoneurotics) as they pass through the Somatotype Performance Test. (With this procedure well established and handled by a smoothly working team of four it would be my guess that it is impossible for a subject to conceal *any kind* of first- or second-order psychopathic tendency. The possible exception, if there is one, would be an individual with a moderate second psychiatric component and with good viscerotonia.)

With respect to secondary *g* the criminals define a dramatic contrast with the gynandrophrenes. The mean for the former is 1.6; that for the latter 3.4. In the persistent criminals of the HGI series there was little of femininity, virtually none of the Peter Pan coyness always encountered in gynandrophrenes and usually encountered in case histories of "criminals" written by psychoanalysts (who almost invariably try to show that the individual was "not really criminal"). In our series there were numerous examples of the "hard-on-the-outside-soft-on-the-inside" pattern, but these were not found among the really persistent criminals. Our criminals meant business, on the whole, and apparently were relatively hard all the way through. This may be an important point. It should not be forgotten that the HGI series represents an extremely well caseworked group of boys. Perhaps we can assume that for this group as a whole the culture in which we live truly exerted itself—put out a best effort—toward rehabilitation and reform. Every one of the 16 in the criminal residue of the series had been sent through the rehabilitative laundry a dozen times or more. Those who remained criminal in the face of all that must have had tough internal resistance to treatment, and it may be significant that among these most toughly resistant ones no softies—no secondary gynandrophrenes—are found. Possibly the conclusion could be justified that where there is secondary gynandrophrenia the internal resistance is less than maximally tough and therefore, so far as criminality is concerned, there is hope. Maybe the psychoanalysts who report on criminality always select cases with secondary *g*.

Next to the criminals, the platoon lowest in secondary *g* is the first in Company A—the feebleminded boys, with mean secondary *g* at 2.0. The third section of this platoon, consisting of the 10 most severely feebleminded, has a mean secondary *g* of 1.6—the same as the primary criminals. Such a finding, insignificant in itself, would seem to support Jung's hypothesis that gynandrophrenia (*anima* in the male, *animus* in the female) may play the role of an enzyme necessary to the development of good intelligence. Except for the Chaplain's Unit the section of gynandrophrenes has the highest average IQ (109) in the series. However, both the Chaplain's Unit and the only other section in the battalion with an average IQ over 100 (Section 3 of Platoon 1 in Company B) shows a very low secondary *g*. The product-moment correlation between *g*, both primary and secondary, and IQ would be low if there is any correlation at all. That the *DAMP RATs* are nearly always bright, in their dilettante way, is undeniable and I would expect a fairly high correlation between *DAMP RATism* and IQ, but in *DAMP RATism* there is at least one other variable in addition to gynandrophrenia and this may possibly be the variable which led Jung to suspect a relationship between gynandrophrenia and intelligence. We have seen enough in our exploration of the constitutional variables, I think, to indicate that a new continent in psychology lies plainly before us, but the real work of exploring these variables has been scarcely begun.

In considering the data for *Primary* and *Secondary t* as given in Table 12 it should be remembered that both of these variables are here expressed in terms of a simple 5-point scale where 3 represents the mean for the general population (1.8 on our conventional 7-point scale) and each unit of variation from 3 represents approximately a standard deviation from this mean. For the HGI series of 200 the mean primary t of 2.6 is thus about .4 of a standard deviation below the mean for the general population, and the mean secondary t of 2.5 is half a standard deviation below. That is our frame of reference for the t component.

The lowest primary t is found in the platoons of insufficiency—2.3 for both the mental and the medical variety, and the insufficiency platoons also have the lowest secondary t—2.1 for the mental variety and 2.3 for medical insufficiency. The criminals, at 2.8, are above the mean for the battalion in primary t and at 2.4 are close to the battalion mean in secondary t. The psychotics are at the battalion mean in primary t (2.6) and are well above that level in secondary t with 2.8. The large psychoneurotic platoon of Company B almost reaches the mean primary t for the general population with 2.9 and is not far below that level in secondary t with its 2.7. The Chaplain's Unit surpasses the mean t, both primary and secondary, for the general population with 3.2 and 3.4 respectively, but that unit has only 5 cases.

The low t of the HGI population as a whole may be of some significance, and the fact that the reservoir of *very* low t is found mainly in the insufficiency platoons rather than among the criminals may shed light on an old controversy in criminology. Lombroso and his brilliant although poorly objectified insights into the constitutional characteristics of criminals have provided two generations of academic social scientists with a sort of push-over whipping boy. When I first taught social psychology in the colleges it was fashionable for a young instructor to get up an easy and very ego-inflative lecture by elucidating to astonished sophomores what a half-wit Cesare Lombroso had been. Lombroso postulated a theory of atavism and a theory of degeneration to explain the differences often observed between criminal groups and noncriminals. The criminals, he thought, presented repulsive or aesthetically inharmonious physical anomalies which were atavistic throwbacks to primitive and inferior breeds of human life. Along with the atavism, and sometimes progressing parallel with it, Lombroso saw "stigmata of degeneration" in the various series of criminals he examined. These stigmata he regarded as indications of degenerative biological failure and devolution—a sort of sliding downhill of the stock. Both the atavistic and the degenerative stigmata were observed by Lombroso to be hereditary and he looked upon these characteristics as indicative of grave and deep-seated biological disorder in our germ plasm. Such a view is so sharply contrasted with the recently fashionable idea that it is "all a matter of postnatal conditioning" that Lombroso has been a fine, almost undefended target for the most forthrightly attack, particularly from young social scientists who read mainly by ear. Had Hooton done no more in his *Crime and the Man* than write his admirable reprimand to the conspiracy to suppress Lombroso from the socio-anthropological consciousness, his book would be worth owning for that first chapter alone. But Hooton is no fanatical defender of Lombroso's claims. He insists only that that marsh has not yet been fully explored. In his words, "The central thesis that the criminal deviates psychologically and anatomically from the normal law-abiding citizen was not proved by Lombroso and the criminal anthropologists, but it has never been refuted."

Hooton saw in a long series of criminals what is very probably the same thing that Lombroso saw. Lombroso tried to give it names—atavistic throwbacks, stigmata of degeneration, aesthetically displeasing variations of body form, skull form, features, limbs, and so on. He supported his designations with profuse but eclectic masses of anthropometric and descriptive data. Hooton ordered his material in convenient statistical categories but I believe that he felt in the end that the essence of the real differences he saw still eluded the categories, as Lombroso must also have felt.

At the HGI, and in various penitentiaries, I too have probably seen the same thing that Lombroso and Hooton saw, and I have felt the same frustration because of profound inadequacy both in descriptive vocabulary and in available statistification procedure to reflect and set down for educational purposes what was manifestly there. The concept of the *t* component is perhaps no more than a temporary makeshift summoned up to meet the frustration. I entertain no notion, and neither does Hooton, that criminals *as such* are any different from anybody else but I am aware, as Hooton has been, that the criminal population as a group is everywhere very kind to us socio-anthropologists and psychologists. It is gracious enough to include in its presentation statistically large samples of something that ought to be interesting and perhaps instructive for us all to look at and study. The process of human change is going on before our eyes, and sweeps us along like helpless drift on the slow current of a mighty river. The HGI population, like Lombroso's and Hooton's populations, is somehow offering an inkling—possibly a definitive clue—as to how and whither the current is running. Our job is to read the clue—into a language that posterity can handle.

Lombroso saw these things, and under difficult circumstances he gave his life energies almost heroically to the task of building a contribution to such a language. As Hooton says, no blame can be attached to Lombroso for not using the modern methods of statistical analysis which were developed later by Karl Pearson and the biometricians. It is true that the contribution Lombroso did make has not grown into a language tool that anybody can handle effectively at the task of describing in differential terms a human personality, but neither has the contribution of anyone else, yet. No tool of language can meet that task if it misses, or fails to lay hold on, the *qualitative* differences in human beings that Lombroso was trying to describe. Nearly all of the conventional text material in the social sciences fails to touch the heart of this problem. To read it is like fishing with no hook, but in a sea where game fish abound. That is frustrating. To read Lombroso is to feel the strike of powerful and dangerous game. Lombroso hooked something of tremendous importance. The tackle he had was insufficient to land it. Hooton went after the same fish with better but still with insufficient tackle. He got a scale or two. A wise and eye-twinkling man, Hooton knows very well that the tackle we now have is still far short of sufficient for the under-taking. But Hooton knows where the big fish lives and if we had ten thousand Hootons we might catch a fish the taste of whose flesh would cure the lust for war and for delinquency.

The *t* component is a very small contribution to the language for which we still must grope. It might be compared to a meer sharpening of the barb of Hooton's hook—a slight thing indeed. Yet the fact may be of interest to future fishermen that the *t* component concept, when applied to a population such as the HGI boys, seems to catch hold of the same general phenomenon that both Lombroso and Hooton have brought near to the surface of consciousness with different tackle.

The most useful finding in the HGI study may be the clear-cut fact that the boys of the lowest *t* present primarily insufficiency and not primarily criminality. This may mean that what both Lombroso and Hooton saw so clearly in their penitentiary populations was the spoor of insufficiency and not that of anything that needs to be called criminality. There may be no such thing as criminality, and I think it is quite possible that we will forget that concept when as a body of social scientists we at length face the meaning and the reality of human insufficiency. If the hypothesis can be tentatively accepted, for purposes of discussion, that Lombroso and Hooton were really dealing with stigmata of insufficiency, i.e., with indications of low *t,* then their findings not only accord well with one another but also with the HGI study, and the three contributions are from somewhat different angles reflections of the same phenomenon. Moreover the three different reflections, even after passing through the refractive media of quite differently trained minds, are in remarkably close agreement. All three center the focus of the problem of crime control unequivocally on the practical matter of selective breeding. If the HGI study offers any particular advance beyond the Lombroso and the Hooton contributions the advance will lie in a further sharpening of the tools of constitutional description. These tools need to be put in the best possible order for in the end it will be their validity and efficacy that will determine the outcome of the inevitable struggle to combat the progress of biological degeneration of the human organism.

In *General Strength* the mean for the HGI population falls at 3.0, which is exactly the assumed mean for the population at large. The platoon of mental insufficiency is of average general strength (3.0) and the platoon of medical insufficiency is the weakest in the battalion (2.5). The psychotics are at 2.7 and the psychoneurotic platoon returns to average general strength (3.1) despite the weakness (2.3) encountered in its sixth section which is composed of 17 gynandrophrenes. The criminals, at 3.9, are the strong boys of the battalion with the Chaplain's Unit not far behind at 3.6.

In *Hand Strength* the battalion as a whole falls off a little to a mean of 2.7. The mental insufficiency platoon is weak (2.4), the medical insufficiency platoon weaker (2.2), and the psychotics are in this variable the weakest unit of the battalion (2.1). The psychoneurotic platoon at 2.8 is above the mean for the battalion, and it may be worth noting that the gynandrophrene section, at 2.6, is the only section in this battalion that stands higher in hand strength than in general strength. The honor of having the strongest hands in the battalion falls to the Chaplain's Unit, at 3.6, while the criminals drop back in this variable to 3.1, well above the battalion mean but far below their high score in general strength. In general strength the criminals surpass the gynandrophrenes by 3.9 to 2.3, but in hand strength only by 3.1 to 2.6.

In *General Athletic Ability* the battalion as a whole falls back to 2.5 with the heavy decrement conspicuous throughout Company A. The platoon of medical insufficiency reaches the extreme low of 1.7, with the psychotics at 1.9 and the platoon of mental insufficiency at 2.3. The criminals at 3.9 are the athletic champions, with the Chaplain's Unit at 3.8 furnishing good competition. The psychoneurotic platoon averages 2.8 in this variable although handicapped by the inclusion of two sections that make a poor athletic showing—the near psychotics (Section 1 at 2.2) and the gynandrophrenes (Section 6 at 2.2).

On reviewing the three criteria of physical prowess—general strength, hand strength, and general athletic ability—it becomes evident that Company A as a whole is far below par in all three while Company B as a whole appears to be above the average endowment in all three. Here again, then, we encounter a strong indication that a delinquent or criminal population needs to be analyzed into its primary constituent elements before any very useful generalizations can be drawn from a study of it. Certainly the first step in such an analysis needs to be one which separates the constitutional weaklings—the cases of insufficiency—from the mentally and physically competent. When this step was taken, the latter group (at the HGI) turned out to be of normal physical size and strength, and somewhat above the normal average in athletic ability. We do not know what the results would have been if the same step had been taken in the Lombroso and Hooton studies, but the HGI findings in this respect may further support the possibility that what both Lombroso and Hooton were reporting was a rich vein of insufficiency in the criminal ore they assayed.

The second analytic or segregational step that we took in the HGI study of criminality—a precipitating out of the psychotic and then of the psychoneurotic cases—did not yield such clear-cut results so far as the criteria of physical prowess go. The psychotics are grossly deficient enough in athletic ability (although not in general strength) but the psychoneurotic platoon contains groups sharply divergent by these criteria and the divergent groups cancel one another out. What that second step did accomplish however was fairly sharp definition of the residual group of criminals and I think that the high level of physical prowess in this criminal group indicates two things: (1) That all of those studies which have reported physical inadequacy of any kind among criminals would have done well to have first precipitated out the cases of gross insufficiency. There are scores of such studies. Lombroso's and Hooton's are only examples so far as that finding goes. (2) That the residual of what is here called primary criminality is probably a small one not only at the HGI but elsewhere, perhaps in all of the penal institutions where constitutional research has been carried out.

At the HGI we found only 8 per cent classifiable as primary criminals. When this 8 per cent was examined apart from the rest of the population there, we found not physical inferiority but (grossly at least) physical superiority. It should follow that if primary criminality (by our definition) had been predominant in the other criminological populations that have been studied, or even if it had been *very* conspicuously present, those populations would not have presented predominantly the criteria of physical inferiority and insufficiency that have almost always been reported. I would hazard the guess, therefore, that primary criminality is comparatively rare in the penal institutions, that only a small minority of the inmates of most of these institutions are residual criminals.

The mean *IQ Scores* within the different units of the HGI battalion are also given in Table 12. The mean for the battalion is 89.2, corrected to the 16-year level. This is theoretically about 10 points below the mean for the general population, since IQ 100 is by definition normal or average, but there is good ground for doubting that the true average for the general population (including the feebleminded) ever was that high, and moreover nobody knows just how much the average IQ in this country has declined since 1916 when Terman attempted to standardize the meaning of IQ 100. In comparing the IQ's of our HGI boys with other reported IQ's it should be remembered too that in many quarters there has been a patriotic tendency toward "mild inflation" of the IQ. Some mental test clincis calculate the IQ on a 14-year basis instead of the 16-year basis, and in general it has commended itself as better business to report high than to report low IQ's. If your IQ has been reported to be 178.4 do not be too certain therefore that you have twice the IQ stature of the HGI average.

The platoon of Mental Insufficiency is by definition of low IQ, with the mean at 68.7. The severely feebleminded section of that platoon has a mean of 59.0. The mean IQ for the medically insufficient is 85.6 and for the psychotics 92.1. In Company B the psychoneurotic platoon almost reaches "normal" at 99.2, being helped in that direction by the gynandrophrene section which has a mean IQ of 109.4. The criminals fall back to 85.8 and the Chaplain's Unit carries the day for *alma mater* with 111.6.

The most interesting item in this series of data is doubtless the rather low standing of the criminal platoon. Here is one variable which does appear to reflect a real inadequacy on the part of the criminal group, so far as the HGI series can be considered representative. Although of normal or superior energy, strength, and athletic ability, the criminals are of significantly inferior IQ. The ancient question will be raised as to whether the bright criminals do not usually get away, and I cannot answer that. Hooton discusses it with some heat. He says (*Crime and the Man*, p. 12) ". . . it is necessary to deal with one stupid, perennial objection advanced against the study of criminals . . . that prisoners represent only the failures of the criminal population. It implies that the inferior physical, mental or sociological qualities of incarcerated felons are not shared by the more clever criminals who escape arrest and conviction."

Hooton scoffs at the objection, and perhaps rightly, but he does not answer it convincingly. He tries to brush it aside with two observations: (1) "More than half of the criminals now in jail have been there before, and most of them will be there again. Hence a large, but indeterminate, proportion of the crimes presently to be committed will be due to the activities of the convicts who are going to be paroled or released." (2) "Again, the presumption that successful criminals are rarely or never convicted is almost certainly incorrect. I doubt that any considerable part of the crimes committed in the United States is perpetrated by persons who steadily pursue antisocial careers without ever falling into the clutches of the law. I do not believe that many clever men commit crimes, and that only a few of the stupid are caught." To some this may sound a little like an avowal of faith in God and the Harvard overseers and at best it does not prove the point, but as Hooton goes on to indicate, it would be no reason to neglect the study of criminals that *are* caught even if we knew that most of the biggest and best ones got away.

In summary, the HGI criminals are pronouncedly ectopenic mesomorphs with about average endomorphy. Psychiatrically they are Dionysian with a mild sustaining paranoia and they are almost aseptically free of the third psychiatric component. They are of moderately short stature as an average. They are of average primary g but of low secondary g, of almost average primary t but of lower secondary t. In general strength and general athletic ability they excel almost conspicuously but they are of only average hand strength. In IQ their mean is at about the level sometimes called normal subaverage.

5. The Parental Backgrounds

One of the frustrations associated with the study arises from the fact that our knowledge of the immediate antecedents of the youths is as it were chopped off with such disappointing abruptness. Whenever I read over a few of the cases there is the same sense of vexing frustration that I used to feel as a small boy when taken into the deep woods on hunting trips. Always we turned back and started for home just when the really exciting part of the adventure seemed ready to begin. And I have found in later years that human life as a whole seems often to culminate in that kind of frustration.

We were able to find out much about the parents of these youngsters but not enough. Information on grandparents is scanty. Back of the grandparents little is known and there are only vague indications. What we did learn of antecedents was illuminating and can be summarized in the simple statement that *on the whole the parents of the 200 must have been fully as delinquent as the boys themselves.* This is to use the concept delinquency in its comprehensive sense and to include medical and psychiatric as well as civil or sociological shortcomings. Table 14 presents a summary of the parental backgrounds of the 200 youths under eleven headings, as follows:

1. BURGEONED. By this is meant simply a conspicuous heaviness of body. Early in the investigation of parental background we began to encounter comments by social agency representatives to the effect that one or both parents—usually the mother—had grown very heavy, were of unusually full-bodied or massive physique, had become grossly obese, were of ample proportions, and so on. Many of these comments from agency records appear in the paragraph on *Origins and Family.* They are of too frequent occurrence to be a statistical accident although conclusions as to possible meaning or significance would be premature. The point of interest is that a large number of social workers—several hundred of them from more than three hundred agencies—reiterated the common impression of a certain *burgeoned* or luxuriantly full-bodied characteristic in the mothers in particular. On reading the case histories of our youngsters and their families, as these are written up in the social agency records, it is difficult to prevent the emergence into consciousness of a kind of mental stereotype of hefty, full-bodied, often blowsy parentage. It is usually the maternal parent that is so described. Early in the study we had the feeling that the social workers *didn't like* the mothers of their clients. We wondered if the frequent vilification of the mother might not be an expression of the current Freudian theological outlook which nearly always finds the mother at the bottom of sin in general. There may be something in this idea and we might have been tempted to dismiss further thought of the "burgeoned mothers" had we not seen a few score of them. Those we saw were a burgeoned lot, certainly heav-

ier, both endomorphically and mesomorphically, than the general population as I know it.

In Table 14 an *M* indicates that the available social records refer to the mother as unusually heavy, coarse, muscular, or obese. An *F* indicates the same with reference to the father.

2. DIED, DECADE OF LIFE. Indicates that one of the parents is known to have died. *M* for mother, *F* for father. The numeral following the letter indicates the decade of life in which the death occurred. Thus *M-4* means that the mother died during her fourth decade.

3. PATHOLOGY OF THE BURGEONED ESTATE (CVR). Pathology commonly associated with the vigorous or burgeoned physique. Usually a cardiovascular-renal picture. A check indicates that there is a history, in one or both of the parents, of organic heart disease, kidney disease, or abnormally high blood pressure with some kind of clinical symptomatology. In medical parlance the *CVR* syndrome usually refers to the presence of an already full-blown complex of symptoms associated with high blood pressure, heart disease, and renal involvement. Here the concept is used in not quite that technical sense but more broadly to indicate that some of the symptoms of the *CVR* syndrome have appeared and that the individual has had medical attention therefor. *CVR* symptoms are in general characteristic of hefty or plethoric people. Pathological hypertension, apoplexy (cerebral hemorrhage), the sudden coronary episode (as distinguished from *angina pectoris*), and nephritis are the principal medical entities associated with what the profession refers to as a *CVR* picture. People presenting early signs of the *CVR* picture tend to be vital, vigorous, overenergized, and possibly overblooded. That is to say, they may have literally too much blood. As a group they present an antithesis to a sector of the population that could be called constitutionally anemic or weak, and their presence in the population probably explains the historically cyclic popularity of bleeding or leeching for relief from many illnesses. For them, such a treatment is undoubtedly beneficial.

4. PATHOLOGY OF THE ASTHENIC ESTATE (PPPPT). Pathology usually associated with asthenic inadequacy. History in one or both parents of weakness, inadequacy, chronic sickness of a general or vague nature, associated with low energy. Usually associated also with low *t*, low blood pressure, and with poor muscular tone. These people are the "neurasthenics." Draper used to call them the *PPPPT*'s (see p. 23). Whatever else may be true of them they are a discernibly different population from the overly vigorous and the burgeoned. If the latter may be compared to tires carrying too much pressure and therefore inclined to blow out early, the asthenics are underinflated. They are the flat tires of the population. All biological dichotomies are too simple, of course. There is an overlapping between the burgeoning-hyperemic family of diseases and the asthenic-anemic family of diseases. Many individuals from the latter group turn up with some kind of cardiac or renal disorder,

and a few present hereditary hypertension along with the general picture of weakness and low energy. There are dyscrasias of predisposition to pathology as well as dysplasias of morphology. Yet science usually starts with dichotomies and there *is* a dichotomy here. It seems to embrace two different directions of departure from a biological balance; a departure in the direction of too big a head of steam, and another in the direction of insufficient steam.

5. PATHOLOGY OF C-SED-T. *C* for cancer, *S* for syphilis, *E* for epilepsy, *D* for diabetes, *T* for tuberculosis. These appear to be the five "more or less constitutional" disorders of a specific and serious nature most prevalent among the parents of the HGI 200. A check in this column indicates that one of the parents has died of cancer, or has died or been seriously and chronically ill with one of the other four entities of the group. The specific nature of the illness in most instances, in so far as is deemed safe from the standpoint of protection of the identity of the persons concerned, is indicated in the paragraph on *Origins and Family*. For this study, the diagnosis of cancer has not been accepted except in fatal instances. Cases of luetic infection (syphilis), epilepsy, diabetes, and tuberculosis have been included only when the records indicate that the condition existed prior to the birth of the youngster in question. In five instances in the series a check in the *C-SED-T* column indicates not one of the specific entities listed but some imperfectly diagnosed condition which has been continuous or recurrent and is strongly suggestive of or seems related to one of the latter. The question as to whether or not a constitutional factor is involved in all of these clinical entities is pertinent to the theme of the discussion but is at present controversial. One of the main objectives of the Human Constitution Series as a whole is to shed light on this question, but elaboration of the matter is planned for a later volume.[4]

6. MENTAL INSUFFICIENCY. Indication that one or both parents are described in social agency records as feebleminded or of low IQ. There is not in all instances documentary evidence that the parent in question was technically feebleminded, although such evidence is on record in many of the cases—this evidence is usually indicated in the paragraph on *Origins and Family*. Often there are no records of mental testing of the parent but merely the recorded opinion of psychiatrists and social workers at one or more of the agencies where the parent has been known. However these opinions are not casual and in the course of the study we did not encounter an instance in which a social worker had made such a commitment regarding a foreign-born parent where a language factor could have induced, in itself, a false impression of mental insufficiency. Social agencies are democracy conscious. They do not often question the *intelligence* of their clients without excellent justification.

7. ALCOHOLISM. Indication that one or both parents have been in some

---

[4] Tentatively called *Introduction to Constitutional Medicine*.

kind of medical or civil difficulty associated with drunkenness. In most cases
—in nearly all of those in which a check is also found in the final column
labeled *Civil Delinquency*—there have been arrests on this charge. Drunkenness is by far the commonest "cause of arrest" for parents of our 200 boys
but that does not mean that alcoholism was the primary problem any more
than it is the primary problem in the case of the boys. Alcoholism is what
appears most frequently on the court records of the parents, and in the final
summary, a generation hence, it doubtless will be the most frequent court
charge of record against our 200. But I hope that this statistical datum will
not lead any reader of the book to conclude that delinquency can be overcome by a campaign against alcoholism. A railroad once employed a statistician to study the causes of accidents and to recommend steps for reducing
the number of them. The statistician found that more people were killed
in the rear car of a train than in any other car. He recommended removal of
the rear car from all trains. His influence was felt, too, in the Volstead Act
of 1919.

8. IRRESPONSIBLE REPRODUCTION.   This means literally what the term implies. Reproduction without responsibility. In many instances it means illegitimacy, or without legal responsibility. These cases are indicated in the
text, under *Origins and Family*. But in other cases it means without personal, moral, or economic responsibility. Where there has been continued
reproduction, with older children already removed from the family because
of parental drunkenness, squalid conditions, mistreatment of the children
and the like, in short where social agencies have already requisitioned civil
authority to remove children from a parent or set of parents *and reproduction has still continued,* I have called it irresponsible or delinquent reproduction. In most of such instances the delinquently reproducing parents
have had institutional sanction—they have had the rationalization that the
law tacitly approved and that some religious institution openly approved
the reproductive delinquency. But this does not mean that the reproduction
was any the less delinquent. It may mean that the law is lax and that there
is a delinquent factor in the religious institutions, but these considerations
are extraneous—they are *in addition to* the delinquency of individuals who
use them to excuse their own irresponsibility. Institutions follow far behind
the growth of knowledge, and one kind of delinquency consists in failure to
be influenced by the latter *despite the institutional support of such a failure.*
This is Promethean delinquency. Failure to obey the law may be considered
Epimethean delinquency. Irresponsible reproduction illustrates both kinds
of delinquency. When it involves departure from the law, it is Epimethean.
When it involves departure from good sense, even though supported by institutional sanction, it is Promethean delinquency.

9. DISTRIBUTION OF PARENTAL DELINQUENCY.   A check in the subcolumn
headed *Insuf.* indicates that one or both parents would score at least 1 on

Insufficiency as this was defined on page 105. That is to say, there is good evidence of a serious mental or medical shortcoming in one or both parents, that this is not healthy parental stock on both sides. A check in the subcolumn headed *Psychiatric* indicates that one or both parents have been under psychiatric observation or treatment, and that there is recorded opinion to the effect that a psychiatric condition of some kind exists. This does not necessarily imply that a parent is psychotic but it does indicate that one or both parents are sufficiently "psychoneurotic" to score at least 1 in psychiatric delinquency as this was defined on page 108. The subheading *Civil* indicates that one or both parents have been known to be delinquent under the law. In the case of parental delinquency of record we do not undertake to make a judgment as to its nature or cause, as we do to some extent in the case of the youngsters. Most of our information on the parents is indirect.

10. TOTAL D, PARENTAL. An estimate of what the score for Total D might have been—taken as an average for the two parents—if we had had the privilege of the same direct contact with them, and the comparatively intimate knowledge of them, that we enjoyed in the case of the boys. This of course is anything but a satisfactory datum. We do not have enough information on these parents and therein lies the main frustration of the project. But we do have some information on nearly all of them and in many cases have had available several volumes of intimate biography. On some of these parents, and on the families from which they come, the social agency records are sufficiently voluminous that the services of an able-bodied man (or gynandroid woman) are required to lift them from the files and carry them to a reading desk. On a few there is only a paragraph or two of general information kindly forwarded from a distant city. For the purposes of Table 14, when the information on a parent has seemed too scanty to permit of a reasonably accurate estimate of *Total D*, no estimate is made for that parent. If our information on *both* parents is too scanty, the estimate is omitted altogether. When the available information on both parents is deemed sufficient for a reasonable estimate the numeral expressing an average of the two estimates is followed by the letters *MF*. If only the mother is included in the estimate, the numeral is followed by *M*. If only the father is included, the numeral is followed by *F*.

11. TOTAL D, FILIAL. Same as *Total D* in Table 11. Repeated here for individual comparison with *Parental D*. In comparing the two *D* scores, parental and filial, it will be borne in mind that we know a great deal more about the children than about the parents, and that lack of knowledge of the fathers is the greatest weakness. In many cases we know only that there *was* a father and that he must have been irresponsible to a greater or less degree. Some of these irresponsible fathers were possibly more delinquent than the mothers, about whom we know. Perhaps if the unknown fathers were included, the total *D*'s for the parents would be higher than they are, or per-

haps they would be lower. This would depend on how many of the fathers went to Harvard.

TABLE 14

THE PARENTAL BACKGROUNDS

Predominant weakness	Company	Platoon	Section	No.	1. Burgeoned	2. Died, decade of life	3. Pathology of the burgeoned estate (CVR)	4. Pathology of the asthenic estate (PPPPT)	5. Pathology of C-SED-T	6. Mental insufficiency	7. Alcoholism	8. Irresponsible reproduction	9. Insufficiency	Psychiatric	Civil	10. Total D, parental	11. Total D, filial
Mental insufficiency	A	1	1	1	M	M-4	√	√						√		3 MF	2
				2		M-4 F-7	√							√		3 MF	3
				3					√	√	√	√	√	√	√	7 M	5
				4	M	M-4	√		√	√	√		√	√		6 M	6
				5		M-4		√	√	√		√	√		√	6 M	6
				6						√		√	√			—	6
				7	M		F-5	√		√		√	√	√	√	7 MF	6
				8	M			√	√	√		√	√	√	√	6 M	7
				9						√		√	√	√		7 M	7
				10			F-5	√		√			√	√		4 MF	7
				11	M F			√		√			√	√		3 MF	7
				12	F					√		√	√			—	8
				13	M	M-4	√		√	√		√	√		√	6 M	8
				14	M			√	√	√			√	√		5 MF	7
				15				√	√	√	√	√	√	√	√	9 M	7
				16						√	√	√	√	√	√	7 M	7
				17	M					√	√	√	√	√	√	7 MF	7
				18			√			√	√		√	√		8 M	7
				19	M		F-6	√		√	√	√	√	√	√	8 MF	7
				20					√	√	√	√	√	√	√	7 MF	7
				21	F			√		√		√	√		√	8 MF	8
				22	M F		F-4	√		√	√	√	√	√	√	9 MF	8
				23	M					√	√	√	√		√	6 MF	8
				24	M	M-4	√		√	√	√	√	√	√	√	8 MF	9
				25	M	M-4	√		√	√	√		√	√	√	8 MF	9
				26	M	M-4	√		√	√			√	√		8 MF	9
			3	27	M F			√		√	√	√	√	√	√	9 M	6
				28	M F			√		√	√	√	√	√	√	7 M	6
				29	M	M-5			√	√	√	√	√	√	√	8 MF	7
				30				√		√	√	√	√	√	√	7 MF	7
				31						√	√	√	√	√	√	5 MF	7
				32			M-3 F-4	√	√	√	√		√	√		8 MF	8
				33			M-4 F-4	√	√	√			√	√		8 MF	8
				34						√	√	√	√			—	6
				35						√		√	√	√		—	8
Medical insufficiency	A	2	1	36	M F	M-4 F-4	√	√	√	√			√	√		9 MF	9
				37				√					√	√		5 MF	2
				38			F-3							√		0 MF	3
				39									√			1 MF	2
				40				√		√			√	√	√	5 MF	3
				41	M	M-5		√					√	√		4 MF	3
				42	M			√			√		√	√		5 MF	4
				43	M F		√			√			√	√		5 MF	5
				44	M							√			√	5 M	5
				45	M		√				√	√		√	√	7 MF	5
				46	M		F-4				√			√		5 MF	6
				47	F			√			√		√			5 MF	6
				48						√		√	√		√	—	6
				49	M		F-5	√		√	√		√	√	√	7 MF	6
				50	M F			√					√	√	√	4 MF	6
				51			M-4	√			√	√	√		√	7 MF	6

TABLE 14

THE PARENTAL BACKGROUNDS (*Continued*)

Predominant weakness	Company	Platoon	Section		1. Burgeoned	2. Died, decade of life	3. Pathology of the burgeoned estate (CVR)	4. Pathology of the asthenic estate (PPPT)	5. Pathology of C-SED-T	6. Mental insufficiency	7. Alcoholism	8. Irresponsible reproduction	9. Insufficiency	Psychiatric	Civil	10. Total D, parental	11. Total D, filial
				52	M F	M-5	√		√				√	√		6 MF	6
				53			√		√			√	√	√	√	7 MF	6
				54	M				√		√		√,	√		5 MF	7
				55		M-4		√	√		√		√		√	7 MF	7
			2	56		F-5	√	√	√			√	√	√	√	7 MF	5
				57	M		√				√		√	√		5 M	6
				58	M	F-6	√	√		√			√	√		6 MF	6
				59	M		√	√	√				√	√		8 MF	7
				60		M-2 F-3				√	√		√		√	—	7
				61	M F	F-5	√		√	√			√	√		7 MF	7
				62	M		√					√	√		√	7 MF	7
				63	M	M-4		√	√	√		√	√	√	√	8 MF	8
				64	M		√				√	√	√	√	√	6 MF	8
				65	M	M-4 F-4	√	√		√	√	√	√	√	√	9 MF	8
				66									√	√		4 MF	6
				67	M	M-5 F-5	√	√	√	√	√	√	√	√		8 MF	7
				68	F	M-4 F-5	√	√		√			√	√		8 MF	8
				69	M F					√	√		√		√	7 M	8
				70	M F	F-6	√		√	√			√			7 MF	9
			3	71	M F				√	√	√	√	√	√	√	8 MF	5
				72		M-4			√	√		√	√	√		7 M	5
				73					√	√	√		√	√		4 MF	6
				74	M	M-4 F-5			√	√			√			7 MF	6
				75	M		√	√			√		√		√	7 MF	7
				76		M-4 F-5			√	√	√	√	√	√		8 MF	8
				77	M	M-4			√	√			√			7 MF	8
				78	M F		F-5	√	√		√			√			7 MF	9
				79	M		F-5	√	√	√				√			7 MF	9
				80	M					√	√	√	√			7 MF	9
				81	M	M-4			√	√		√	√			8 MF	9
				82	M				√		√		√			7 MF	7
First-order psychopathy	A	3		83						√			√	√		7 MF	6
				84	M					√			√	√		5 MF	6
				85		F					√	√	√	√		8 MF	6
				86			√				√	√	√	√		6 MF	8
				87	M		√				√	√	√	√		6 MF	6
				88		M-4 F-5	√	√		√			√	√		8 MF	7
				89						√		√	√		√	—	8
				90	M	M-4	√	√		√			√	√		5 MF	8
				91		M-5	√	√	√		√	√	√	√	√	8 MF	9
				92	M		√						√	√		7 F	7
(A, cont.)		(3, cont.)		93	M F				√	√	√	√	√	√		8 MF	7
				94				√			√	√	√	√		7 MF	8
				95				√			√	√	√	√		8 MF	8
				96	M		√	√				√	√	√	√	9 M	9
				97				√			√			√		3 MF	9
				98	M							√	√	√		7 MF	8
				99								√	√	√		4 MF	8
				100	M F		√						√			3 MF	9
None	B	Chaplain's Unit		101												0 MF	0
				102												0 MF	0
				103	M F											1 MF	0
				104		F-3										0 MF	0

TABLE 14

THE PARENTAL BACKGROUNDS (Continued)

Predominant weakness	Company	Platoon	Section	No.	1. Burgeoned	2. Died, decade of life	3. Pathology of the burgeoned estate (CVR)	4. Pathology of the asthenic estate (PPPPT)	5. Pathology of C-SED-T	6. Mental insufficiency	7. Alcoholism	8. Irresponsible reproduction	9. Insufficiency (Distribution of Parental Delinquency)	Psychiatric	Civil	10. Total D, parental	11. Total D, filial
				105								√				1 MF	0
Second-order psychopathy	B	1	1	106	M F	M-5							√			3 MF	2
				107		F-6		√					√	√		5 MF	4
				108	M F						√	√	√			6 MF	6
				109				√	√		√	√	√		√	8 MF	7
				110							√		√			5 MF	7
				111	M	M-4 F-5	√		√		√	√	√			6 MF	6
				112	F			√				√	√	√		6 MF	6
				113	M	F-5	√						√	√		4 MF	6
				114	M F	F-5	√	√					√	√		8 MF	6
		2		115		F-7			√				√	√		4 MF	1
				116	M	F-4				√			√	√		5 MF	1
				117	M	F-5	√						√	√		3 MF	1
				118								√			√	2 M	2
				119	F	M-5 F-5	√				√	√	√	√	√	5 MF	2
				120								√				3 MF	2
				121	M		√						√	√		3 MF	3
				122	M	F-6	√		√				√	√		6 MF	2
				123												0 MF	2
				124		M-4			√		√	√	√		√	8 M	3
				125			√						√	√	√	3 MF	3
				126								√				3 MF	3
				127	F	M-4	√						√			3 MF	3
				128	M		√				√	√	√		√	5 M	4
				129	M	M-4 F-4			√		√	√	√			5 MF	4
				130		M-4		√	√		√	√	√			6 MF	5
				131		M-4 F-5	√	√			√	√	√			8 MF	5
				132	M	F-4	√				√	√	√		√	6 MF	6
		3		133	M		√									1 MF	1
				134		M-4 F-5				√		√				—	3
				135								√	√		√	3 MF	3
				136	M	M-4	√				√	√	√			5 MF	3
				137	M F		√						√	√		3 MF	3
				138								√			√	—	4
				139							√	√			√	5 MF	4
				140										√	√	4 MF	4
				141	M F	F-4	√					√	√		√	5 MF	4
				142	M		√					√	√			3 MF	4
				143	F											2 MF	5
(B, cont.)	(1, cont.)	4		144	M	M-4	√				√	√	√		√	8 M	5
				145		M-5	√				√	√	√		√	6 MF	5
				146		F-3	√	√	√		√	√	√		√	8 MF	6
				147	M F		√				√	√	√	√	√	6 MF	6
				148								√			√	7 M	7
				149								√			√	4 MF	5
				150		M-4	√		√			√	√		√	—	5
				151	M		√				√		√		√	5 MF	6
				152	M	M-4	√	√					√	√		7 MF	6
				153	M		√								√	6 MF	6
				154		M-3		√	√		√	√	√		√	5 MF	6
				155	M	M-4		√		√	√	√			√	7 MF	6
				156	M		√				√	√	√		√	6 MF	6
				157							√	√	√		√	4 MF	7
				158			√				√	√	√		√	7 MF	7

TABLE 14

THE PARENTAL BACKGROUNDS (Continued)

Predominant weakness	Company	Platoon	Section	No.	1. Burgeoned	2. Died, decade of life	3. Pathology of the burgeoned estate (CVR)	4. Pathology of the asthenic estate (PPPPT)	5. Pathology of C-SED-T	6. Mental insufficiency	7. Alcoholism	8. Irresponsible reproduction	Distribution of Parental Delinquency			10. Total D, parental	11. Total D, filial
													9. Insufficiency	Psychiatric	Civil		
				159	M	F-4									✓	6 M	7
				160						✓	✓	✓	✓	✓	✓	7 MF	7
				161								✓		✓	✓	4 MF	7
				162	M F		✓		✓				✓	✓	✓	7 MF	7
				163	M	F-5	✓		✓	✓	✓	✓	✓	✓	✓	8 MF	7
				164	F	M-3	✓			✓				✓	✓	4 MF	8
			5	165	F	F-5	✓			✓				✓	✓	5 MF	7
				166	M		✓			✓				✓	✓	5 MF	8
				167		M-4 F-5	✓	✓	✓	✓				✓	✓	7 MF	8
			6	168	M F		✓				✓	✓	✓		✓	5 MF	1
				169												0 MF	2
				170							✓			✓		—	3
				171	M	F-5								✓		5 MF	3
				172	M									✓		3 MF	3
				173												2 MF	4
				174		M-4 F-5	✓		✓				✓	✓	✓	7 MF	4
				175	M											1 MF	4
				176							✓			✓		—	5
				177		M-4	✓				✓			✓		6 MF	6
				178	M		✓				✓		✓	✓	✓	8 M	6
				179										✓		3 MF	6
				180				✓						✓		4 MF	3
				181	M								✓	✓		5 M	5
				182				✓			✓			✓	✓	5 M	5
				183	M				✓	✓		✓		✓	✓	5 MF	5
				184	M	M-6	✓		✓	✓	✓	✓	✓	✓	✓	7 MF	7
Primary criminality	B	2		185	M F	M-5 F-5	✓		✓			✓			✓	6 MF	5
				186							✓	✓				6 MF	6
				187	M					✓	✓	✓	✓		✓	7 MF	5
				188		F-5			✓	✓	✓	✓	✓		✓	7 MF	7
				189	M	M-4	✓		✓	✓	✓	✓	✓			6 MF	4
				190	M						✓					4 MF	5
				191	M F							✓				3 MF	5
				192	M										✓	5 MF	6
				193						✓	✓	✓	✓		✓	6 MF	6
				194		M-4 F-4	✓		✓	✓	✓	✓	✓			8 MF	7
				195										✓		—	7
				196				✓			✓	✓	✓	✓		8 MF	7
				197							✓	✓	✓			—	7
				198										✓			8
				199					✓		✓	✓	✓			8 MF	7
				200	M F				✓		✓	✓			✓	6 MF	7

Table 14 is, I think, the *pièce de résistance* of the HGI study. It speaks for itself, requires no elaborative comment. The indication is simply that the parents of the series, taken as a group, were delinquent in very much the same way that the boys are delinquent, and apparently to about the same degree. This aspect of the study can be summarized in the generalization—after all not very revolutionary from a biological point of view—that like tends to produce like.

The medical and mental insufficiency, the psychiatric manifestations, the alcoholism, the irresponsible reproduction, and the civil delinquency encountered in the boys are all reflected in about the same way in the parents. Indeed, as one glances down the eleven headings in Table 14 the question arises naturally as to whether the boys ought ever to have been called delinquent at all. They certainly are not delinquent with reference to their origins, but on the contrary seem to have reflected the latter with commendable rectitude. What the boys are they appear to have come by honestly, and with this consideration in mind it may be worth a moment's attention to contemplate briefly the individual headings in the table.

1. THE BURGEONED CHARACTERISTIC. In the platoon of mental insufficiency 18 of the 36 mothers, and 7 fathers, are of sufficiently hefty persuasion to have elicited social service comment on the fact. In the platoon of medical insufficiency the phenomenon is even more dramatic—30 of the 46 mothers and 10 of the fathers. Among the psychotics, 8 of the 18 mothers and 3 fathers qualified. For the mothers of Company A this is quite a remarkable batting average, 56 out of 100. In Company B the phenomenon is still encountered although not quite so dramatically. There, 44 of the 100 mothers and 18 of the fathers impressed social workers with their burgeoned qualities.

This phenomenon of the burgeoning overgrowth of human flesh, together with what appears to be a complementary phenomenon of asthenic failure of the flesh, raises questions of great interest to students of delinquency and medicine alike. Here may lie some of the explanation of the continuum between medical and civil delinquency so prominent in the HGI study and so clearly implied in both the Lombrosian and the Hootonian reports. The topic is a difficult one but in the present study it has so consistently commended itself to attention that Chapter 5 will be devoted to a discussion of it.

2. DIED, DECADE OF LIFE. Twelve of the 36 mothers and 8 of the fathers of the platoon of mental insufficiency were known to have died before the study was closed—11 of the mothers and 4 of the fathers before the age of 40. In the platoon of medical insufficiency the record is even worse. There, 14 of the 46 mothers and 15 of the fathers are known to have died. Three of the mothers and 1 of the fathers of the 18 psychotics were dead at the closing of the study. Thus for Company A as a whole 29 mothers and 24 fathers were known to have died. In Company B 24 of the 100 mothers and 24 fathers had succumbed. For the battalion as a whole, 53 mothers were known to be dead and 132 were known to be living—a mortality of 29 per cent. Fifteen mothers were unaccounted for. Of the fathers, 48 were known to be dead and 96 were reported as alive—a mortality of 33 per cent. Fifty-six fathers were unaccounted for.

Thus the known over-all parental mortality at the closing of the study was about 31 per cent. Almost one parent in three was known to be dead, with another 71 parents unaccounted for, when the mean age for the 200 youths was about 26. How these figures compare with figures for the general population I do not know, as I have no data available for the comparison, but doubtless such data exist and perhaps someone will make that comparison. We would then have one kind of rough index of the medical insufficiency of the parents of the 200 youths. Another such index could be derived from following up these parents until all had died, and by then comparing their mean longevity with that of other groups. The present indication is that the result would be striking. Of the 53 dead mothers, 43 are known to have died before the age of 40, and only one is reported to have lived past 50. That in this study we were dealing with short-lived stock is certain, but a quantitative measure of just *how* short-lived it is could be had only by arranging for somebody to sit out the entire drama.

3. PATHOLOGY OF THE BURGEONED ESTATE (CVR).   Among the 185 mothers and 144 fathers on whom we were able to get *some* medical information —329 parents in all—the spoor of the CVR killer had been reported in no less than 82 instances. Forty-four of these 82 parents were already dead, although not more than 10 or 11 of them (by the best guess we could make) from the CVR cause directly. The heaviest CVR morbidity was reported among the parents of Company A (45 cases) and 25 of these came from the parents of the platoon of medical insufficiency. Oddly enough the CVR spoor was picked up only twice among the parents of the 16 primary criminals, in Company B, and only four times among the parents of the 17 gynandrophrenes.

4. PATHOLOGY OF THE ASTHENIC ESTATE (PPPPT).   Once the concept of asthenia is established in your mind you find yourself recognizing the signs of "poor protoplasm poorly put together" as readily as the signs of measles. Yet this is a condition difficult to objectify and statistically it is not a very satisfactory item. The trail we try to follow here is that of the chronically ineffectual weakling (flat tire) with more or less endless vague complaints and "neurasthenic conditions." Medically it is not so sharply defined a trail as that of the pathology of the burgeoned estate, but in many instances the picture is painted so dramatically (in the agency records) that it cannot be missed. The striking thing about this condition is that 44 indicated instances of it are encountered among the parents of Company A, and only 13 instances among those of Company B. The parents of the 46 boys in the platoon of medical insufficiency must have been an asthenic lot, since 26 of them qualify under this heading. In sharp contrast, not one of the parents of the 16 boys in the platoon of primary criminality is so described. Asthenic weakness in the parentage seems clearly to be associated with the insufficiencies in the offspring (and with hebephrenic psychopathy), not with primary criminality.

5. PATHOLOGY OF C-SED-T.   Ten of the 185 known mothers and 6 of the 144 known fathers had died of cancer at the time of the closing of the study.

The ten mothers had died at a mean age of 42, which is young for cancer. Unfortunately we do not know the exact mean age of the mothers at the closing of the study, but we know that it was in the neighborhood of 49 or 50. (The mean age of the mothers at the time of birth of our 200 clients was between 23 and 24—which is young—and the boys as an average were about 26 when the study was closed.) Since the mortality of many forms of cancer is higher in the fifties than in the forties, it is probable that more than another 10 of these mothers will have died of cancer and that the cancer death rate among the mothers will be above 10 or 12 per cent. That might indicate a statistical relationship between cancer and the population with which we are dealing, although it would not follow that the relational factor is necessarily associated with civil delinquency. It would be far more likely to be associated with the burgeoned estate, since 9 of the 10 mothers who had died of cancer, and 5 of the 6 fathers, were also described as burgeoned people. It may be significant, too, that 11 of the 16 cancer deaths—7 mothers and 4 fathers—were among parents of Company A. Cancer may be not merely a correlate but a criterion of insufficiency, and there may be gold in the bleak hills of constitutional record keeping.

The trail of syphilis was not often crossed, or at any rate was not often recognized, in this study. Only five times did we encounter the specific statement in the social records that a parent had been diagnosed as syphilitic. There seemed to be "hints" in quite a number of other instances but for purposes of the record there were only 4 instances of syphilis among the mothers and but 1 case among the fathers. This may indicate a relative scarcity of that disease in Boston, or relative efficacy of the conspiracy to avoid mentioning it.

Ten cases of parental epilepsy are recorded, 7 among the fathers and 3 among the mothers. This also is perhaps too low a figure. The social records wax eloquent on the frequency of occurrence of both syphilis and epilepsy among near relatives of a client but tend to avoid mentioning specific instances among the clients themselves. It is possible that the two-to-one predominance of epilepsy over syphilis indicates no more than that the latter is about twice as unmentionable as the former.

Nine cases of parental diabetes are reported, 2 mothers and 2 fathers from Company A, 3 mothers and 2 fathers from Company B. Since little if any social stigma is attached to diabetes this is very likely an accurate census of the condition. Nine cases among 329 known parents is nearly 3 per cent, which would be high for the general population but (for so small a sample) probably not significantly high. There may be little relationship between diabetes and *general* medical insufficiency, and it may be significant that 5 of our 9 cases occurred among the parents of Company B, where medical insufficiency was least conspicuous.

Twenty-six instances of parental tuberculosis are recorded, 18 from the parents of Company A and 8 from those of Company B. The platoon of medical insufficiency yields 11 records of this disease among the parents. In comparing such data with other medical statistics, however, it should be remembered that tuberculosis is a peculiar customer and an uncertain tenant. About 98 per cent of persons—nearly everybody—will show some traces of (early or late) pulmonary tuberculosis if a sufficiently careful postmortem examination is made. Yet only a comparative few ever develop clinical symptoms of the disease and in perhaps no two of these does tuberculosis behave in exactly the same manner. Possibly only the very serious or fatal cases (in the parents of clients) would be likely to get into the social history records. What we can say here of tuberculosis is that at least 26 of the parents were known to have clinical cases of it, and that more than two thirds of these were Company A parents. Tuberculosis appears to be associated with insufficiency and with the asthenic estate. Seventeen of the 26 cases of parental tuberculosis are listed as also presenting pathology of the asthenic estate.

If the five entities of the C-SED-T pathology are considered as a group, at least one parent of each of 63 of the 200 boys could claim membership in the fraternity. That is, 63 of the boys, or almost one in three, had one or two parents who presented serious instances of one or more of the five diseases indicated. Thirty-two of these C-SED-T parental delinquencies came from Company A and 31 from Company B. Oddly enough, the platoon with the highest parental C-SED-T batting average in Company A was the platoon of mental (rather than of medical) insufficiency. The parents of that platoon of 36 yielded 15 C-SED-T involvements, and the parents of the platoon of medical insufficiency, which has 46 soldiers, also yielded 15. Thus the two insufficiency platoons, between them, contributed about half of the C-SED-T parentage, but it would be difficult to explain why the parents presenting the highest degree of this kind of *medical* insufficiency should have produced offspring with the highest degree of *mental* insufficiency. One answer to such a puzzle would be the (perhaps overly) simple one that the relationship between the two kinds of insufficiency is closer than we have supposed—or even that these two manifestations of insufficiency are only events in a continuum.

Another point of interest is that the platoon of primary criminality, with only 16 soldiers, yields seven instances of C-SED-T parentage. This is actually the highest incidence for any platoon in the battalion and is surprising because the boys themselves are a vigorous and outwardly a rather healthy lot. Is it possible that they are not really a healthy lot in the long run, that despite a heavy endowment in elemental vigor they are a comparatively short-lived fraternity *and somehow know it?* That therefore they tend to embrace easily the philosophy expressed by the formula "a short life but a merry one"? Anyone who has read the cases carefully will recall how frequently this particle of wisdom cropped out among the brighter and more articulate of the persistently troublesome youngsters. It is certainly not impossible that the Irish philosopher Shaw was right when (in *Back to Methuselah*) he attributed human delinquency and frustration in general to the *unnecessary* shortness of the life span. It was Shaw's point that the difference between what the maximal life span could be (if we were to do our best) and what it is, is the true measure of human delinquency; that other manifestations of delinquency are superficial symptoms. This is a point of view which ties medical practice intimately both to the sociology of delinquency and to religion, and we shall follow out that trail a little further in Chapter 6.

6. MENTAL INSUFFICIENCY. Sixty-three of the 200 boys have at least one parent described in the social agency records as of defective mentality, or feebleminded. Fifty-one of these 63 are Company A boys and this seems to be quite a striking demonstration of the hereditary nature of one kind of insufficiency. Twenty-three of the 36 in the platoon of mental insufficiency are known to have parents who are also mentally insufficient, and in the platoon sections where the mental insufficiency is moderate and severe, respectively, the record becomes really dramatic. Twenty-two of the 23 boys in those two platoon sections are known to have parentage of defective mentality. In the platoon of medical insufficiency also the record is dramatic enough. There 22 of the 46 boys have mentally defective parents, and 18 of these instances of mentally defective parentage come from the second and third platoon sections (moderate and severe medical insufficiency) which include 27 boys. We see then that two thirds of the boys in the series whose difficulty is moderate or severe medical insufficiency have mentally insufficient parentage, and all but one of the twenty-three boys showing moderate or severe mental insufficiency have mentally insufficient parents. Here is a pretty clear showing of a close hereditary relationship between two quite different manifestations of insufficiency, and these data were partly responsible for our initial formulation of the concept of *general* insufficiency as one of the primary factors in what has been called delinquency.

It is perhaps odd that only 12 of the boys from Company B, as compared with 51 from Company A, have parents known to be mentally insufficient, while the pathology of C-SED-T is about equally distributed between the parentages of Company A and Company B. It would seem to follow that medical insufficiency is more contributive to civil delinquency than is mental insufficiency, while the latter is more genetically determined than the former. Our markedly feebleminded boys were almost certain to have at least one feebleminded parent, but the feebleminded parents were apparently less prone to produce offspring delinquent-other-than-mentally than were the medically insufficient parents to produce offspring delinquent-other-than-medically. In other words medical delinquency seems to be a more insidiously dangerous factor in a population than does mental delinquency. If this observation is sound in general, our attitude toward delinquency and our whole conception of social psychiatry needs thorough revision. The tendency since the first World War and with the development of mental testing has been to carry most of our sociological eggs in the IQ basket (and more recently in a sort of paper bag of environmental determinism). But it may be that attention to simpler and more specifically organic factors such as the pathology of the burgeoned and the asthenic estates, and of C-SED-T, would be better for the eggs.

7. ALCOHOLISM.   Among the 185 families where enough is known about the parentage for *anything* to be recorded (in the agency records), alcoholism is referred to as "a serious factor" in exactly 100 instances—50 of these from the parentage of Company A and 50 from Company B. This is remarkable. If you were to spend a week reading those agency records you would probably gather the impression that the parents did little else than drink, fight, and fornicate. It is remarkable too that the mothers are not far behind the fathers in getting themselves referred to as drunkards. Fifty-eight of the mothers and 79 of the fathers are categorized as alcoholics in agency records or court records, but in trying to interpret such a datum two things should be remembered: (1) that Boston, with its Irish government, is actually quite an alcoholic city; and (2) that to be labeled alcoholic in that city is (perhaps for that reason) not a very serious derogation.

The common and in some cases almost constant court charge for a wide range of civil offenses, particularly against persons of the right religio-political persuasion, is "drunkenness and disorderly conduct." There are cases in our series of parental records where even manslaughter (if it wasn't murder) has been covered by that charge. The art of seeing that a relatively innocuous charge goes on the record, in the case of a member of one's constituency, is an important art among local and ward politicians, although probably no more so in Boston than in other large cities. In Boston it so happens that the charge of drunkenness is almost the unanimous charge of choice. I should say, therefore, that we know little about the true incidence of alcoholism (medically defined) among the parents of the series, and that this item should be considered merely as is. A check in column 7 means that at least one of the parents has been seriously troublesome and that for purposes of the record the fact is blamed against the commonest cerebrotoxic drug.

8. IRRESPONSIBLE REPRODUCTION.   This is the commonest and probably the most important actual delinquency in the backgrounds of the population represented in the Study. At least 57 of the sets of parents of Company A, and 50 of those of Company B were guilty of irresponsibile reproduction by the criteria indicated on page 766. These are not exacting criteria, and are not dependent on any fine hairsplitting of moral issues. They are simply: (1) illegitimacy; (2) continued reproduction after civil or social agencies had

found it necessary to remove older children from the parents, or otherwise to intervene and to subsidize or partially institutionalize the parents themselves.

At the time when our first investigations were made, for the most part during the first two years of the Study, the parents of the 200 boys were known to have produced at least 741 other children, or 941 in all. Most of these parents were at the time still young enough to reproduce, and were continuing merrily to do so. Also a goodly number of them had remarried and were again (or still) breeding in their new family units—we did not attempt to follow out any of those parental side trails. Further, there was no way of knowing how much reproduction, legitimate or otherwise, these parents had accomplished that was not listed in the official records. In the light of all these factors it would probably be a safe assumption that the parents of our 200 HGI boys produced well over 1,000 offspring. Many of these offspring will have populated the colleges and not the jails. Will the colleges give them erudition, or will they give the colleges delinquency? It is a nice question and a final answer is not implied, for we may possess educational resources not yet assessed.

Of the 941 offspring known to be produced by the parents of the HGI battalion, 487 were from the parents of Company A and 454 from those of Company B. In Company A the parents of the platoon of mental insufficiency (36 soldiers) tallied 150 offspring, those of the platoon of medical insufficiency (46 soldiers) 249, and those of the psychotic platoon (18 soldiers) 88. In Company B the parents of Chaplain's Unit (5 soldiers) produced 14, those of the psychoneurotic platoon (79 soldiers) produced 339, and those of the criminal platoon (16 soldiers) produced 101. Thus the highest rate of breeding was among the parents of criminals, with the parents of both kinds of insufficiency and those of the psychoneurotic platoon not far behind. Taken as a group, the parents of criminality and those of medical insufficiency (62 family units) were known to have produced 350 offspring, or 5.65 per family unit. This is Dionysian reproduction.

The fact that the parents of Company A were outbreeding those of Company B, and particularly that it was in the platoon of *medical* insufficiency that so high a reproductive rate was encountered, may be of more than passing interest. Why should these medically insufficient parents have been doing so much breeding? One complacent explanation of our well-known and profoundly disturbing differential breeding rate has been that the more uninhibited breeders must be more vigorous, or more fecund, or somehow healthier, and that therefore it is "all right"; that nature or Mr. G or somebody has the matter in hand and is looking out for future biological interests better than we could hope to do it ourselves. But here is one piece of evidence that the most prolific breeders—in a laissez-faire breeding situation—are anything but vigorous or healthy people, that they are in fact biologically as well as economically and mentally a sort of marginal caboose of society often requiring institutional intervention in order to be kept alive themselves. Do they breed, then, because they are better breeders or because they are less inhibited, which is to say, because they don't know any better? This too is a nice question and one to which we will return in Section 5 of Chapter 6.

9. DISTRIBUTION OF PARENTAL DELINQUENCY. In Company A the trail of parental insufficiency was so fresh and plain that our scouts and outrunners were able to document its presence in no less than 91 of the 100 sets of parents. In Company B also there were 62 manifest instances of it. In the two insufficiency platoons of Company A, with their total of 82 soldiers, mental or medical insufficiency was reported in the parentage in all 76 of those instances in which anything at all was known of the parents. That gave us food for thought and seemed to suggest two conclusions with respect to insufficiency: (1) That whatever insufficiency is, it tends to breed true; (2) That our youngsters who presented insufficiency as a factor in their delinquency came by it honestly.

Psychiatric delinquency in the parentage was reported 58 times for Company A and 42 times for Company B, although only twice among the 16 sets of parents represented by the platoon of primary criminality. Criminality thus appears to be more closely associated with medical insufficiency than with psychiatric difficulties in the parentage. Fifteen of the 18 sets of parents of the psychotic platoon presented a history of psychiatric delinquency, and 40 of the 79 sets of the psychoneurotic platoon yielded such a history. Psychiatric difficulties were also encountered among 43 of the 82 sets of parents of the two platoons of insufficiency. Thus it is clear that a relationship exists between insufficiency and the psychiatric disorders, but what is not clear—and for this study can never be clear—is the extent to which the psychiatrists who had contact with those parents were confusing the insufficiencies with what here is called (first- and second-order) psychopathy. This is a distinction which can be made sharply, but it is dependent on a good mental and social history of the patient and on the ability of the doctor to make an accurate constitutional diagnosis.

Fifty-two of the known sets of parents of Company A, and 51 of those of Company B, present a record of civil delinquency. There is of course no way of knowing what proportion of the true parental delinquency appears on the records available to us, but for statistical purposes we know that at least the number of families indicated had parental delinquency of record. It is in the platoon of primary criminality that the highest parental delinquency of record occurs—13 instances out of a possible 16—and the lowest incidence is found in the psychotic platoon—6 instances out of 18. The incidence for the platoon of mental insufficiency is distinctly higher than that for the platoon of medical insufficiency—25 out of 36 as compared with 21 out of 46. Parents of feebleminded delinquents, whom we have seen almost invariably to present feeblemindedness themselves (p. 768), appear to be about 50 per cent more likely to have a record of criminal delinquency, than parents of delinquent youngsters who are medically insufficient but not feebleminded.

10. TOTAL D, PARENTAL. The point of interest here lies in the remarkable agreement between total parental and total filial delinquency throughout the entire series. This may be the most significant feature of the Study. Disregarding those cases where not enough is known of the parents to assign a Total D, Table 15 gives the mean Total D standings, parental *versus* filial, for all the platoons of the battalion.

TABLE 15

THE MEAN STANDINGS IN TOTAL D. PARENTAL VERSUS FILIAL

	Mean total D, parental	Mean total D, filial
Company A, Platoon 1 (mental insufficiency)	6.78	6.90
Company A, Platoon 2 (medical insufficiency)	6.16	6.27
Company A, Platoon 3 (the psychotics)	6.41	7.59
The Chaplain's Unit (environmental delinquency)	0.40	0.00
Company B, Platoon 1 (the psychoneurotics)	4.93	4.69
Company B, Platoon 2 (the criminals)	6.15	5.92

If now we were to consider delinquency in terms of a delinquency quotient (DQ) in which the numerator would be the Total D of a youth ($\times$ 100), and the denominator would be the averaged Total D of the parents ($\times$ 100), it might be assumed that a DQ of 100 would be "normal," or par for the situation into which the youth was born. With such a conception in mind a glance at Tables 14 and 15 will reveal that the DQ's of most of our HGI youths must have been just about dead normal. The average DQ for the 200 was in fact 100.04. As a group those 200 boys were neither better nor worse than their parents but were reflecting with astonishing accuracy the same level of life and usefulness that had been attained by the parents, even though about half of the boys had been reared apart from their parents.

This is not a chapter of interpretation but it might be well at the end of it to pause and ask ourselves the question, What does this remarkably accurate reflection of the parental level of delinquency mean? Does a biological population, like water, tend to come to rest at its own level and are efforts to improve the conditions of human life *while disregarding biological humanics* therefore mainly a waste? I do not mean to prejudice an answer unduly, for the plain fact is that we are not quite in a position to give an answer. No profession among us has yet gone about the business of looking at human populations with such a possibility intelligently in mind. But I think there is enough indication of a positive answer to the question to justify heart-searching meditation on the implications of a biological humanics. Therefore the remaining chapters of this book will be mainly an exploration of ideas not on what might be done about individuals already delinquent but on what seem to be the underlying correlates and causes of delinquency.

CHAPTER 5

BIOLOGICAL DELINQUENCY
THE BURGEONED AND THE ASTHENIC
ESTATES

1. The Burgeoned Mothers and the Social Workers

The frequent appearance of the coarse-heavy mother in the background of the play was one of the curious sidelights. Among the 185 mothers concerning whom the staff gathered what seemed to be sufficient information to record a rating on Total D, there are 100 who are described either by our own social workers or by those of other agencies as hefty, muscular, burgeoned, gross, obese, or the like. That this was not entirely a matter of prejudice or hostility-to-the-mother on the part of social workers we know from having seen some 60 or 70 of the mothers. Among those we saw there were power-houses fearful to confront.

One of our own social workers on the project, who was something of a communicant of the psychoanalytic church, many times called attention gleefully to "The Mothers." "Now take a good look at *that* one," he would gloat, "and tell me if the boy wasn't rejected." I would have to agree with him that Freud's over-all description of the family did present realistic elements, and that in all likelihood the mother in question did reject her off-spring and was rejected by them. I would then proceed to point out that behind the rejection might lie good biological reasons and that the job was to study those deeper causes of difficulty. But with my Freudian friend this only got me into a kind of flypaper which in childhood I had encountered also among Christians. I recall asking my Christian betters how Mr. G got the way *He* was and being told that the question was not only impious but irrelevant. The psychoanalytic social worker seemed to feel the same way about underlying biological causes or concomitants of rejection, fear, insecurity, jealousy of parents, intrafamilial warfare, and so on. These things *were* and that was enough for him.

But some of us found the burgeoned mothers of great interest as biological phenomena. And the fathers too. Less was known of the fathers of the principal actors in the drama than of the mothers, or at any rate less was said. It was true that in many instances the fathers were unknown, but in many others the fathers must have been as well known as the mothers. However, the social service records usually were written around the activities of the mother, with the father playing a minor or peripheral role and getting comparatively little attention. We wondered whether this was part of the reason why only 39 fathers had impressed the social agencies as being unusually burgeoned as compared with 100 mothers. It certainly would not be the only reason. Women do get fatter than men, and by our social conventions are constrained to dress so that what they are shows better. After the years of "youthful slimness," especially in stock of low or average *t* component, women show whatever grossness or blowsiness may be in them more conspicuously than men do. Perhaps this was the main reason that so many of the mothers looked full blown to social workers. Possibly the only safe conclusions are, (a) that these mothers were of more or less hefty somatotype and (b) that they were not of very high *t* component. This would be only to say that the mothers were to that extent of about the same morphological patterns as their offspring.

At the Inn we had for a time a social worker who seemed to feel a peculiar antipathy to the burgeoned characteristic. He was about a 2–3–5 with a sharp, quick mind and an even quicker tongue. In the course of interviewing mothers of our youngsters—it will be remembered that Dr. Hartl had several thousand boys at the Inn, not merely the 200 in the series—this social worker gathered the impression that the mothers were very much of a type. "Another of those all-body-and-no-soul females," he would comment, and then he would seem to feel better.

2. The Burgeoned Estate in the Clinical Population

The problem of the burgeoning of human flesh is of more than academic interest. Insurance companies have for generations collected statistical indications that the hefty organisms are inclined to be short-lived. The medical profession is aware of a strong predisposition among the hefties to such diseases as diabetes, nephritis, hypertension, cardiac breakdown, and apoplexy. Nearly all physicians admonish their patients to watch their weight and physicians usually have weight charts hung in some conspicuous place about the office. But unfortunately the vast accumulations of actuarial statistics and of medical notations have been made without any differentiation between the two primary components of morphology that contribute to massiveness. A pronounced endomorph or a pronounced mesomorph can be equally massive and in the middle years of life either may become obese. All but possibly a quarter or so of the somatotypes can become obese.[1] The

---

[1] As is the case with pigs—a species now selectively bred in captivity so that nearly all of its members grow obese at the drop of a bucket of swill. By selective breeding we doubtless could do the same thing with the human species.

fact that an individual is heavy means little if his constitutional pattern is not known.

At the Presbyterian Hospital, in New York, a branch of the Constitutional Research Project has for some years been carrying on studies of a number of different disease groups; that is to say, of people presenting the same kind of illness at the clinics. Standardized somatotype photographs have been taken of several cumulative series of patients.

The mothers of the Boston youths seemed burgeoned. As one colleague at the Inn put it, "they stuck out in the northwest." When a few years later this same colleague visited the Constitution Clinic at Presbyterian Hospital to watch the population there for a time, he ejaculated "Why those are the same women we interviewed in Boston!" He had seen a few cases of peptic ulcer, some diabetics, a number who had cancer, several gall bladder cases, and other miscellaneous clinical entities. They reminded me of Boston too, although I was not able to put a finger on a satisfactory specific reason. I had a feeling that if I *could* put a finger on just what was causing the resemblance I might thereby define a clue of acute importance both in medicine and in the study of delinquency. Indeed the more I have looked at the civilly delinquent and the medically delinquent, the more forcibly has it been driven home that the two aspects of the problem of delinquency are in a continuum.

My Boston colleague decided that one principal characteristic in common between the Boston mothers and the Presbyterian Hospital population was t component. They all had low t, he said, and he fancied that he could make out also in both groups an asthenic characteristic in common. He finally summarized the common description thus: *"They are burgeoned northwesterners with asthenic stigmata and low t."*

I took him one day for a long ride on the New York subway system and asked him to point out the individuals crossing our line of vision who answered to all of these descriptive criteria. The hunting was excellent. "This one, that one, those three over there, the fat one now glowering at me," and so on. The New York subway system is an anthropological paradise. I have often experienced there an ecstasy which must be related to that felt by coin collectors when they dream of taking a bath in Brasher doubloons. You see things in those subway trains thought of which will keep you warm of winter nights.

The hunting in the subways was so rewarding that I decided to "objectify" the study a little. On one trip I took along what is called a double recording hand counter. This is a gadget with which you can keep the count on two cumulative series by pressing appropriate push buttons. We reviewed two consecutive thousands—a thousand men and a thousand women—from the subway population, making a decision in each instance as to whether the individual did or did not qualify as a "burgeoned northwesterner with asthenic stigmata and low *t*." That is to say, whether the person could qualify as a BM-PH (Boston Mother-Presbyterian Hospital) type. My friend may have been too exacting a judge. He credited only 36 per cent of the women and 29 per cent of the men with making the grade on this rigorous test. One afternoon I took him to Grand Central Station, found comfortable seats near the main line of flight and readily bagged another thousand of each sex. At Grand Central the scores were lower; 22 per cent for the women and 18 per cent for the men. This was, apparently, a less delinquent population and if my colleague's ratings of overt delinquency on the basis of the BM-PH syndrome are to be relied on there is hope for the species. If only about a fifth of the general or Grand Central population are manifestly delinquent (by long-range inspection) and only about a third of the subway population, matters may not be as bad as the radio and the newspapers and the automobile noise would indicate. Perhaps the delinquent fifth, or the delinquent third, are responsible for a very disproportionate amount of the New York radio and automobile noise.

But it should be remembered that my colleague was looking at his population sample with their clothes on; in fact they were more or less dressed up for public inspection. It is difficult to make out the asthenic characteristic and low *t* when people are covered up with clothes. Indeed it may be that the principal function of clothes, in our present culture, is to cover up asthenic weaknesses and low *t*. I am not certain that, under standardized somatotyping conditions, *two* fifths of the Grand Central population and *two* thirds of the subway population would not have qualified at the BM-PH level. It is possible that the great achievement of our period will have been an unprecedented aesthetic deterioration of the human carcase, i.e., a general lowering of the *t* component. This achievement may constitute the principal contribution of modern medicine, brought about indirectly, of course, through keeping people alive indiscriminately. It may also constitute the principal criterion of delinquency.

3. Burgeoned Delinquency versus Asthenic Delinquency

Mental hospital patients (Figure 7, p. 70) present a morphology which as a whole is strikingly different from that of the Presbyterian Hospital groups. Further, the distribution seen in Figure 7 is probably illustrative of male mental hospital populations in general, since it can be virtually superimposed on the distribution for a large series of 3,800 such patients in New York state hospitals whose somatotype photographs were taken in 1938 (p. 56). In the mental hospitals (at least where the diagnosis *dementia praecox* or *schizophrenia* predominates) we do not find the predominance of heavy bodies seen at Presbyterian Hospital and also seen, apparently, in the parental background of the 200 boys in the Boston series. Figure 10 (p. 73) points up the matter even more sharply. These are the 85 from the Elgin series for whom, according to the Elgin hospital records, the third (hebephrenic) psychotic component was most strongly predominant. They are found mainly in the southeast segment of the somatotype family, and so consistently so that the correlation between ectomorphy (third morphological component) and the third psychiatric component, for the Elgin series, was +.64. The hebephrenes are usually ectomorphs, but even more conspicuous than the ectomorphy is an overwhelming asthenia.

Figure 8 (p. 71) indicates where the 12 patients dwell morphologically whose diagnoses at Elgin reflect strong predominance of the first psychiatric component. These live in the west and northwest and the morphological differential between the manic-depressive psychotics and the hebephrenes is a dramatic one. The latter seem to present something like a morphological antithesis not only to the expressional (cerebropenic) psychoses but also to a large medical population not ordinarily regarded as psychiatric at all. Peptic ulcer, gall bladder disease, and especially cancer may seem a long way removed from psychiatry. Yet there is one kind of correlational bond between all of these entities and the expressive psychoses. Both they and the latter are found in the same morphological territory, and this is the territory in which the human body burgeons out in a kind of brash luxuriance which may be not unrelated biologically to the phenomenon of Dionysianism. There seems to be also a psychological antagonism between the burgeoned side of the human distribution—which is the west side in general, both southwest and northwest—and that population which lies in the east.[2]

[2] 'This is not quite an expression of the dichotomy between Jung's extraversion and introversion because introversion, strictly speaking, means extreme cerebrotonia or cerebrosis. That phenomenon is to be found not in the east in general but in the extreme southeast peninsula of the distribution. The extreme ectomorphs are encamped out on that point and they are not effectively antagonistic to anything. They are tightly con-

A phenomenon so persistent in early constitutional observations that I made it one of the definitive characteristics of cerebrotonia[3] was an almost universal resistance to disease, or freedom from disease, in active, well-developed ectomorphs—i.e. in ectomorphs showing none of what I have later termed the asthenic characteristic, and usually presenting secondary strength in the second component. At a convention of the Grand Army of the Republic in Chicago I was astonished at the high proportion of mesomorphic ectomorphs among those octogenarians and nonagenarians. Those long-lived men were by no means extreme ectomorphs, but they had a generous endowment of that component, along with nearly as much, possibly quite as much, of the second, and most of them were endopenes. Also they had consistently high primary *t* and a conspicuous freedom from asthenic characteristics. There were few if any burgeoned somatotypes among them. They were what people used to call clean-cut, and possibly that term can be translated into *freedom from both the asthenic and the burgeoned characteristics.* Such men are rare in the general medical clinics. Perhaps they present one kind of antithesis to medical delinquency.

In addition to those psychiatric disorders in which the predominant psychiatric component is the third, there is another common clinical entity which in the minds of many clinicians has been associated with the asthenic estate. Tuberculosis is a puzzling disease. Clinicians have felt that tuberculous populations present a "constitutional factor" but have been unable to define a clue to the common constitutional characteristics. So far as the somatotype goes, I am satisfied that no such clue has been present. That disease seems to be just about indiscriminate of somatotype. You see the whole somatotype range in the tuberculosis wards, and I think you see it about normally distributed. Yet the term *phthisic habitus* is persistent in medical literature, and comes down from the Greek physicians. Nearly every medical school has one or two "intellectuals" on its staff who devote a lecture or two, in the course of the four years' training of medical students, to constitutional differences. A principal feature of these occasional lectures on constitution is often an elaboration of the meaning of *phthisic habitus.* The concept is usually identified with ectomorphy or with Kretschmer's asthenic type, and the term tuberculous diathesis is sometimes invoked to indicate weak, thin, inadequate people—pale, anemic people of poor muscular tone and of low general resistance.

In civil and Army hospitals and elsewhere I have had an opportunity to look at a number of thousands of tuberculous patients and to speculate on

---

strained, more or less closed up like molluscs at low tide. In order for active antagonism (fight) to transpire, a fairly good amount of second component must be present. A 1–4–5 or even a 2–3–5 can muster up vigorous antagonism and this is often directed toward those biological opposites (to endopenia) that lie in western territory.

[3] See *Varieties of Temperament,* chap. 3.

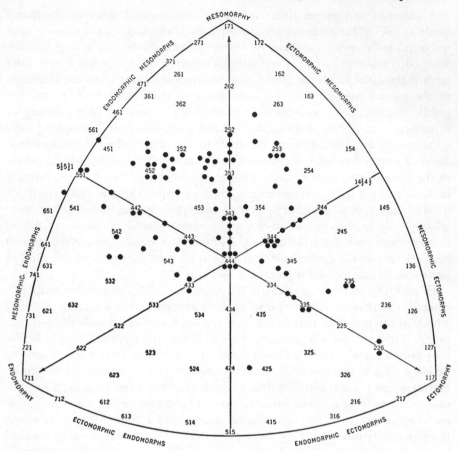

FIGURE 44. Somatotype Distribution for Pulmonary Tuberculosis. 100 Men.

who they were. That they had something in common always seemed manifest. Certainly there was a tuberculous look, but whether that was constitutional or a product of the disease was difficult to say. They looked asthenic, in the sense in which I use that term but not in Kretschmer's (ectomorphic) sense. They rarely looked burgeoned, even in the postinfectious stage after being overfed and fattened—they then looked merely fat. Far from being ectomorphic, they seemed to me in general to suggest asthenic mesomorphy, if anything.

During World War II Dr. C. W. Dupertuis and Dr. George Draper had occasion to study a group of tuberculous patients in an Army Air Forces hospital, and they took somatotype photographs of 100 of the men. The somatotypes of these 100 are shown in Figure 44. For comparison study also the distribution of somatotypes in Figure 45, which presents 3,000 aviation

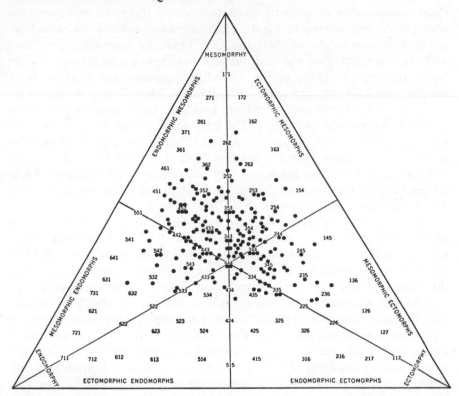

FIGURE 45. Somatotype Distribution for 3000 Aviation Cadets Who Had Successfully Passed the Air Corps Physical Examination. Each dot represents 30
cases.

cadets who at the time of being photographed (by the writer) had just successfully passed a rigorous test of good health and physical competence—the
Army medical examination for admission to pilot training.

Here then are two groups from Army aviation, one with pulmonary tuberculosis and one illustrating perfect health. The two distributions are
sufficiently similar to indicate a strong likelihood that tuberculosis is not
related to somatotype. Among the tuberculous patients there is no tendency
to pile up heavily in one segment of the distribution. There is to be sure a
dearth of mesopenes among the population, but there is this same dearth in
the control series (Figure 45). Mesopenes were rare in the Air Forces, and
extreme endomorphs were almost unknown there—they were rejected as
overweight. (A few of the latter were to be found in the medical and quarter-
master corps, however.)

Contrary to popular medical supposition tuberculosis seems decidedly not
to be a disease associated with ectomorphy as such, but does appear to be

closely associated with asthenic characteristics. In the series of somatotype photographs represented in Figure 44, conspicuous asthenic characteristics can be made out in almost every instance. These are most often associated with the thoracic region and with the legs, but there are no regions of these bodies that escape. Many of the tuberculous patients are asthenic mesomorphs who *look like* catatonic schizophrenes. They look as if the Potter must have started with mesomorphy in mind but forgot some ingredient essential to the proper flowering of the mesomorphic bud. In short these tuberculous patients as a group look remarkably like some 30 or 40 per cent of the boys we photographed at the Inn. Most of the latter were not known to have had active tuberculosis, but they may remain good candidates for it. (If any of them do develop tuberculosis we shall doubtless hear that it was the disease that made them look that way.)

For some twenty-odd centuries, at least, medical men have been looking at what I suppose have been asthenic somatotypes and have been calling them by such a name as *phthisic habitus*. I think one of the most pertinent problems in the medicine of the future is going to be to find out just what this asthenic factor is. In hebephrenic and catatonic schizophrenia it is always seen. In tuberculosis it is usually seen. In the case of hebephrenic schizophrenia, early photographs of patients that develop that psychosis appear (in my experience) uniformly to show the characteristic. Whether or not this can also be said of tuberculosis I do not know, but many psychiatrists have commented on an apparent affinity between tuberculosis and psychiatric disorders in which the hebephrenic component is predominant. The asthenic estate may be a factor comparable to the burgeoned estate in the investigation of medical delinquency.

In the asthenic estate the organism appears to have stopped short of a full elaboration or full flowering of some of its tissue, perhaps of all of its tissue. What is possibly the same sort of curtailment is seen in other animals, notably in dogs. A few years ago I spent a vacation with a friend in Hot Springs, Arkansas. We took many long walks about the environs, which consisted largely in vast accumulations of shacks occupied by what seemed to be squatters or indigent citizens of varying degree, both white and Negro. One thing they all had in common was dogs—swarms of them—and remarkable dogs they were. I had been pondering the asthenic estate as it was manifested in South Boston, and here it was again. Those dogs, both in face and in body, looked so pathetically like the human drift of South Boston on a Saturday afternoon, and in particular they so suggested the tag-end 30 per cent of our HGI series, that my companion stared aghast.

There was the same dwindling of extremities, the postural lassitude or inertia, the lack of molding in the body, the disharmony and asymmetry of all proportions with frequent flaccid obesity, the lack of identity-with-breed of any kind and the sense of a chaotic mongrelism. We sat musing for a long time one afternoon in the shade of a hackberry. Distributed about in various attitudes of semiparanoid repose were the canine contingents from two or three neighboring front yards—possibly a dozen and a half dogs. With fragments of two frankfurters they had been bribed into such silence that, with careful improvement of opportunities, conversation could be carried on. We had been trying to scale the asthenic component for each individual dog, and also, since we were both amateur students of breed in dogs, had been trying to make out probable ancestry and to trace possibilities of consanguinity. One shaggy fellow really stumped us. He was shaggy only in spots. His face had the innocuous benignity of Britain's late Prime Minister Chamberlain and he had a flat, almost hairless tail like a muskrat. It dragged like a muskrat's tail, even when its owner as a whole was in a state of activation. The forequarters were contracted and yellow, of about 3–2–5 somatotype, but the hindquarters were tremendous and shaggy. Except for the muskrat tail he looked like a 3–6–2 in the fourth region. The legs were much too long in the distal segments, with the front ones virtually amuscular. My companion, with more of wistful affection and empathy than of fun in her voice, mentioned how obviously urgent was the need for psychoanalysis. You could *see* the conflict protruding in three dimensions. We went back to the hot dog stand and bought Roland a whole frankfurter, and wondered if dog marriages too are made in heaven.

There are asthenic dogs, hens, birds, trees, plants, and even asthenic leaves of plants, as well as brash and burgeoned examples of all of these organisms. Life, or organic chemistry at the level we call life, seems to be confronted by a delicate problem of balance. In the ordering and catalyzing of those transformations of structure which constitute growth and development, and in the creation of that pattern of catalyzing which is called the gene pattern, there is apparently this same problem of balance, with a good chance of sliding off fatally, as from a rooftree, into the burgeoned or into the asthenic estate.

4. Delinquency May Reside in the Cellular Morphogenotype

The problem of balance is one of which biologists have been aware, and biological attention has for some time been directed particularly to the cell in the hope of picking up a clue to the control of that kind of balance which avoids both delinquencies—the burgeoning delinquency and the asthenic delinquency. At one level of consideration the cell is the biological unit of structure. What an organism as a whole is and does is what its cells are and do in much the same way that the activity of an army is the activity of its individual soldiers.

Immunologists know that resistance to disease is a characteristic not invested, as a rule, in a particular organ or group of cells, but carried in all the cells of the body. The cells of different organisms are unlike the bricks of different buildings. Two buildings may contain bricks from the same mold but every cell in an organism is a direct lineal descendant from ancestors which for innumerable generations have been developing characteristics and acquiring adaptations of their own, or have possibly been degenerating and losing adaptive qualities. A cell is a living thing with personality. Whatever the asthenic estate is at bottom, and the burgeoned estate, these are without doubt expressions of the personality of the cells of the individual, and they without doubt reflect processes which have been going on for a relatively long time—a long time at any rate from the point of view of the life of an organism. For the cells of an organism to become grossly delinquent it may be that more time is required than we suppose, although severe disturbances in nutrition and severe toxicity will for the time being change some cellular personality radically.

Better understanding in this field is in the future but it may not be far in the future. Biologists have not yet taken a good look at cells, as they have not yet taken a good look at somatotypes. Recent developments in microscopy may greatly help the business of seeing. When it becomes possible to see cells in somewhat the same perspective as that in which we are now accustomed to seeing the human organism as a whole, it may be that the personality of cells will throw light on the personality of organisms. This may lead to a kind of psychology—or orderly description of human behavior—in which the problem of delinquency will further merge with that of medical pathology. For it may be that the delinquency that matters in life is cellular, and not only cellular but deeper, within the genetic structure. The cell might then be an important way station in a study of delinquency, and Dr. Nolan Lewis' famous aphorism "Cancer is paranoia on the cellular level" may contain a rare insight.

We might say that biologists have scarcely as yet looked at cells from the standpoint of their differing personalities in different organisms. There is no reason to suppose that the same primary components cannot be made out in cells that are present in the organism as a whole, and if this should turn out to be the case it will doubtless follow that secondary components will also be seen. It may be found that what we have been calling the t component in the organism as a whole is more manifest and more objectively scalable in the cellular elements that make up the organism. The asthenic and burgeoned characteristics might become as conspicuously objective, for biological scientists, as such a variable as stature is now.

Once a methodology for looking at organisms systematically becomes habitual the detection and scaling of components of variation can revolutionize human life. The cell may offer hope to biological humanics along the same general line as that in which the somatotype seems to hold promise, by presenting a descriptive frame of reference through which to steal a march on the morphogenotype. If the concept of a morphogenotype is applicable to the body as a whole it very likely is also applicable to every cellular unit within the body. That is to say, each cell should have as good a right to a genetically transmitted predisposition toward a distinctive and classifiable pattern as does the body *in toto*. It may be possible to describe such patterns in cells by more satisfactory devices than such a concept as the somatotype offers. The differential structure of cells can perhaps be expressed in terms of, or correlated with, the structural chemistry of organic compounds. In the other direction, it may also be correlated with the morphogenotypes of the organisms that the cells compose. That may seem remotely theoretical in a book concerned with the nature of delinquency, but our inquiry is in fact aimed at *the nature* of delinquency. The method of inquiry has been that of looking at the personality as a whole, structurally and behaviorally. But there may be another way of getting to the same place by sailing in the opposite direction. Or, better, by extending a pincers movement in both directions simultaneously.

We have not yet begun to look at cells from the point of view of their relationship to the morphogenotype, but when we do begin to do so there may be dramatic developments in the way of understanding both the cells and the morphogenotype. Our classification of diseases is in some respects a very unsatisfactory one. We seem not to have got back yet to the fundamental processes involved in disease. There may be basic cellular idiosyncrasies underlying not only the so-called constitutional diseases but also the responses of the organism to the common infections and to all of the exigencies of physiological existence.

In cancer we see cells dividing too easily, too fast, and they seem to have lost touch with headquarters. They appear to have forgotten who they are and how to behave. Instead of dividing to reproduce and to replace functionally their own ancestral type, as respectable cells in a developed organism are supposed to do, they throw off the genetic yoke and burst into a wild orgy of reproduction which gets ahead of the blood supply, encroaches on other tissues, and results finally in destruction of the whole organism. These cancer cells appear to express one kind of biological delinquency. They have thrown off controls which the organism cannot afford to relax. In a sense they might be compared to criminals who disregard social controls which society cannot afford to disregard. They have lost or escaped from or broken down certain inhibitory restraints which it is fatal to lose. Perhaps we could call such cells *positively* delinquent. In some other maladies the tissues seem to be *negatively* delinquent; the cells atrophy, fail to maintain their place in the marching order, and despite an apparent abundance of available nutriment they wither and die without replenishment. In response to the presence of toxic substances or invading organisms, or other forms of irritation not usually or not normally over-whelming, these negatively delinquent cells appear to fail. They surrender too easily to the enemy. They seem to lack vitality.

In a dichotomy of positive and negative cellular delinquency there might be the beginnings of a useful approach to pathology. Nearly all classifica-tions begin as dichotomies, and possibly speculations of the sort indicated in the preceding paragraph are a sign of the times in medicine. The profes-sion was fascinated if not obsessed for two or three generations with a sort of joyous bug hunt, but that is largely over now. In the zestful adventure of ordering and systematizing virtually a new world of causative agents the teachers of medicine often forgot—or could not find time to remember—that it takes more than the causative agent to produce a disease. A disease is a bargain arrived at—a deal—between causative agent and reacting host. Medical attention will return inevitably to the consideration of con-stitutional or relatively deep-seated differences in prospective hosts. The cell may offer a convenient vehicle for such a return.

If cancer is indeed associated with a kind of cellular exuberance it may be that the exuberance is reflected in the morphogenotype of the organism as a whole and also, possibly, in something like a cellular morphogenotype. That the women who develop carcinoma, in the clinical population I have observed, do present a kind of full-bodied morphological exuberance is a fact. I do not believe that their somatotypes are always to be found so dra-matically in the northwest as was the case with the Presbyterian Hospital sample, but they are, on the whole, morphologically burgeoned people. Does this mean that the morphogenotype might yield a clue to the nature of cancer if we knew a little more about the relationship between cellular personality and the morphogenotype?

5. Cancer and Hebephrenia May Contain a Major Clue to Delinquency

If we could bring together for somatotyping, by the method of the stand-ardized photograph, a really representative sample of the cancer patients of the country, and could approach the question of what *is* cancer by thus as it were asking a population sample of perhaps ten thousand to *show* us what it is, we might pick up an important clue.

Cancer patients are usually open, objective people. They are open minded and open hearted. In short they are extraverted, but it is a little more specific than that. They are usually *benignly* extraverted, in contrast with the strained and often hostile extraversion of personalities with a con-spicuous second psychiatric component (paranoid). Cancer patients are generally among the most cooperative and willing of a hospital population. Dr. George Draper, one of the most articulate observers among modern clinicians, long ago pointed this out. It may be said that cancer patients have tried hard enough, and uncomplainingly enough, to show doctors what is the matter. In talking with them I have sometimes experienced one feeling that religious people are always relating: a feeling of being in an exalted presence, or in the presence of motivation nobler than is usually encountered. In talking with people who knew that they were dying of cancer, and had made peace with it, I have had the feeling that the patient knew something important and beyond ordinary conscious knowledge but could not transmit it because there were no words for it. The body seemed to be trying to talk:[4]

Cancer patients are as a rule cerebropenic. They lack the signs of cerebrotonia and of cerebrosis. Their difficulty seems to present something like a biological antithesis to the difficulty which gives rise to the third psychiatric component. There is a marked antithesis between cancer and hebephrenia. Cancer is very rare in association with a predominant hebephrenic component. It will be difficult to prepare data reflecting the degree of the negative correlation between cancer and this component because of the almost universal nonoperationality of psychiatric diagnosis;[5] and such data will perhaps not be very meaningful until the need for operational

[4] Perhaps that sounds like romanticizing and I surely have no desire to invoke a mysticism. The matter may admit of a simple explanation. As medical people know, every now and then somebody rediscovers "the unconscious" and then we have a new insight into psychology. This rediscovery of the unconscious is probably always made by an individual of horizontal dissociation (*Varieties of Temperament,* p. 64), that is to say, somebody who is temperamentally somatotonic and so is, so far as the conscious focus is concerned, more or less out of touch with what is going on in his own body. Such people get "sudden insights" which I believe are really but a matter of getting back into touch with themselves, or of resuming a conscious rapport with what is going on inside, i.e., in their bodies. Probably persons with reasonable cerebrotonic strength never lose this rapport in the first place, and that may be why they experience difficulty in understanding what their more extraverted or more feebly inhibited friends mean by "the unconscious." Not many decades ago the literature of philosophy reflected in nearly every issue of its journals the same difficulty in a controversy over the nature of the "conversional experience," which is really, I suppose, the experience of being suddenly restored to the unconscious—that is, to one's own body. On page 4 I have ventured the somewhat radical suggestion that the body *is* the unconscious.

[5] In one mental hospital where we have been doing research on the psychoses I was told by the Clinical Director that there were four hebephrenic patients with cancer. I hunted up the patients and reviewed their psychiatric histories, translating the diagnostic history in each instance to the quantitative formula described in Chapter 2. Here are the four patients:

Somatotype	Psychiatric Index
4–5–2	4–4–2
5–4–1	5–3–2
3–6–2	4–4–2
4–4–3	5–4–3

In each of the four instances the third was actually the weakest of the three psychiatric components, as I reviewed the histories from the hospital records. All of these patients had at one time or another been called hebephrenic schizophrenes by some hospital officer, and that was, in their cases, the diagnosis which had stuck. But all four of them had also been called catatonic schizophrenes, three had been called paranoid, and three had been called manic-depressive. It was almost a stenographic accident that these patients were on the records as examples of hebephrenic schizophrenia, and the fact is no reflection on the diagnostic acuity of the hospital staff. It is a reflection on the custom of continuing to use, for official diagnosis, a nonoperational typology.

psychiatric diagnosis is met by an accepted schema for the quantification of primary psychiatric components.

The hallmark of the third psychiatric component is the asthenic estate. This relationship is so pronounced and so constant that I am not sure that the third psychiatric component is not *an expression* of asthenia. In cancer the asthenic characteristic is rarely seen, and I think it is almost never pronounced. The cancer people are burgeoned, the hebephrenics are asthenic; and this is one of the most clearly marked biological antitheses encountered in constitutional research. It may be, therefore, that cancer and the third psychiatric component are overt manifestations of two opposite kinds of cellular imbalance; the one an example of a biological exuberance that has got out of hand and so destroys the life balance, the other a kind of biological impoverishment or dying down which likewise fails to maintain the balance on which continuation of life depends. These processes may be of a chemical nature which we shall some day refer to as "simple" or they may depend upon a complex shifting of ionic interrelations which lie beyond human control. It is possible that both are part of the poorly understood mechanism by which the organism maintains adaptive efficiency in the flux in which it exists, that is to say, they may be integral to the evolutionary process. In a very broad sense biological evolution may consist in three essential elements: an element of thrust, or burgeoning advance; an element of retreat or inhibition; and an element of equilibration.

The organisms especially susceptible to cancer and those especially susceptible to hebephrenia may represent two biological fringes or extremes, respectively, of thrust and retreat. This may be nothing more mysterious than an instance of the universal counterbalance between the second (somatotonic) and third (cerebrotonic) components. The secret of continuance of the evolutionary process in organic life may lie in a kind of symbiotic development of these two components in balance, and biological delinquency may be in a measure definable in terms of the various kinds and degrees of failure to do it. From such a point of view cancer might be viewed as an ally, or as a protection against perpetuation of one kind of grave biological error. Hebephrenia might also be considered an ally against an opposite error, and the whole series of disease processes which have been regarded as more or less constitutional, or hereditary, might be reviewed in quite a new light. It is an old saying in medicine that the patient's symptoms are the doctor's best friends. Perhaps our constitutional ailments are only symptoms of biological delinquency.

6. Relation of Dysplasia to Delinquency

One general class of delinquent failure may be reflected in the burgeoning of structure, another general class in asthenic failure of structure. In the former case it would be the inhibitory third component that apparently is lacking. In the latter case the difficulty seems to lie in the second component although not always in a lack of it. The asthenics appear to express qualitative failure of the organism rather than a specific, quantitative failure of the second component. The behavioral manifestations of delinquency make sense to some degree in terms of such a dichotomy. Nearly all of the delinquency encountered in this study can be classified either as insufficiency of expression or as insufficiency of control. The manifestations of asthenia can be looked upon as insufficiencies of expression; the positive misbehavior delinquencies, for the most part, as insufficiencies of control. The first difficulty with so simple a classification is that most of the delinquent individuals show both kinds of delinquency, both in their structure and in their behavior. Among the 200 boys mesomorphy is the predominant component to a conspicuously greater degree, apparently, than in the general population. At full physical maturity the 200 will be on the whole a burgeoned population, as its parents are. Yet in much of its structural detail it is also an asthenic population, as its parents may well be too.[6] Almost half of the 200 boys show asthenic characteristics of sufficiently striking degree that they need to be mentioned in the brief summary of the presentation shown by standard somatotype photography.

It may be that an important clue to the personalities of people who get labeled delinquent lies in an incompatible *mixture* of asthenic and burgeoning characteristics. The public outlook on crime and toward criminals presents a remarkable history of ambivalence, or of pendulum swing between the protective attitude natural toward weakness and the vengeful attitude natural toward strength. There may be a reason for this. Perhaps sociologically there are two main kinds of delinquents, those in whom insufficiency is the predominant factor and those who, essentially strong, yet carry some unassimilable asthenic characteristics. Public feeling about delinquency would then rather naturally alternate between the two poles of mothering concern and righteous indignation, as it in fact seems to do.

The problem of delinquency may thus be related to that of dysplasia, and the positive aspects of delinquency may arise to a considerable degree from a too vigorous protesting, on the part of an essentially vigorous organism, against the dysplasias with which it needs to compromise in order

[6] It is a kind of sociological crime that we lack somatotype photographs of the parents. Possibly the parents would present the same asthenias as their offspring. Then we might have a biological clue to delinquency and something like a beginning toward an operational humanics. Another sociological crime may consist in failure to follow the offspring of these youngsters by constitutional photography. This could be done at the present time only over the dead bodies of many dominating figures in both the Christian and the Freudian priesthoods. The two conflicting priesthoods are in nearly perfect agreement on one essential point, which is suppression of the study of biological heredity in the human scene. Both fear (with a desperation which I think is quite unwarranted) lest the broom that sweeps away the cobwebs of a mysticism should sweep the priestly spider too.

to make sense of itself. Certainly it can be said that what little success I encountered in trying to "reform" some of the subjects of the study, or in trying to stimulate them to see the light concerning themselves, seemed to take its origin in most instances from a discussion of the obvious dysplasias presented in the photograph. At least a dozen of the boys in the series seemed to change their pattern of behavior more or less after being shown their own structural dysplasias which appeared to be fatal to mesomorphic ambitions. *Pari passu,* several seemed to desist from somatorotic violence upon being brought to realization of their comparatively great strength and muscular competence.

If delinquency is related to dysplasia it by no means follows that dysplasia in general can be considered a *cause* of delinquency, but there may be a statistical association between delinquency and the particular kind of dysplasia that involves an incompatible mixture of burgeoning strength and asthenic weakness. An organism with that kind of dysplasia may be on the toboggan from optimal biological balance *in both directions at the same time.* The problem may then be a simpler one than seems to be implied in the way I have stated it. It may be statable in terms of segmental energy potentials, and some of the segments involved may be of sufficiently discrete structural integrity that when adequate description of the morphogenotype is achieved an operational segmental classification of structure will be practical. If this is the case the study of dysplasia may offer more than a faint trail—perhaps even a broad highway—to an attack on human genetics. On such a highway the problem of delinquency would shrink to the consequence of one of those fading markers often seen along highways indicating the site of some nearly forgotten historic event. If delinquency should offer a clue leading to the release of serious scientific energy in the study of the morphogenotype, delinquency might be among the most useful of our present pastimes, and the delinquent youngster then might be a citizen of foremost value.[7]

[7] But the problem may not be so hopefully approachable. Little is actually known about the behavioral autonomy of bodily segments. The reflexologists—a group of psychologists who at one time had hopes of describing the learning process in terms of "conditioned reflexes" and in that way putting psychology on an operational basis—discovered that it is easier to conceive of a reflex than to write a useful taxonomy of reflexes. The reflex psychologists tried valiantly to build a science of behavior with units (reflexes) which cannot be abstracted from the behaving structure. So they tried to forget about the behaving structure. Their efforts to construct a psychology while ignoring the behaving structure is historically comparable to the story of medicine before systematic attention was directed to anatomy, and comparable also, I think, to the contemporary story of speculations on human genetics (p. 33). To get at the problem of dysplasia optimally it is necessary to face the same potentially fatal dilemma that seems to have been disastrous to the reflex psychologists. They had either to find a way of identifying their postulated behavioral units with demonstrable segmentation of the behaving structure—and thus build from purely structural foundations—or try to build a psychology in the abstract. They elected the latter alternative, assumed a *hypothetical* behaving segment, and then proceeded to conjure with it wildly, disdaining the organism. There resulted an edifice of undoubted interest to reflex psychologists but of little value to biological humanics.

DYSPLASIA AND CONFLICT. The fact of overt structural dysplasia may possibly offer a key to such a flooding of the general problem of conflict with new light that problems like delinquency will disappear like dirty snow in spring. But for this to happen it will be necessary to describe dysplasia systematically—taxonomically. The reader is already familiar with the exceedingly small step that has been taken in that direction by the Constitution Project. Dysplasia is initially defined as structural disharmony between different gross regions of the body. The concept is operationally useful only in so far as one employs a segmental differentiation of bodily regions which does actually reflect and reveal dysplasias. The segmental differentiation used for the purposes of the statistics presented in *Varieties of Human Physique* is a rudimentary one, postulating only five bodily regions (p. 19). The astonishing thing is that even so crude a beginning toward a segmental taxonomy does appear to reflect dysplasia with some statistical reliability. That is to say, it reflects dysplastic distribution of strength in the three primary components within five gross segments of the body. But I think this degree of revealment of dysplasia is about comparable to proving that you can measure stature in yards. It is probable that the dysplasias revealed by so rudimentary a segmental differentiation as a fivefold one are of academic interest only. They did serve to demonstrate that dysplasia is there, and they help a little at the beginning of an individual analysis. But this is not a delicate enough tool for coping with problems of psychological conflict where any elaboration at all of mentality is present.

Dysplasia is manifest in the different segments of an arm or leg, in the hand and foot, even in the different phalanges of the fingers and toes. It is also seen in the two sides (right and left) of the various body segments, especially in the two sides of the face. Probably the greatest complication of dysplasia of the external morphology is encountered in the features of the face. In the nose, for example, there is a somewhat independent variation of somatotype in the proximal, middle, and distal segments. Possibly the differentiation can be drawn more finely than that. Maxillary and mandibular structure both show a range of variation on which, in large part, some of our anthropological classifications of race or breed have rested. All of these variations can be expressed as local dysplasias. Many of them "breed true" or appear by inbreeding to have become established breed characteristics. Everybody is familiar with family foreheads, Jewish noses, Negro lips, and so on. The palate and teeth have long been productive hunting grounds for dysplasia and in these structures the ranges of variation are so well mapped that several approaches to somatotyping have been made by the dental profession quite independently of our own approach.[8]

There are dysplasias in the structure of the skin in different parts of the body and in the various appendages of the skin, such as hair and nails and

[8] For a provocative presentation of this problem, see Ryan, E. J.: *Psychobiologic Foundations in Dentistry*. Springfield, Ill., 1946.

sense organs. It is not uncommon to find mesomorphic skin and mesomorphic hair in some regions of the body, with ectomorphic skin structure elsewhere. Since the nervous system is also an appendage of the skin it is not improbable that similar dysplastic variations in nervous and brain structure exist, although no work has yet been done on that problem so far as I know. Internal organs form a continuum with externally manifest structure and certainly show the same sort of dysplastic variation seen at the surface of the body. Beginnings have been made toward the description of cardiac dysplasias. It has become popular, especially in psychiatric literature, to comment on dysplasias in the external sex organs and on autopsy to report these dysplasias. Dysplasia is clearly a concept applicable to any organic structure where different components are more or less in balance and more or less in competition for dominance. Analysis of dysplasia in an individual case could be continued, theoretically, all the way to the cellular structure and perhaps beyond that.[9]

In the two earlier books in the series, and for the most part in this one, we have been discussing dysplasia mainly as it applies to disharmonious arrangement of strength in the primary components—endomorphy, mesomorphy, and ectomorphy. But there are also secondary components of structure, and these too show segmental variation. Pigmentation is a good example of a secondary component showing sometimes dramatic segmental variation. We have said little about pigmentation in the constitutional studies that have been published, although it is a conveniently quantifiable characteristic. The reason for neglecting it is simply that I have not yet noticed a crossing of that trail with any other that seemed important. The student of constitution is always faced with a problem similar to that of a bird dog in the woods. There are many crossing trails, but not all can be followed and only a few lead to game. The dog has the great advantage of his nose. The constitutionalist has only his paranoid component.

[9] I think that nearly all so-called "systems" of character analysis by physiognomy, phrenology, hand reading, and so on depend on more or less intuitive (and perhaps unconscious) judgments arising from the dysplasias manifest in the subject. Even the analyses based on handwriting may depend in large measure on this factor, for handwriting is really an athletic skill arising from coordination primarily of arm and hand muscles but secondarily of all the postural muscle systems of the body. The trouble with the systems of analysis just referred to is simply that the system never goes back far enough. The characterologists are as a group too impatient or too lazy. They grasp a fragment of truth and rush eagerly to the bank with it, to cash it in. No analysis of the dysplasias or of the behavior of one segment of the body taken alone, even if done thoroughly and well, can offer a sound basis for analysis of the personality. Before interpretive value can be attached to even a good analysis of local structure it is necessary to know the somatotype, and thus to approach as closely as possible to a knowledge of the morphogenotype. Once this is done I think that both interest and value may inhere in many of the characterological approaches now so disdainfully and on the whole rightly scorned by all who have "taken" Psychology 101. These approaches have been trying to dig out the woodchuck of dysplasia, but the digging has been done with an ice cream spoon. Characterology may possibly be defined as *lazy* constitutional analysis.

DYSPLASIAS OF GYNANDROMORPHY. Dysplasias of gynandromorphy are common and appear to be a major cause of frustration in mesomorphs. One of the commonest dysplasias is that in which the fifth and possibly the fourth regions are gynandroid, with the other regions perhaps fiercely masculine. This dysplasia is the *bête noire* of athletic coaches and of fathers who have invested hope in the athletic prowess of sons. It also may be at the bottom of much unhappiness in the individuals themselves, in a culture which places a premium on athletic performance in the male. These tough-looking individuals who have nevertheless a gynandroid caboose are fatally handicapped in nearly every branch of athletic competition except swimming. They are often first-rate swimmers but they cannot compete with the nongynandroid male at running, at fighting, or at any of the games involving hard bodily contact or prolonged muscular endurance. These are the boys, undoubtedly, whom the psychoanalyst Alexander has called hard-on-the-outside-soft-on-the-inside. He considers this a common delinquent "type" and I am sure he is right. Good examples of it are seen among our 200 (Nos. 47, 85, and 120). I believe that several of the 7 or 8 killers whom I have had the opportunity of meeting and studying would show the characteristic but I have never had a chance to test that idea by taking somatotype photographs.

Gynandroid dysplasias are of course not limited to the part of the anatomy that goes over the fence last, although in the male they are most dramatic in that quarter. There are, for example, powerful athletes who show no manifest departures from masculine extreme mesomorphy except in the first region. In common with a number of other morons I have had a lifelong interest in major league ball players, especially the great and the famous. (For years I hopefully hunted for a major leaguer, other than a pitcher, who would not be a six in mesomorphy, and never found one.) Enos Slaughter of the Cardinals has a face and neck that are gynandroid but there are no other manifestations of *g* component and he has been one of the best in the game. Ted Williams of the Red Sox shows this same dysplasia but as he is a big man the 6 in mesomorphy also manifests itself conspicuously and in general. It should be obvious, then, that *g* in the first region is one dysplasia that does not seriously handicap a ball player.

I think that the most painful of all gynandroid dysplasias, in a growing boy in American democracy at any rate, is that of feminoid arms. This dysplasia is common, and is perhaps growing more common. Such an individual simply cannot fight, cannot throw, and from what is often his point of view, cannot do *anything* except perhaps produce a violent temper tantrum, which he often does.

If dysplasias were all-or-none phenomena, which you have or don't have, that would be one thing and life might be simple enough not to require constitutional psychology. But the worst thing about dysplasia is that it is often insidious—just faintly present and not sufficiently for an honest and overt announcement of its presence. Then it can really get youngsters into monkey traps. The youth who has the coordination, the reaction time, the energy, and the "heart" for top-flight athletic performance of some kind but has just a slight gynandroid dysplasia in his running gear may spend the first half of his life trying to find out what is the matter, and the second half trying to drown out the memories of the frustration. It is detection of the faint dysplasias that constitutes one of the fine points, I think, in analysis of personality.

DYSPLASIAS OF t COMPONENT. The gynandroid dysplasias as a group are fairly obvious. Less obvious but perhaps even more important psychologically is another kind of dysplasia in a secondary component—the t component. Many persons are thoroughbred, perhaps "overly thoroughbred" or too fine drawn in one region of the body but coarse and poorly put together in other regions. An individual so constituted is really born into an aesthetic monkey trap.[10] He has overfine discrimination and is *at the same time* coarse or undiscriminative. Worse than this, from the standpoint of his social adaptation and his "success with people" he may be both attractive and repulsive in the same situation. For such a person it is sometimes nearly impossible to find a social level or to feel at home in any kind of social setting. Many marriages come to grief through incompatibilities arising from dysplasias of the t component, and perhaps the worst thing about these dysplasias is that they cannot, as a rule, be explained or even indicated to those who present them most dramatically. It is not an altogether safe thing to talk about the t component, even in the abstract, in a democratic society, for it smacks of not being democratic.[11]

[10] For those familiar with *The Promethean Will*, a fifth panel monkey trap.

[11] And perhaps it isn't democratic. I have never been quite sure on that point. Can you stand off and look at yourself and other human stock in the same naturalistic way that you look at any kind of biological stock? Can you size up and "judge the points" of a specimen of human stock—yourself, for example—without feeling any more "undemocratic" about it than you would if you were looking at dogs or roosters? Can you do this and be democratic? I do not know, because I do not know what emotional and conceptual responses that term evokes in your mind. For myself, it would be undemocratic not to be able to do these things, and it seems to me that there must be a certain prudishness or possibly a superstitious arrogance in a mind not prepared to stand up to that simple test of earthiness and biological good humor. I am perhaps as intolerant of the outlook that would set the human organism apart, or on a different plane from other organisms, as the most zealous democracy-shouters are intolerant of such social pruderies as particularly irritate them.

To be afraid of the t component, or to be prudish or squeamish about it, is in my opinion equivalent to being afraid of biological democracy. The t component is really another word for biological quality. Now biological quality is a concept that human beings cannot afford to throw away. The original idea of democracy, and the idea of it still dominant in the minds of some who have called themselves democrats, is that biological quality is a goal ultimately attainable by the whole breed of us. I should therefore include in a definition of democracy a sense of fraternity and equality with all life, but also a profound reverence for biological quality. If in human life we have somehow in the name of democracy lost that reverence for quality, then we will probably throw life itself into the democratic wastebasket.

Dysplasias of the *t* component, and especially incompatibilities between primary and secondary *t*—which also are dysplasias—are common throughout the HGI series. They show, to a degree, in the original photographs but cannot be seen well in the half-tone reproductions of the photographs, and are obscured too by the necessary blocking out of the features. *Secondary t* is by definition that aspect of *t* that you do not see in a photograph. In the HGI series there is such a dramatic range of *primary t* that it can still be made out even in the worst of our photographs.

What the relationship is between *t* and the phenomena that in this book are referred to as the burgeoned and asthenic characteristics, respectively, is a question of some interest. We are in an early pioneering phase so far as systematic exploration of human personality goes. These concepts can develop only by trial and error. A good guess may be that the characteristics in question are really *t* phenomena; that texture or quality is in the cellular structure of the organism and that both asthenia and burgeoning are but outward macroscopic expressions of variations from a biological balancing which is likewise and similarly reflected in the aesthetic harmonies of cellular structure. Burgeoning may be definable as a general coarsening of cellular structure, without good architecture. Asthenia may be a general falling back from pattern, or an architectural recession and shrinking of the cellular structure.

The most curious thing about the asthenic and burgeoning characteristics is that both are often found in the same organism. There are well-established breeds of people who show burgeoning in some segments of their structure and asthenic "degeneration" in other segments. In some oriental stocks, for example, a deliberate effort has been made for centuries to encourage what seems to be an asthenic degeneration of the feet in women, while at the same time a degree of burgeoning robustness or even rotundity is prized in other bodily regions. Binding of the feet of females is still practiced in parts of China, to try to ensure tininess of structure. This curious practice seems to have its origins in an identification between aristocracy and fragility of structure, perhaps between aristocracy and ectomorphy of high *t* component. If that *is* the origin of this persistent human taste, the story presents a good example of a biological monkey trap which may be of wider dissemination than is realized. Ectomorphy of high *t* component, especially in women, has long stood as a sort of stereotype for biological aristocracy. The catch is that high *t* must in the beginning always have meant *first-rate performance*. If we believe in a structure-function continuum, high *t* means functional efficiency of the first order and this is its *basic* operational meaning. Beauty of structure and beauty of performance are one conceptual continuum and any separation of the two is a sign of biological bad health prodromal to the closure of a monkey trap. (This is one special instance of the body-mind monkey trap.)

BOTH THE ASTHENIC AND THE BURGEONED ESTATE MAY START AS BIOLOGI-
CAL COUNTERFEITING.   I have seen Chinese women with small, deformed
feet which far from being examples of high *t* component ectomorphy were
good examples of low *t* component asthenic degeneration. And they had
been taught to be *proud* of such feet. It was, in their family, a mark of aristocracy. Their mothers and grandmothers had had similar feet. Somehow,
back at the beginning of the monkey trap, somebody had apparently confused asthenic degeneracy with high *t* component ectomorphy. Perhaps it
was because the two had a certain element of fragility in common. Now that
mistake would never have been made with horses. Nobody would for generations maintain a breed of horses with uselessly degenerate lower extremities.

In this country too there is a strong trace of the same misanthropy, especially in the South, where it is sometimes fashionable to make quite a fuss
over the minuteness of the female extremity. There are, either in consequence or *pari passu,* thousands of American females whose feet, and usually
hands also, present more or less vestigially degenerate structure and function. In this instance also the taste seems to have begun as a kind of worship
of what has been considered quality of structure, or high *t* ectomorphy.
There are also women who show the latter characteristic, women of both
physical delicacy and first-rate performance. In the South they are not uncommon but even there the asthenic counterfeit is now commoner, I think,
than the genuine article.

The monkey trap seems to lie in a failure to restrain asthenic counterfeiting of high *t* ectomorphy, and it may be that ectomorphy in the human species is a luxury which should be prohibited until man becomes a biologically
responsible organism trustworthy with such dangerous luxuries. The real
potency of the monkey trap resides in our bisexual reproduction. Everybody
wants fine, aristocratic-looking women, and since everybody is not an expert
student of biological counterfeiting, some get stung. This still would not be
so bad except for the fact that the asthenic characteristics are transmitted to
the next generation of both sexes. Then every possible sort of asthenic dysplasia crops up in men and women alike, and the termites are in the biological foundations. It is thus that ectomorphy may have got us into trouble.
A remote ancestral twinge of pure ecstasy over the light efficiency of a finely
chiseled nymph; a little carelessness with the biological currency; and now
Casper Milquetoast and about half of the HGI series, not to mention a civilization increasingly delinquent in its hands and feet.

Among the Hottentots and among several native stocks of Africa there is
a curious fad for feminine *steatopygia,* which may be defined as a dysplastic
burgeoning of the buttocks. Literally *stea-* refers to fat, but steatopygia is by
no means all fat. It is an overdevelopment of muscle, fat, and connective tissue—a burgeoning in general—and is not confined to the buttocks but usu-

ally includes the thighs and also, in some degree, the entire fourth region. I have discussed the question of steatopygia with both Negroes and Jews, in whose stock there are strong traces of the phenomenon. Some of these people had been culturally indoctrinated with the same appreciation of it that had been felt by their antecedents. On one point they have been in agreement. The nexus of the attraction is not fat as such, but what is called, rather, "comely development." There is an ancient intuition that women well developed in their equatorial south produce better children. Asked *better in what sense?*, my friends have almost invariably replied, stronger, healthier, more vigorous children.

This answer may or may not reflect the true origin of the fashion. If it does, here seems to lurk the same kind of monkey trap that has produced our astounding crop of asthenia. In this instance, though, the lure was not aristocratic ectomorphy but good, earthy, endomorphic mesomorphy. What those ancestral Negroes saw, apparently, was that the women well endowed with endomorphic mesomorphy, especially in the fourth region, produced the huskiest offspring, and did it with the least fuss. The burgeoning of the buttocks (and thighs) was probably but a conspicuous concomitant of a general emphasis on ampleness. But in the course of time it was no doubt to be expected that so prominent a structural sign might come to be taken for the quality with which it had been originally associated, and might so come to displace that quality. The trap is now ready to close. The machinery for biological counterfeiting is set up and lubricated.

We begin to see in what burgeoning may actually consist. As I use the concept, it refers to a gross enlargement of structure *which does not serve a biological purpose but may be inclined, rather, to hinder the purpose it seems to serve.* The fatty burgeoning of the buttocks and thighs now so often observed in American Negroes, Jews, and to some extent in other stocks of both sexes, is quite possibly a product of biological counterfeiting not essentially unlike that reflected in the asthenic degeneracies. It is not uncommon to encounter in American cities Negro and Jewish women so grossly obese, and so burgeoned both laterally and to the rear that they require the whole of a bus or streetcar seat intended for two. But these are not the prolific producers of offspring whose biological efficiency in that department long ago set the jaws of the trap. These burgeoned women generally produce defective children or, when the burgeoning is extreme, none at all. There are many Negroes, and people of other breeds, whom our complex urban civilization seems to have swept so far from their biological moorings that they have lost the biological orientation necessary for distinguishing between real coin and the most grossly counterfeit article. I think it is people like that who prize for its own sake nonfunctional burgeoning of the buttocks as well as that flaccid asthenic degeneracy of southern and other women which is so offensive to people who love nature.

Both the asthenic and the burgeoning perversions of biological structure, then, may sometimes owe their perpetuation to human failure to distinguish between good and counterfeit biological coin. Both probably tend to get established in the germ plasm at the start as dysplasias associated with some kind of superior performance, and therefore are highly prized. But the human organism lives for so short a time that its transmission of even elemental biological wisdom from one generation to the next is defective, and the responsibility for selective reproduction of the species—now that the medical profession has largely removed that responsibility "from nature"—has been proving too much for us. If we keep the luxury of the medical profession, therefore, we evidently are going to have to train specialists for the conscious control of reproduction.

DYSPLASIA OF t COMPONENT IN THE CLINICAL POPULATION. I have mentioned only a few of the commonest asthenic dysplasias, and only one of the conspicuous dysplasias of burgeoning. Actually both of these phenomena are of almost endless occurrence. Ride in the subway and look at noses, ears, mouths, jaws, shoulders, chests, bellies, extremities, trunk-limb proportions. Watch all these structures in action as well as in repose. You will see an endless parade both of burgeoning departure from good t structure and of asthenic falling away from it. Your grandmother may have told you that the secret of good manners is the averted eye. But he who walks with averted eye walks into biological monkey traps. The first step toward biological humanics lies in development of a thoughtful, searching eye.

An even better place than the subways to look for the phenomena of dysplastic delinquency is the nearest medical clinic. There you see a selective population in which the factor of selection may be reflected to a considerable degree in these very dysplasias. In the United States about 85 per cent of the population never come to hospitals as patients except for normal childbirth, for an episode or two of acute infection, or for final leave-taking in old age. In 1938 something like 95 per cent of the total days of hospitalization were being expended on 11 per cent of the population. An interesting question is, just *who are* the people making up this 11 per cent?[12]

One observation is that those who constitute the chronic hospital population, both in consequence of somatic disease and in consequence of

[12] To find out in a statistically satisfactory manner would not be very difficult although it would require coordination between a large number of hospital administrators, doctors, photographic technicians, and people trained in constitutional analysis. The results of the study of the hospital material would have to be compared against similar results obtained from the study of statistically valid samplings from many segments of the general population. An enterprise of the latter sort could be carried out as a mere detail or side project in connection with the regular census-taking procedure. But it could not be done satisfactorily by an individual or group of individuals working without governmental cooperation. Incomplete or inadequate data bearing on problems of this kind are worse in some respects than none at all. From hasty and abortive surveys inaccurate information gets out into the main arteries of propaganda and confusion grows worse confounded. Yet before surveys of any sort are made there have to be pioneer observations.

what is called mental disease, are singularly rich in both kinds of the *t* component dysplasias we have been discussing. The burgeoning dysplasias are seen dramatically in such illnesses as the carcinomas, gall bladder disease, and the expressive psychoses. The asthenic dysplasias are conspicuous in tuberculosis, rheumatoid arthritis, and above all in the hebephrenic psychoses. In many instances of carcinoma and gall bladder disease the individual seems burgeoned as a whole unit. In hebephrenia the picture of complete or overwhelming asthenia is often seen. But in many, possibly in most, clinical entities there are often strong indications of both a burgeoning and an asthenic process going on at the same time. Striking examples of this are seen in patients with persistent peptic ulcer. As Figure 40 (p. 788) indicates, the peptic ulcer people are on the whole mesomorphs. Also they are on the whole vigorous and hearty, overly active mesomorphs. Many of them tend to burgeon, especially in the first two regions. But along with the burgeoning there are nearly always patent asthenic dysplasias, and these are seen with remarkable frequency in the fourth and fifth regions. An asthenic disharmony in the structure of the legs is so common in peptic ulcer that at the Constitution Clinic we have sometimes spoken of *peptic ulcer legs*. These are usually of good length, in contrast with the peglike underdeveloped legs typical of schizophrenia, but are gynandroid, are of relatively weak muscling, and are inclined particularly to be weak or hollowed in the inner aspects of the thighs. When this hollowing of the inner thighs is presented, with comparatively delicate but poorly proportioned distal segments of the gynandroid legs, together with a big chest and thick neck and signs of hyperactivity, the medical delinquency to think of first is peptic ulcer. The ulcer without the asthenic deficiency in the lower part of the body is apparently a rarity, although this asthenia is common without the ulcer and other asthenias are also common *with* the ulcer. For examples of morphologies suggestive of peptic ulcer, study the photographs of Nos. 53, 129, and 142.

On watching quite a number of hospital populations from a constitutional point of view I have sometimes felt that there may be a general factor of medical delinquency which is reflected in the organic structure, and that this factor may be measurable. The life insurance companies have in their concern for the "overweight" state of affairs long been sensitive to a spoor of the overblown or burgeoned characteristic. But the asthenic dysplasias may be equally important. They are not reflected in the weight or in the somatotype, and are not too well reflected even in the standardized photograph. To gauge them accurately you almost have to see the individual move and perform. But then, you generally have to do that to arrive at a medical diagnosis, or to judge a dog properly.

When the asthenic dysplasia is manifestly present it interferes with grace and with efficiency of bodily movement. Possibly the best of all tests for traces of asthenic dysplasia is to dance with a person. In dancing you immediately get the feel of either kind of departure from a good primary t component if any trace of either is present. If later burgeoning is on the calendar there is a ponderousness or lack of lightness of muscular movement which cannot be concealed in the dance. If any asthenic interference is present there is a muscular lifelessness or lack of suppleness, or wooden quality, which no amount of practice and training can remove. It is nearly as difficult to conceal the asthenic quality from an observant dance partner as for a cross-country runner to conceal a wooden leg. Indeed, the two kinds of concealment are of somewhat the same nature. I am not sure that the dance, in some form or other, has not served as useful a function in human mating as in that of other species.[13] Possibly if marriages in general were cradled on the dance floors of the nation, after the prospective brides and grooms had been well instructed in constitutional analysis, a more effective attack on medical delinquency might be implemented.

THE LONG-LIVED PEOPLE ARE FREE FROM DYSPLASIAS OF t. There is another fragment of indirect evidence that a relationship exists between what we have been calling t component and medical delinquency. This is the fact that there appears to be a positive correlation between t and longevity. One of the most neglected of the obviously important branches of medicine is systematic study of the outstandingly healthy, and of those who have shown by long lives free of disease that they have good resistance to the common pathologies or disintegrative influences. Very little has been done in this field. A good project would be one in which constitutional analysis were carried out for a few hundred of those who have in this way demonstrated a biological superiority. On page 795 is mentioned a peculiar similarity of structure noticeable among the last surviving veterans of the Civil War, and I may add that, in our culture at least, a similar phenomenon can often be seen in other people who have arrived in their eighties and nineties without much balking of the biological machinery. *These people almost uniformly present a high primary t component* and I think that is their most conspicuous common trait. They show gross bodily dysplasias, so far as the general distribution of the primary components go, but this is not incompatible with high t.[14] I have seen a number of healthy old people who because of these primary dysplasias would scarcely have taken the blue ribbon at a human stock show—if we had such a thing—but the kind of secondary dysplasias that I have been describing as the burgeonings and the asthenias are certainly not common in "successful old age." The mean primary t in a

[13] Almost any treatise on natural history will be found rich in accounts of elaborations of the dance that seem to play a part in the mating of birds and of animals at nearly all levels of the complexity scale. For many flying insects the chief business in the final or mature phase of life appears to consist in a more or less elaborate dance which eventuates in mating.

[14] The great tennis player Tilden, for example, is grossly dysplastic but of high t in every region. In the first two regions he is about 1–6–3, while in the fifth region (legs) he is about $1\frac{1}{2}$–$4\frac{1}{2}$–$4\frac{1}{2}$.

series of 50 healthy persons past 80 observed in 1940 by the notebook method and rated for that characteristic, was 2.4. This is on a scale where the mean for the general population falls at 1.8 (p. 22) and that for a college population of 4000 fell at 1.96. If observation at such a preliminary level is worth anything at all the phenomenon of primary *t* may be an important structural correlate of long life.

One other characteristic of long-lived men seems to be a good balancing of the second and third components. In my experience it is rare to meet a healthy octogenarian male who presents a marked lack of either mesomorphy or ectomorphy, and even rarer to meet an extreme mesomorph or extreme ectomorph in that age range. I have never seen an extreme endomorph of either sex who was "doing well" past 80. The long-lived people often "weigh about the same" all their lives.

In women the picture is a little different from what I have observed in men. In women ectomorphy seems to be less important for longevity and there appear to be quite a number of endomorphic mesomorphs who do well at the extreme age ranges. These are not infrequently ectopenes who, had they been male, would almost certainly have blown out a cerebral or coronary vessel or would have run into renal vascular trouble, long before reaching 80. The female constitution appears to keep the pressure down, or lends a degree of elasticity not possessed, in general, by the male even when the latter is markedly gynandroid.

Medically, in the human male the least delinquent organism seems to be about a 2–4½–4½ of high primary *t* and of average or slightly under average stature. The longest lived men would be called by the average observer lightly built, clean-cut, and as an average, slightly undersized. To this picture I will add one more detail which may be more hazardous. I think these men have good general coordination and that they are naturally good at such exercises as walking and dancing. That of course does not mean that they necessarily *like* dancing, or know that they would like it.

Probably the same general description would hold for the medically *least* delinquent females. I think I have encountered more ladies of that pattern, living healthily in their eighties and nineties, than of any other pattern. But among the healthy old ladies there is also a generous sprinkling of solider, chunkier physiques, likewise free from the *t* component dysplasias and, I think, of good coordination. It is almost as unusual to find very large women among the ranks of the medically innocent in old age as very large men. For biological superiority the optimal size of the human organism appears to be somewhat less than the mean size, and this raises a question that may have a bearing on modern pediatrics.

OUR PEDIATRIC PRACTICE MAY BE DIRECTLY CONTRIBUTIVE TO MEDICAL DELINQUENCY. During the past three or four decades pediatrics has become a very popular branch of medicine, and pediatricians naturally vie with one another for the lucrative trade. By and large the most rewarded of the pediatricians are those who guide the mothers most successfully in the stuffing of the babies. One up-and-coming pediatrician with whom I went to medical school recently told me that the schedule we learned for "normal weight gain" in babies is out of date. We were taught that an infant of vigorous good health should triple his weight in the first year, or should weigh about 20 or 21 pounds at age 1. But those babies whose corporational destinies are now being presided over by my friend are doing better than that. *They* weigh, on an average at the end of the first year, 25 pounds, and some of them do still better. The secret, my friend says, is to *feed 'em*. Fill 'em up full, especially with bananas and vitamins. Let 'em eat all they want whenever they want it. None of this old-fashioned schedule stuff. "Anyhow that schedule business tends to create friction between the mother and the baby and probably leads to complexes. Not that I go for all that Freudian psychowhatever stuff, you understand, but some of the mothers do, and anyway there may be something in it, you know."

Pediatrics has fallen into step with a fad for the burgeoning of children. There has been really a Dionysian orgy of eating (as well as of drinking) in this country during the past couple of generations. It seems to be one aspect of a general throwing off of restraint and is, I think, a religious phenomenon at bottom. We have been stuffing our young to make them grow *bigger*. Stature at Harvard has increased about three inches since 1900 and stature in the United States armed forces increased more than an inch between the two World Wars. Weight has increased nearly proportionally—probably more than proportionally if the weight of the college boys and of the soldiers had been recorded at middle age instead of in early youth.

It would be of interest to know the consequences or correlates of such a "forced draft" burgeoning of human flesh. What is actually involved is apparently a burgeoning or blowing up of individual cells, not an increase in the number of cells. It amounts to a kind of wholesale cellular burgeoning, and there may be a question whether we are thereby lowering cellular resistance to those medical delinquencies which appear to be especially associated with the burgeoned state. If this is what has been happening there should be within a few generations a detectable rise in the incidence of cancer, and possibly of other so-called constitutional diseases, along with a fall in the longevity of the comparatively healthy.

If burgeoning and asthenia are comparable, as they seem to be, to the two slopes of a roof, each falling away from an efficient biological balance, it may be that the two states are more intimately related than has been supposed, and that any environmental influence tending strongly to precipitate one of these conditions is also, in the long run, a stimulant to the other. In that event a promiscuous encouragement of the burgeoning process would be also the precipitant of a bumper crop of asthenia, together with medical and psychiatric delinquencies associated therewith. The achievement of extending Harvard stature (and future girth) by several inches is without a doubt a triumph of some kind. But it may be a costly triumph if the cost must be reckoned in additional millions of cases of hebephrenia, manic-depressive psychosis, paranoia, malignancy, cardiovascular disease, and in brief all of those life-shortening conditions which are not controllable by such bug killers as penicillin and the sulfa drugs. We are rushing about very blindly in medicine. Instead of pausing to take account of stock and to set up machinery for a kind of record keeping that in time would reveal what we are doing, we have been plunging into fads and have been inclined to boast of achievements that are at best equivocal. This may be delinquency.

CHAPTER 6

THE SOCIAL PSYCHIATRY OF DELINQUENCY

1. What Then Is Delinquency?

The task undertaken was to write psychological biographies of 200 youths more or less delinquent. Having read a number of treatises on delinquency I was at the outset aware that we would encounter a nearly insuperable difficulty in defining the concept. Most of those who had written in this field had either ignored altogether the matter of defining their subject or had waived the problem with a legalistic definition: to be delinquent was to be caught at breaking laws. This is one kind of circumlocution that is indicated by the term "begging the question."

If you were to live for a time among the more or less professedly delinquent youngsters at the HGI you would soon come to understand that every theft or act of illegal aggression is an *executed judgment* either against individuals or against society. Sometimes the judgment is made and executed lightly, sometimes with the highest degree of cogency. It would seem therefore that there can hardly be such an entity as delinquency, judged on the external or objective manifestations alone. What we call delinquency will always involve at least two more or less independent variables; the consequences and the justifications of the act, and neither variable is simple. It would seem, further, that unless you are prepared to fall back on some supernatural or mystical theology for the foundation of your ethics, and are ready to take the consequences in the coinage of a nonoperational social philosophy, you are constrained to make peace with the idea that every delinquent act must be judged in terms of its own relationships. A dozen or more dictionary definitions of delinquency, hunted up by an obliging student, boiled down readily to two ideas. To be delinquent was: (a) To break laws; (b) to be a disappointment, usually to some abstract entity like Society, or Mr. G, *by deviating too far from an expected performance.*

On a little reflection it is clear that by both criteria most of the American population would have to be called delinquent. The question might even be raised as to whether law itself may not often be a precipitation of delinquency, law being theoretically an expression of the will of politically dominant agglutinations of people themselves only too patently delinquent by the second criterion, and often enough so by the first. In the best circles law is always suspect. Nearly all, possibly every one of humanity's most revered legendary heroes, from Prometheus to Jesus Christ and Robin Hood, have been so delinquent under the law that their lives were legally forfeit. The legal criterion of delinquency, useful enough in meeting the requirements of Ph.D. theses in sociology, would in fact be adequate only in a static society where legality is foreordained and where the main purpose of life would then be conformity to omnisciently established law. There are men, I know, who think we live in that kind of society, but they are growing fewer and less articulate. With their departure the legal criterion becomes less definitive, and as it does so the power of Zeus yields more and more both to Promethean fortitude and to Dionysian revelry.

The second criterion of delinquency, that of the disappointing performance, may retain more meaning. The difficulty of course is—disappointing to *whom?* If you have made peace in your mind with the probable reluctance of Benevolent Omniscience to participate in the business of being disappointed, and you had better, you have to face the awful possibility of your own responsibility for human affairs, even for delinquency. Then you are the one with the moral obligation to feel disappointed, and delinquency is behavior disappointing to *you.* Another difficulty of definition is this: The criteria of biological delinquency may remain fairly constant throughout time, yet may not be even positively correlated with those of sociological delinquency in twentieth-century American democracy. In our habitual thinking there are not yet any operational ties between biological and social science. Here may lie the root of the difficulty in defining delinquency, and this may be the reason why correlations between specific traits and delinquency or between almost anything and delinquency seem nearly a waste of time. The job in this prepsychological period is not to try to correlate things with what cannot yet be operationally defined but to set up criteria for definition. For the present the most direct step toward definition of delinquency may lie simply in an operational description of individuals who by various agencies have been labeled delinquent.

After spending some portions of a decade thinking about delinquency, living intimately with it, and now and then attempting to define it, I grew aware that a book on the subject would be a fool's venture unless it were also a book on behavior which was not delinquent, and I am afraid there will never be a way of defining delinquency satisfactorily except in terms of the whole performance of any individual who is to be called delinquent. That is why the basic method employed here has been primarily biographical rather than primarily statistical. Within the biographical fabric there is a closely woven pattern of quantification which renders the study to a degree scientific or objective, but an effort is also made in this study not to wash away the sociological baby in statistical soapsuds.

It should not then be necessary to labor the point further that delinquency is never quite an either-or phenomenon, that nobody can be wholly delinquent or wholly nondelinquent, that all scales or quantifications of delinquency, including those used in this book, are good only with reference to the time-place-person-and-circumstance of their origin. With this assumed, the nearest I can come to a definition might be this: *Delinquency is behavior disappointing beyond reasonable expectation.* That is not so much a definition as an emphasis on the difficulty of definition. Delinquency is a phenomenon varying at both ends—at a disappoint*ee* end and a disappoint*er* end. But any student of natural science is aware that many things which cannot be satisfactorily defined can nevertheless be classified and scaled. Art, for example, beauty, heroism, life. These things, like delinquency, have variables at both ends—a plea*see* end and a plea*ser* end. Beauty is form that is pleasing beyond ordinary expectation. Art *was* something like that but has recently become something else—possibly a delinquency.

So I have no apology to offer for trying to scale and to quantify delinquency even though I cannot define it. It is possible that by systematizing (making scientific) the biographies of a sufficiently extensive series of labeled delinquents valuable information on the general subject can be revealed. Information valuable, I mean, for a future biological humanics. If in your own scale of values this is insufficient justification for a book, and if yet you are tolerant of "art," I would submit this study as an experimental exercise in the art of biography.

2. Why Statistics on Delinquency Have Been So Worthless

In the Army during the last war I had for a time as a messmate an officer who expressed much curiosity over the study of delinquency, on which he had heard I was working. The subject was one that concerned him closely, he said, because he had inherited an interest in a very active manufacturing enterprise. As an employer of men and women he was deeply concerned in their welfare. It was important to maintain high morale in the business organization he helped direct. It was especially important to detect and eliminate delinquent individuals, to "find the rotten apples before they could spoil the whole barrel." "Preventive sociology," he called it. Punishment of delinquency was a matter to which this major had given considerable thought. He was not old fashioned. None of your eye-for-an-eye and tooth-for-a-tooth business for him. In fact he didn't really believe in punishment at all, he said. Having been to college and become a liberal he believed in reform—rehabilitation. The thing to do was find out what made a man tick. To study the man, analyze him, and then "give him a break."

That was the sober or as it were the official statement of the matter. But the major was not often sober and with alcohol his opinions about delinquency were different. Then there was nothing he hated so much as a thief.

Reform and rehabilitation were now all very well—for those in "honest" need of it—but you can't cure a thief that way, or a liar. The only thing to do with that kind of a sonovabitch is nail him up on the barn door. We simply can't have that sort of thing and we've got to fight people like that, as we do the German bastards, with any weapon we can get hold of. "I hate a liar. When I find out that a man's a liar I'm through with the guy. The hell with him."

I knew the major for six months, probably talked with him fifty times. Perhaps I failed to make out his philosophy justly but in its essentials it seemed to be about this: Life is a sort of struggle for survival, and for the better automobiles and women and places in the sun, with no playing of favorites. What a man can get is rightly his so long as he plays the game in accordance with certain rigidly fixed rules. Life is very much like an organized sport, with established rules of quite detailed nature. To succeed illustriously one must attack the opposition with vigor. Indeed one must override, knock out, maim, render prostrate, and in general annihilate the opposition. But it must all be done according to the rules. To break any of the rules, and be caught at it, is just a little worse than running up a low score (bank account).

We returned in our discussions now and again to the subject of delinquency. My friend developed a hypothesis. A cure for delinquency might be found, he suggested, in universal athletics. Let every youngster learn to play competitive games. Substitute gymnasiums, sports programs, and directors of athletics for much of the police and social service machinery. Make the kids rule conscious. Indoctrinate them with the idea of sportsmanship. Let them learn to obey the rules of the game by playing games. He pointed out that he had learned sportsmanship that way, in school and college, and that although he had had delinquent impulses, like all normal fellows, he had learned to curb them by playing the game. As time went on he warmed up to the subject. Once (with the help of alcohol) he decided to put his second five million into a "project." He would set up a model school for underprivileged and delinquent boys. It was to be a place where the youngsters would be taught athletic games, and not much else. The major is a 3–6–2.

The business in which the major's family exercises an interest is that of manufacturing and selling razor blades. One day he gave me some packages of blades, explaining that these particular blades were unusual. They were made of specially treated steel which rendered the steel harder than that ordinarily used. The blades would shave better and would last much longer, I was informed, than even those regularly manufactured by the company. I accepted the blades with gratitude and found that in fact they did retain their edges remarkably. One day I asked my friend why his company didn't make *all* their blades that way. The answer was simple and to the point. To make them all that way would spoil the razor blade business. Blades of this particular kind of hardened steel are too good, would last too long. The company was spending vast sums advertising; educating people, by suggestion at least, to use a new blade every day and to throw away yesterday's blade. The resulting enormous volume of business had produced stabilized employment for hundreds, and stabilized profits too. The distributional aspect of the thing was also important. To make the blades last longer would slow down sales, thus working a hardship on retailers. Business in general would suffer. The value of the company's stock would fall.

The company had bought out a patent in connection with this hardening process, but that was just to prevent the process from being used by other manufacturers of lower ethical standards—there are always sonsabitches around, you know, who will take shortcuts even when obviously against the general welfare. Buying up the patent was one of those expenditures for public good that a big company has to make all the time. We never get credit for that sort of thing, of course, but it is part of life, like helping old ladies across the street. Vigilance is the price of survival, etc. You'd be surprised at how much the company spends every year just to keep things stable and right in the razor blade business.

The company sells shaving cream, too. You'd be surprised at the cost distribution on a tube of shaving cream. On a 50-cent tube (the highest retail price of which is actually 33 cents) the cost of the shaving cream itself is about half a cent. The container and packing costs two cents, average transportation costs are about a cent, national and other advertising five cents. To maintain a fair profit level on a sale the company has to nearly double the cost, so the company gets about 16 cents for a tube of its shaving cream. The difference between this amount and the price you pay at the drugstore (which sells the "50 cent tube" for 33 cents) is the cost of wholesale and retail distribution.

Returning to the razor blades, their cost of manufacture is, or was in 1941, a little less than seven cents per hundred. After passing through a series of cost increments approximately similar to that which applied to the shaving cream, the blades finally cost the retail purchaser about $2.50 per hundred. The user of the shaving cream pays sixty or seventy times the manufacturing cost for a unit of this vitally important product, while for his razor blade he gets off a little easier. That costs him only about forty times its manufacturing cost.

Not being either a cost accountant or in the razor blade business, I offer no guarantee of the accuracy of these figures. They are merely the figures the major gave me in support of his defense of the public spiritedness and rigorous honesty of his House. His presentation of the matter was punctuated by reiterations like these: You see, we play the game. It's living up to the rules of the game that matters. The company don't give a damn for profit—it's an ethical company. Sportsmanship wins. Everybody gets a break with us. We'd rather drop a million and be able to look the Referee up Yonder in the eye than make ten million by some dishonest dodge.

Now the nearly incredible point I want to make is that the major *was sold* not only on the nondelinquency of his razor blade racket but on the essential integrity of his own motivation and on the nobility of his objectives. In his own mind he was playing the game according to the rules and he was pretty sure of his rules. Yet the racket he expounded is fully as *delinquent* a racket, in its total effect on the human drama, as any other swindle. The worst effect of the swindle lies not in the fact that the public gets cheated, by forty to one, but that it gets miseducated to like it and to regard such legalized cheating with complacency as "good economics."

In the course of daily conversations for upwards of a decade with young men who had been labeled delinquent it was impossible for me to fail to be aware that most of them, too, were playing according to rule and were fairly sure of *their* rules. Throughout the presentation of the biographies I have many times emphasized the point that the boy in question seemed, like the major, to be at ease with his own conscience. That is to say, he seemed to be playing a role which from his point of view called for the very sort of activity which others would label delinquent.[1]

On talking with the major it would be difficult to regard him as individually delinquent, by any definition of delinquency that would make sense. For he was perfectly adapted to his society, successful, and considered a good officer. But I did experience the feeling, poignantly, that the society to which he was adapted must be delinquent, by *every* definition that would make sense. Certainly it had to be delinquent economically. The razor blade story alone should be sufficient evidence of that. Sociopolitically it was delinquent. A good test of that delinquency would have been to ask one hundred officers of the American Army to explain just what were the objectives and causes of the war in which they were engaged. An analysis of the answers would perhaps have convinced the hardiest optimist of an approaching fact of sociopolitical chaos. In the sexual-reproductive field there could be little doubt of general delinquency. When a species suddenly quadruples its numbers, overrunning a planet as cockroaches uncontrolled may overrun a kitchen, and does this wildly, without any parallel development of measures for qualitative control of its reproduction, such a species is stampeding toward the status of vermin. When that delinquency is complicated by the development of measures tending to defeat nature's normal defense against the very contingency of overpopulation, the species is truly sowing the teeth of the

[1] There are some exceptions in the series. Some of the misbehavior boys even when we first knew them were aware of being out of character and felt that they were somehow headed in the wrong direction. These were readily recognized, usually at the first interview, and in most such cases we seemed to know intuitively that the prognosis for "reform" was good. But among this group the stronger and more interesting personalities were conspicuously absent.

dragon of war, and war is one price of just such delinquency. Delinquency in the fourth panel[2]—religious delinquency—has been sufficiently manifest. In substance this is failure to impart educationally an over-all system of values conducive to the biological betterment of the species.

We come then to some conception of the difficulties, at least, in defining delinquency. From the point of view of personal adaptation to his society it might in a day's search be hard to find a man less delinquent than the razor blade major. Yet from the point of view of long-run adaptation of human society to the earth, which is the fourth panel point of view, this man seems to express the essence of delinquency. For he is a waster—an unchastened accelerator. He is a leader, vigorously accelerating what looks like a stampede toward biological catastrophe. In the fourth panel he is delinquent as all getout.

It may be that students of delinquency, failing to take into account the inherent delinquency of institutions, have never got to the heart of delinquency at all. It will be recalled that a number of the boys among the 200 were so well fortified in their imputation of a general social delinquency that we could make no headway against their argumentative armor. Some of these boys stated their cases more effectively than I (at least) could state the case for the defense. I often had the feeling, when talking with the more intelligent among these delinquent youths, that the ground I was holding against them was not in human fairness tenable ground. Practically it was tenable, of course, because police power and military power, along with majority opinion, were on that side. But I had the uneasy feeling that *we* might

---

[2] In *The Promethean Will* (Chapter 6) the whole complex of considerations bearing on food supply and on matters of immediate biological sustenance was reviewed as the *first panel* of mind. These things come first. Without oxygen and other food human life can be sustained only for minutes. The second most immediate need seems to be one for a protective social arrangement, a social order. This is what makes feasible the long human period of infantile helplessness with resulting elaboration of development. Also it makes possible specialization of function in many directions. The whole complex of awareness involved in protection of social interrelationships may be conveniently referred to as the *second panel*. Reproduction and sexuality appear to constitute the third most pressing consideration in human affairs. The complex of arrangements and awareness growing up around this elemental problem may be embraced by the term *third panel*.

The first three panels of mind thus take shape inevitably from the three basic biological needs—for sustenance, for social protection, for reproduction. In varying degrees these three basic panels are shared by human beings with many other animals. There is nothing distinctly human about the three basic needs. But with the comparatively enormous development of the human forebrain there comes into existence a remarkable intensification—if not the first beginnings—of a fourth need. This grows out of awareness of the implications of time. The whole fabric of awareness of time, and of the consequent struggle either to forget time or to find orientation in that new dimension of thought, is what is meant by the *fourth panel* or religious panel of awareness. The first panel is economic, the second sociopolitical, the third sexual, the fourth religious. The fourth panel may be distinctively human. At any rate the monkey traps associated with it appear to be distinctively human.

be the delinquent ones; that we were in a way bearing false witness and were using false weapons. I often felt that if by some act of magic our debate with the boy—with the boy presenting his case against society and with us presenting the grievance of society against him—could be held before unbiased judges who had never lived in such a society and so were tarred with none of its inherent delinquency, we might lose the debate hands down.

It was really because of this feeling that I decided to write a book on delinquency.

My friend the razor blade major presents a healthy and perhaps normal example of what used to be called the point of view of rugged individualism. To him life is not only an organized sport with specific and immutable rules but it is a sport at which he is in a sense well gifted and knows it. He radiates success and confidence. He is perfectly "adjusted" although to a society that is on the toboggan. In order to be meaningful the concept of delinquency would seem to need to embrace the behavior and all of the overt and covert commitments of such a man; that is to say, the pattern of institutions in which such a man is caught. There are minds among us to which the major's razor blade racket is disappointing *as far beyond reasonable expectation* as is the robbing of drunks. It is true, of course, that statistically there are no grounds on which the fraternity of delinquency can be extended to include the major but this may be the principal reason why statistics on delinquency have been so nearly worthless.

3. The Way of Dionysian Predation Is a Happy Way of Life

I have lived among quite a number of different groups of people, flocculating as they have along numerous cleavage lines, and some of the groups have seemed to enjoy life after their own fashion. But I have a somewhat unhappy suspicion that no group of them all has been fundamentally happier than the first two platoons of the HGI series. Those boys were on the whole having a good time. If you will read over the first 82 cases with the question in mind as to whether or not the individual was able to meet his situation with an adaptive pattern—that is, a pattern adaptive *from his point of view* —I think the impression will grow in your mind that most of the boys were successful. If you could have seen and lived among them, after first recovering from the initial shock of their superficial appearance, the impression would perhaps grow stronger. The youngsters must be judged against their own standards and criteria, if they are to be judged at all. They were doing pretty well at finding a way of life that served their own purposes, and they had fun, probably more fun than average or ordinary people have. They were more interesting than ordinary people are. If they were to be compared, individual for individual, with the social work profession that with manifest bewilderment was trying to ride herd on them, I think that the boys had the better of it—especially the feebleminded and the medically insufficient ones. They seemed more lighthearted. Certainly they were more fun-loving and they had more humor than their social workers had.

I do not mean to imply that all this would be true of some other feeble-minded and medically insufficient population. The observation is specific to the population under discussion. Those youngsters had something else besides their mental and their medical insufficiency, some quality that made them float on the muddy flood instead of sinking waterlogged into the sediment, as do the majority of human personalities. The power of floating may be nothing more mysterious than Dionysian buoyancy. Perhaps they were floating on life because they had the Dionysian don't-give-a-damn point of view. I have had alcoholic friends who said that the only reason they sought that drug was because it gave them that euphorial sense of floating over the surface of things instead of sinking into the mud of life. Were they but trying to snatch little time fragments of the very quality with which our delinquent and insufficient first two platoons were by temperament so well endowed?

The comparatively brighter and more competent ones among the first two platoons, and more noticeably among all the platoons of the second company, presented another quality along with the Dionysian buoyancy, or perhaps it is but another aspect of the buoyancy. This is the quality of unabashed or unashamed predation. In the minds of most of the youngsters who looked on themselves as "takers" (rather than as workers or servants of society or whatnot) there was no doubt as to what life was for. "The world is my oyster. I should worry," was the favorite rejoinder of No. 126 to every frontal or flank attack on his position. He was Dionysian by temperament and predatory in outlook. To him predation was the normal outlook on life and he was no more ashamed of being predatory than is a marsh harrier. Now quite an important question, for anybody who would understand delinquency, would be this: Is predation a normal outlook for the human species? Is it the normal way of life *for some members* of the species? Are some men and women so endowed, morphologically and temperamentally, that it is quite as normal for them to seek to prey upon others and to seek to live off others without "contributing" as it is normal for some of the rest of us weaklings to seek to live as workers, public servants, research scientists, prostitutes, preachers, and so on? Our society is organized on the premise that the question is superfluous, that an affirmative answer is self-evident. I do not mean that you will find public protocols recognizing the predatory element in any current attempt at a social *apologia,* any more than you will find public recognition of the sexual element in a Methodist hymn.

The youngsters at the HGI seemed to be more realistically aware of the essentially predatory philosophy underlying the social structure than were those who had been—and still were—attempting to reeducate those youngsters away from such a philosophy. I many times had the feeling, in talking with the boys, that I was in a false position. I felt sometimes like an envoy of a *dishonestly* predatory enterprise sent to decoy and to trap into a kind of slavery those free spirits who had thus far managed to elude the snare. Years before, I had felt that way when acting as a duck-shooting guide for week-end sojourners to whom the hunt was generally more venerean and Bacchanalian than Nimrodian. There came a time at last when my sympathies were wholly with the ducks, and there is no denying that in the HGI study I felt in the end less closely identified with the reformational aspect of the enterprise than with the reformees. This was not because the youngsters were intentionally more honest than the rest of us—most of them certainly were *not* intentionally honest—but because they were, I think it is possible, more wise. They saw human society in a truer light and were more truly engaged with life than were most of their elders who were professedly engaged in dealing with "delinquency" but in fact were concerned mainly with their own security and righteousness.

4. But Abortive Predation Is Delinquency

The boys, the honestly delinquent ones at any rate, had tossed security and righteousness to the four winds and had undertaken a sincerely avowed life of predation. But *their* predation was abortive. They labeled it predation and usually it came to naught. Meanwhile predation labeled otherwise could be observed blossoming into luxuriant growth all around them. I think that a thesis could be defended to the effect that, apart from the insufficiencies, a principal pattern of delinquency among the HGI boys was abortive predation—predation not quite carried to full term.

For the predation there were the best of precedents. The clue to delinquency must then lie in the abortiveness. Those boys were delinquent because they tried to reflect a predominant and exemplary Dionysian pattern of exploitative irresponsibility but were habitually last in getting over the fence out of the apple orchard. Their attitudes were right. Their execution was poor. That is to say, their attitudes were right from the point of view of the marsh harrier, quite wrong from that of the habitually harried. The difficulty seems to lie in the fact that the human species still plays the role of both hunter and hunted, as it has from time immemorial. Born into a society like that, one must choose from what amount to only three alternatives: (1) To live exploitatively, or off surplus wealth. To do this one must either be born with "advantages" or with the strength or cunning to seize and hold advantages. (2) To live exploitedly and like it, rationalize it however one may. (3) To effect some kind of compromise, to run as it were with both the hare and the hounds.

Obviously the first and second alternatives represent radically divergent paths of life and undoubtedly in the course of time give rise to radically different patterns of temperament. The Dionysian pattern, when in mild or normal degree, may represent a perfectly natural expression of the joyous irresponsibility of the exploitative outlook. The resignational pattern which *in extremis* becomes hebephrenic jettisoning may when in milder degree represent a natural acceptance of exploitation. This is humility, self-abnegation, "love of peace."

Possibly the most suggestive finding in the HGI study is the clear-cut predominance of the first psychiatric component throughout the series, together with a remarkable absence of the third—the resulting psychiatric picture being an exact opposite to that usually found in the mental hospitals. This may throw some light on the fascinating question of the underlying nature of that residual in delinquency which is not a product of recognizable insufficiency. Since the delinquent youths reflect almost uniformly a Dionysian pattern of temperament it may be that their persistent "aggressions" against society are natural expressions of very deep-seated personality characteristics to which they can claim biologically honest title. Perhaps the persistently criminal boy is expressing not so much a "psychogenic resentment against the mother" as a Dionysian reaction which is almost as much a product of his constitutional design as the way he walks. I would not go so far as to insist that every predatory attempt on the part of an individual is a necessitous expression of a predatory factor in his constitutional make-up, but I would suggest that the level of persistent effort at predation reached by the HGI boys who present primary criminality could probably not have been maintained without a strong temperamental predisposition toward predation. The fact that the predation was in these instances chiefly abortive or unsuccessful seems to add weight to the suggestion, for those boys during most of their lives had been subjected to the strongest conditioning *against* predation that a virtual army of advocates of docility could bring to bear. The boys had the impetus to ride out all that conditioning, to defy the psychological "law of effect," and to maintain a persistency of pattern despite repeated and painful failure to make good in the pattern. Even though the mood for predation always eventuated abortively the mood was maintained against all manner of discouragement.

This same phenomenon of mood perseveration in the face of environmental circumstance that would seem objectively to contradict the mood is seen in all phases of the range of psychiatric conditions referred to as manic-depressive psychosis. Such mood perseveration is one of the diagnostic criteria for that label, but in less dramatic degree it is a constant characteristic of the Dionysian temperament. Now the persistent criminals in the HGI study were so distinctly Dionysian in temperament that among the 59 who were given a score of at least 1 in primary criminality 45 presented a psychiatric index in which the first component was either predominant or co-predominant with the second. Fourteen of the 16 in whom primary criminality was finally considered the predominant factor in the delinquency (the second platoon of Company B) were predominantly Dionysian in their psychiatric indices. This does not mean that to be Dionysian is to be delinquent, any more than to have wings is to be a hawk, but it may mean that the Dionysian characteristic was an essential ingredient in that HGI delinquency which was not a product of insufficiency; i.e., the "criminal" delinquency.

Two factors then were fairly consistent in this criminal delinquency: (1) A persistent appetite for predation, and (2) the Dionysian temperament, which implies identification with the constitutional northwest and may also explain a certain euphorial buoyancy which to the puzzlement of many seemed so often to characterize the population of the Inn. The appetite for predation and the Dionysian temperament are not, in general, so far as I know, positively correlated traits. They may be negatively correlated in the general population. But in this particular HGI population both were conspicuously present. For this group, with only two or three possible exceptions, we may add as a third constant factor the continued unsuccessfulness of the attempted predation. (Among our 200 there are two or three who now give promise of achieving *successful* criminal careers and of holding honored posts in Boston political affairs. One of them might someday be a national figure.) These exceptions may constitute the vital nucleus of the study. They may be the real criminals, while the rest are only of the many who were called but not chosen. If that is so our society may be a criminal society, for it is certainly predatory and it is at present in a Dionysian phase.

So far as the HGI population is concerned we can include the factor of the unsuccessfulness of the predation in our endeavor to build up an operational conception of criminality. Conventionally and conveniently, criminality is unsuccessful predation. All of the criminals you will find in jail are unsuccessful. But if you have a mental nose for the faint and difficult trail of a biological humanics rather than for mere objective statistics, you will long ponder the question whether criminality is always unsuccessful. And if it is not, can we find a clue to the nature of successful criminality in the study of a few score—or a few thousands—of unsuccessful criminals? If we can, there may be a social psychology in our future.

Does an unusually persistent appetite for predation coupled with Dionysian irresponsibility spell criminality? When you add a high IQ, vigorous health, energy, and cunning, is the outcome successful criminality, or merely success? I cannot answer these questions. They are really religious in nature, for how you answer them depends upon what you make of life, and on how vigorously you can project your will into a fighting interest in the remote, as opposed to the immediate, consequences of your present commitments. If your concern is more immediate than remote you are happily free from what I mean by the fourth or religious panel of consciousness. You will then be more concerned with being successful than with trying to decide whether your particular variety of success is of the same motivation as criminality. But if your concern is more with remote than with immediate developments —if in short your mind has got itself entangled in the time dimension of the adventure of life, and is thus a religious mind—you may find yourself pondering with great interest the nature of predation and the nature of Dionysian irresponsibility.

I remember a visit to Munich in 1935 in the company of a British friend. We watched for a whole afternoon some singularly Dionysian cavortings on the part of one Hermann Goering and a few thousands of his cohorts. I suggested that here was a situation which must be dealt with *in kind*; that energy unleashed in that somatotonic manner can be met or controlled only by a counterforce of equal leverage power. In short, that somatotonia is sensitive only to somatotonia, that it does not stop but must *be* stopped.

My friend was one of those many moderns who had been mildly infected by both the psychoanalytic and the pacifist virus. No, he said, it is no good to try to stop those Nazis. Far better to let them express it. If we should show hostility to them, or a firm hand, we would be criminally responsible for untold horrors and frustrations. Give them what they ask, he suggested, and before long they will be generous too. Then there can be no war. It takes two to make a quarrel, you know, and if we refuse to quarrel, the combative impulse must die down for want of fuel. I recall suggesting that it might be not a combative impulse but a predatory impulse that was astir in the Nazi bonnet. That elicited the idea that the problem is economic; then what we should offer the Nazis was not the threat of war but help—money, economic planning, and so on.

On that same trip I renewed an earlier acquaintanceship with a native German of Munich who had been an officer in World War I. Fifteen years before, he and I as about-to-be-demobilized youths had discussed together the problems of war and peace, and had solved them all. Now we met again for a pleasant evening in a Munich beer parlor. "Why are you Germans stirring up another war?" I asked him. "*Another* war!" he ejaculated in apparently genuine astonishment. "Since when has there not been war?" I suggested that I thought we had buried the hatchet fifteen years before. "Ah yes," he seemed to grow wistfully thoughtful, "yes, you buried the hatchet— in Germany's back."

I had not been at all prepared for anything like that, for I felt what amounted almost to an affection for that upright, honest-faced German who had lost two brothers in the earlier war, not to mention his own youth. I asked him to elaborate, to explain just how Germany had been struck in the back and by whom. He was delighted to oblige. We talked for five hours, and I learned as much from that lecture as from any I ever attended. I learned that we English-speaking people are a degenerate, rundown stock, a kind of coupon-clipping remnant from a once vigorous and powerful line that has gone to seed. We are not realistic. We established a vast world empire but we only half did the job. A predatory race by nature, we set out to conquer and to organize and live off the human species as a whole. We got the jump on our near relatives, in particular on our German cousins, through our fortunate relationship to the sea. We capitalized on that and for a time gave promise of supplying the order and discipline and centralization of final authority without which the world obviously cannot get along. That was about three centuries back. But by the end of the eighteenth century it had begun to be clear that we were a false alarm. Our acquisition of a feebleminded Hanoverian prince for a king had been a bad sign. The blundered debacle of the American Revolution was another. We showed fear. Fear of France, for example, and so we sloughed off America with its promise of a New World in the West, as a juggler with too many balls in the air might let one or two go. We had started as heroic conquerers, had deteriorated to romanticists, then to jugglers, and later to shopkeepers and "businessmen." In the nineteenth century we had fallen as far as human degeneracy can go—to the mental state of pacifism. At that term my German friend made a face like the one Aunt Mary used to make when she stepped in something very undesirable around the barn. It was his climax of anathema. We once heroic, warlike, and predatory Anglo-Saxons had degenerated to pacifistic bleat. Having whipped half the world into order and into a dependence on us for the military and the police power which it needed next to bread, we now began to make hebephrenic noises and to indignify the high destinies of mankind with a juggling game of politics carried on obviously for the comfort and welfare of our own flesh. That was a German mind picture of our Anglo-American society.

Germany had exercised the restraint of a cheated but loyal and grieving cousin, but Germany at last could stand it no longer. The time for German heroic action was ripe and overripe and Germany had long seen the need, had been preparing to save the family bacon, which was the Nordic bacon. Germany had (in 1914) sprung into the breach, warlike and resolute. What did her English-speaking cousins do? Why, they buried their hatchet in Germany's back. Out of spite, malice, unreasoning jealousy, insane pride, fratricidal paranoia. Lacking the will and the resolution any longer to hold the ancient hereditary estate against the corruptive and disintegrative forces which are natural to a large estate under senile ownership, we Anglo-Saxons finally capped our doom by lacking the wit to trust Germany.

Well, the Germans had learned their bitter lesson. For a generation they had been prostrated—bled white. But now they were coming back. And this time they would know how to deal with England and America. They were going to handle us with firm hands, as doctors deal with recalcitrant patients. They had to. We must be got out of the way for a time, while Germany put the house in order. The world was turning into bedlam and it was obvious that we were incompetent to do anything about it. Germany had inherited a tough job. Nothing was going to be asked of America except that we try to keep our mongrel side show out of the center ring. Britain was to be treated with gentle firmness, like a favorite but somewhat spoiled mother-in-law. She probably would be pensioned to her island. My friend was insufficiently close to the Nazi inner council to have all these details quite at hand but he knew the general tenor of his country's intent. He wanted all the world to know that intent. Open, honest, single-tongued dealings had always been Germany's policy, at least in so far as the responsible element of her population was concerned. If politicians at times departed from the ideal of simplicity and trust, well, politicians were a necessary inconvenience in an incompletely developed society. They were like backhouses. My friend did not want personal association with such characters as Hitler and Goebbels and Roosevelt, he said. Men like these were liars and morally unclean. Perhaps they had to be liars, he was not sure; but Germany was willing to "use the facilities" which politicians constituted because there were no better ones available. The end would justify the means.

Twelve years later I was trying to lay down the hull for this present book, having returned for the second time from a humble role in a war against Germany, now in a mood far contrasted with the youthful exaltation and hope of the 1919 homecoming. My German friend who clearly had meant to help save the world was a discredited delinquent. All of his brother Germans (who had supported the war) were delinquent before our law—they had waged a war of unsuccessfully aggressive predation—and I had sentenced myself to the task of trying to make sense of the idea of delinquency. I could see that the Germans were delinquent, all right, and also the British and the Americans and the whole raggle taggle of world population that has ever been caught at abortive predation. That we have all embraced grave delinquency on a huge scale history attests.

If the Germans were delinquent in resolving to take over the conduct of world affairs by force, and in proceeding therefore to wage vigorous war, we too had been delinquent in our efforts of the same nature. We (our immediate ancestors) for some reason bogged down about halfway and left at our high-water mark the abortive carcase of the British Empire. And every other effort on the part of a breed of people to conquer and rule first its immediate and then remoter neighbors must be reckoned an act of delinquency—for all these efforts have thus far failed. In short, having indicted the Germans for their attempt to conquer and rule the human world, we indict every breed that has ever undertaken predatory conquest. We might maintain that our own predation was beneficent and benevolent while that of the Germans was maleficent and malevolent. We could then qualify predation, rating some predation good and some bad, some innocent and some criminal. But the crux of the difficulty would remain. It grows out of the fact that government is by nature predatory and has always been predatory, yet has never been predatory with complete success. From the beginning of biological time a high premium has been placed on successful predation in the organic world. We humans have always lived by predation and as a species have been so successful at it that now rather suddenly we have found ourselves in undisputed possession of a world. But there is a catch—a monkey trap. The remarkable predatory success of our ancestors won us a world but now that we have overrun the whole of it with our own spawn to the swarming point, we are confronted with the dilemma of having no brake against still further spawning except the continuation of that same competitive predatory struggle that has brought us to where we are. We seem therefore to be caught in a predatory death struggle *with ourselves,* and have begun hysterically to label that very predation criminal. Other species on the Pellet, victims for ages of our ruthless predation, might now chant with glee the old saw about when thieves fall out. We are in fact caught in a hell of a monkey trap, and before long we may stir up a *real* war. We may have to. There may be no other way to get a world government which cannot be adjudged criminal.

Hebephrenic nuclei throughout the human population raise periodically the wail for pacifism. Let us *now* have peace and let us love one another and smell the flowers, they cry. Let us compromise all controversies and thereby abolish predation. Some, aware of the inevitable implications of such a proposal, suggest general adoption of a vegetarian diet. I know one vegetarian who would like to enforce abstinence from eating meat on the ground that human predaciousness cannot otherwise be stopped in the world. He is right, I suppose. If we continue to exploit other species there probably is no logical way to draw the line at exploiting one another, since there are greater differences within the human species than between what is human and not human. But even if this were not so there could be no hope of a general pacifism unless the whole population were to be placed simultaneously under a common and powerful governing influence, and this will first require a brutally predacious world conquest which will not fall short— a predation not abortive. World government can never happen spontaneously because everywhere there continues to be involvement in the competitive struggle, and (in the end even more serious from the point of view of such a hope) there are differential birth rates which are scaled in the wrong direction.

5. Back of Predation Is Irresponsible Reproduction

The stocks and breeds that through earlier competitive success have arrived at a point where the suggestion of a mutual jettisoning of the predatory impulse might have at least an intellectual appeal are those stocks that have already jettisoned their most lethal competitive weapon. That is to say, they have given up in the struggle of competitive reproduction, lowering their birth rate as compared with previously less favored competitors. Thus the heaviest reproduction is now taking place in those human ranks which in comparatively recent times have been at the tail end in the competitive struggle for survival and power. This appears to be a reversal of the natural arrangement through which the long process of evolution has taken place, and is a by-product of a world situation in which one species has succeeded in achieving an overwhelming power over all its rivals.

Under normal or natural conditions reproduction is a consequence of success in the hard test of staying alive against rigorous competition. In the present situation, which is purely a human arrangement and is to an increasing degree a consequence of unregulated competitive activity on the part of the medical profession, reproduction has been made so easy and so safe that even the weakest and least gifted of the species can spawn. The consequence is that these not only participate in but tend to monopolize the spawning business. Except for a very small statistical percentage everybody has "sexual desire" and a greater or less desire to expand his own flesh reproductively. Similarly, everybody desires food and a few other elementals. But the relatively more gifted and more conscious organisms *also* develop interests other than those of food and of expanding their flesh. Where reproduction is made so easy that the most evolved stock, in order to maintain a superior reproductive ratio, would have to drop its other interests and compete with comparatively inferior organisms that do not develop other interests to a comparable degree, the better stock tends to ignore or to neglect the challenge of competitive reproduction. This is merely to say that bad reproduction drives out good.

In consequence, under conditions both soft and unregulated, our best stock tends to be outbred by stock that is inferior to it in every respect. And I mean inferior *in every respect*. It is the fashion in some academic circles to assure students that the alarm over differential birth rates is unfounded; that these problems are merely economic, or merely educational, or merely religious, or merely cultural or something of the sort. This is Pollyanna optimism. Reproductive delinquency is biological and basic.

There is another conventional argument for failing to face the problem. It is contained in the thesis that where reproduction is free and universal, and encouraged equally, it must be the more fertile individuals who produce the greatest number of offspring. These then, far from being inferior, make up in one sense a superior sector of the population. They are superior with respect to fertility, and this must be an important superiority for the future of the species, so all is well after all and let us listen to the symphony. This is a reassuring thought for academic people, many of whom have no intention of competing in what they call the reproductive rat race but feel a little guilty therefore. It is nice for them to be able to say "That is somebody else's specialty." But the notion probably has no basis in fact. The parents of the 200 in the HGI series produced 941 known offspring, plus an indeterminate number not reported in records available to us. This is a considerably faster rate of reproduction than was indulged in by Vassar graduates of comparable age during the same period, but if after reading these cases you think that the HGI mothers were in some way healthier, or *more capable* of producing offspring than the Vassar girls, I am afraid that your opinion casts reflection on my reportorial effort.

After following the histories of these HGI families for a decade, and after interviewing and observing quite a good sample of the parents in question, I should say that the evidence favors a quite different hypothesis; that instead of being more fertile the HGI parents were expending a greater proportion of their energies on uninhibited or irresponsible sexuality. It is possible that if 200 Vassar girls selected at random were to volunteer to spend twenty years at a sociological experiment in which the object is to try to get pregnant as frequently as possible—or even to try to have as much sexual intercourse as possible without particularly caring whether or not pregnancy results—the Vassar girls would *far* outstrip the HGI mothers in the number of offspring produced. This would be a crucial experiment for sociological theory, and it might be a great thing for Vassar. The girls will have to be subsidized, but it should be remembered that the HGI mothers *were* subsidized. They were subsidized with money from the public treasury, with the best medical attention, with housing and food in many instances, and with almost constant attention from a profession likewise subsidized to make a business of aiding and abetting this kind of reproduction ("family welfare") in every possible way and at almost any cost. It sounds fantastic. It is literally true.

Under these circumstances the remarkable thing may be the comparatively *low* rate of reproduction in that half of our population which economically, medically, and intellectually is the second half. Such data as are available indicate that the second half of our population is producing *barely more than double* the number of offspring produced by the first half. If it had a fecundity equal to that of the first half it might perhaps quadruple the productivity of the latter.

The plain fact seems to be that in reproduction as in economics Gresham's Law holds. Bad money drives out good, and bad reproduction drives out good. Whether or not the Vassar graduate *can* compete successfully with the HGI mother at reproduction is a point to be settled only when a satisfactory contest can be arranged. It is a fact that under conditions now prevailing they are not so doing, and the more general fact is that our whole human society has a differential birth rate scaled in the wrong direction. This means that we are not evolving now but devolving. We are therefore scheduled for such inconveniences as social chaos, wars of increasing and crescendic violence, general frustration, and the confusion necessarily attendant upon the pathology of increasing urbanization and loss of zest in human life. All this we have already earned by irresponsible reproduction in the recent past. No amount of regret or prayer or pacifism can cancel that debt, and nature generally collects her debts. Pacifism might be defined as the expression of a hebephrenic wish to escape the consequences of delinquent reproduction already committed. This delinquency is everybody's for since we all participate in the future unless we die out, the one thing that is everybody's responsibility is guardianship of the quality of the reproduction of his own time. If that responsibility is shirked, war is perhaps the least ungentle of natural punishments.

We cannot by now declaring how much we would like to have peace escape the devastating wars of the next few generations, nor do I think that a morally responsible person should want to escape them. *That* punishment is needed for without it the delinquency would continue. We have quadrupled the human population on this Pellet explosively, within less than a half score of generations, and while doing so have manifested an increasingly Dionysian irresponsibility, not only for such an unprecedented quantitative burgeoning of human flesh but also for the quality of it. This we have done after taking that very responsibility into our own hands. The health and quality and the ultimate survival power of our stock are now entirely in our own hands. We have by the development of medical and other science taken these things over, and we no longer have the power either to drop the consequent responsibility or to escape punishment for the delinquency of failing to live up to it. This is an alarming truth, so alarming that the main energy of our religious profession is being spent in a hopeless, pitiful struggle to fight it down and to shout it out of consciousness.

6. Behind Irresponsible Reproduction Is Religious Delinquency

In the long run a society is only as good as its religion, i.e., as good as its institutions for securing and improving its future. The priests of religion in our culture have been so heavily engaged in fighting the thought of a biological humanics that as yet they have not found the strength or the heart to *tackle the problem* of any kind of humanics. The profession of religion is for the time being caught in a monkey trap of supernatural theology, but the *function* of religion is to carry and to some extent to institutionalize responsibility for the biological future. Now I may be even more of a fool than I sometimes think but I retain a certain childish faith in the long-run religious function. This is what I believe has brought us *up*. It seems probable that the underlying motivation behind man's long climb to the top of the biological procession has been the forebrain function of imagining a future. That is the essence of the religious function and is the principle underlying the fourth panel of consciousness (p. 826).

There is nothing necessarily any more mysterious about imagining a future, or more provocative of "mysticism," than about undertaking movement through space. The fourth or religious function comes into being as the organism begins to develop a power of adapting to the time dimension of experience. The locomotive function, which is much older, came into being when early ancestral organisms first began to develop a power of adapting to the spatial dimensions of experience. Meanwhile the time dimension was always there, but we did not begin to possess any power of conscious adaptation to it until a special structure for imaging (imagining) began to take shape, as muscles for locomotion had once begun to take shape. Dr. E. J. Kempf calls this special forebrain structure the *projicient mechanism*,[3] thus naming it for its power of *projecting,* and he develops the idea that now we have got it we have to live with it. It is an instrument for imagining a future or, figuratively speaking, for projecting awareness into the dimension of time. It is not impossible that a carnate organism on this Pellet would be better off without such an instrument, and absence of it would yield the added advantage of a great saving in liquor bills, but until cerebrectomy (or lobotomy) becomes as routine and as general as, say, circumcision, the forebrain will no more let us forget the fourth panel than the gut will let us forget the first. So long as there is a forebrain there will be a "religious urge" in human life as surely as there will be hunger. This means, of course, unlimited opportunity for fourth panel delinquency, for there is no more reason to suppose that the human forebrain is necessarily infallible in the search for truth than is the snout of a dung beetle. The truth which each pursues is in the natural order of things conditioned upon its own organic outlook. But the dung beetle has the easier problem. The truth which he seeks, being more easily recognized as such, is less susceptible to theological obscuration and he thereby enjoys relative immunity from the delinquency of fourth panel monkey traps.

Religion, as I use the term, has to do with the further development and exercise of power over the future. The organic structure on which such a power rests is the projicient forebrain, and religion is thus the one function that is peculiarly human. The forebrain is what we as a species have gone all out for, as external armor and mesomorphic mass were the main reliance of the giant armored reptiles. But it is a good thing to remember that the forebrain is virtually a new biological experiment, and if time were called *now* in the game of Life on this Pellet, our score as compared with that of the giant armored reptiles would be almost infinitely small. We have not in fact really scored at all, yet, in comparison with their score. They ruled the earth presumably unchallenged (certainly unchallenged by us) for at least 80,000,-000 years, perhaps for a far longer period. Our ancestors were doubtless here

[3] Kempf introduces this concept in one of the most thought-provoking monographs in the psychological literature. *The Autonomic Functions and the Personality,* Nervous and Mental Disease Monograph Series No. 28. 1921.

through all that time but only as a form of life which to the saurians was insignificant and hardly worth the trouble of eating. To the armored reptiles we were possibly about what some of the shier, more furtive rodents are to us now—small vermin living in inaccessible holes and crevices.

We have got the upper hand today, but we have not yet held it long. Indeed we have not yet held it long enough to have forgotten entirely a fear of the more powerful carnivores who were our late rivals. Bears, lions, the late sabre-toothed tiger. And in some of the older human legends there are traces of a dim but terrible recollection of what must have been the last remnants of those great reptiles to whom we were vermin that hid in holes— dragons. There is no evidence that we as a species were any particular shucks on the earth until very recent times. There are traces of our presence, in a structural pattern approximating our present structure, at least a half million and possibly a million years back, but it is only with the development of modern weapons that we have got the upper hand enough to come out into the open places and begin to overrun the earth with our own spawn. By modern weapons I mean implements harder and heavier than wood and stone. Explosives are ultramodern.

A simple and operational definition of religion would be *concern for the comparatively remote implications of present behavior.* The etymological origin of the term is obscure. Some authorities trace it to a Greek term which implies the function of (social) binding together; others trace it to a Greek verb referring to lawmaking. Both of these concepts point rather to the sociological devices by which the fourth need is met than to the basic need itself, which is need for orientation in time. That is to say, neither gets back to the basic meaning but both refer to the necessity of establishing social cooperation or social implementation before the need can be met. The fourth function, by harnessing the potential power of social agglutination, establishes a linkage of present life both with the past and with the future. This has been called the time-binding function.

There is almost universal confusion over the concept of religion because of an attempted preemption of that term by adherents of supernatural cults and by addicts to theologies and mysticisms of many sorts. Probably the average American of today, on hearing the word religion, thinks at once of some Christian sect, of churches, and of Mr. G. Actually there is no more justification for identifying religion (the function of orientation in time) with the idea of Mr. G or with other theological conceptions, than for identifying sex with the idea of the harem. Both ideas, that of Mr. G and that of the harem, are attempted answers to fundamental biological problems. Religion is probably just about as much older than the Mr. G concept as sex is older than any particular idea of what to do about it. The idea of God, as an attempted evasion of the human responsibility for facing up to the fourth need, may have been infesting the human mind for a few hundred—or even a few thousand—generations, but this is too short a time to be of any long-run consequence and it is my optimistic view that in the normal exercise of the religious function we can recover from theological monkey traps as surely as the individual organism recovers from measles.

Since it is reasonably apparent that the underlying problems of human life are religious, and that the problem of delinquency must be therefore at bottom a religious problem, it is essential that in this book we *stay out* of *one* monkey trap. That is the monkey trap of confusing religion with theology.

As I use these terms religion is concern, earnest or wholehearted concern, with the comparatively remote future; that is to say, with consequences of present behavior that lie far beyond immediate consequences to the present organism. Religious development involves surrender or abnegation of self but without hebephrenic jettisoning of the energy that is contained in the self. It is an attempt to invest that energy in a greater biological future. This is a difficult undertaking for it calls for close navigation between two fatal alternative temptations. One temptation is the Dionysian Scylla, who whispers *take the cash and let the credit go;* indulge the present biological self, which is the here and now, and live for the full burgeoning and glorification of *this* flesh. More operationally expressed this seems to be a suppression of the third component, an instance of the same pathological cerebropenia which we first encountered in more easily recognizable dress on page 46.

The other temptation is the hebephrenic Charybdis who whispers of the relief from *throwing away the biological self* and yielding up the biological future in a chaotic ecstasy of mystical delusion. Pretend that the biological lifestream is not the reality. Pretend that structure and behavior are not a continuum in human life. Pretend that instead there is something different—spirit, soul, ghost, God, anything. In short, pretend a dualism and dissociate from biological reality. Then nothing biological matters. Biological humanics is a dream and so is life. You live in the other (pretended) world and you can people that with everything from Mr. G to the ghost of your grandmother. Indeed, you can pretend two other worlds, a heaven and a hell, one for the ghosts you like and one for your mother-in-law and such.

There we have what appear to be the two principal devices of delinquency by which the human mind tries to escape facing the fourth panel of consciousness. Nor is it very surprising that so weak and new a thing as human mentality should often fail at so hard a test. After all, what mind we have did not in the first place evolve in the service of fourth panel objectives but in the service of the viscera and somata of ancestral organisms. To us the fourth panel is new, and although in the face of crowding from our own now flagrant overpopulation, and in the face of the pathological predicament of urbanization we can now no more escape the reality of the future than we can escape the reality of hunger, yet our minds are so constituted that for a long time yet we will fight the reality. If we win that fight we escape from the predicament, to join the noble company of the giant armored reptiles that were, and the long line of their predecessors who have performed on and vanished from the central stage of this planetary theater. For to fail now to grow a religion that will produce a biological humanics which will return nobility to human life will be to bow off that stage with what might be commendable promptitude. We can probably wipe out "civilization" with astonishing alacrity, now that so much earnest attention is being devoted to the quality of lethal weapons. Perhaps we have been attending to the weapons for the same reason that a desperate and hopelessly outlawed man attends to the provision for the means for suicide.

The two religious delinquencies most urgently in need of counterbalance seem to be those opposed Dionysian and hebephrenic theologies by which we have been trying to drown out what in another and perhaps too romantically religious book I called the voice of Prometheus. Here let it be called, instead, a desire to stay on the stage for awhile yet and to work out further the theme of the drama. The difference in the metaphor may indicate nothing more significant than advancing senility.

On page 821 we got so far as to call delinquency disappointing performance. Possibly we can now take a further step and define delinquent performance from the point of view of the fourth panel. There will of course remain the problems of defining and dealing with delinquency from the point of view of the first panel (property relations), the second panel (sociopolitical implementation), and the third panel (individual sex and reproductive activities), but all of this is apparently secondary to the main problem of getting an underlying structure into the fourth panel. What a society does about property, familio-political alignments, and sexual intercourse may be of about the same level of importance as what a carpenter does about his tools. If he takes good care of his tools and keeps them in fine order, that is to the good and there is a chance that he is a good carpenter. But the proof of it will be found in what he builds. If we handle our problems of economics intelligently, achieving excellent production and distribution of food and other goods so that everybody is well fed and clothed and housed and happy and eager to go to work, that is to the good, but is not in itself particularly good. We may still be a highly delinquent society. To devote your life to economics or to social or sexual considerations is like devoting your life to the care of tools. Perfectly honorable and necessary, and if your economics is of the trying-to-give kind rather than of the trying-to-get kind you are at any rate not economically delinquent. But you may still have shirked the responsibility of facing the really difficult decisions and alternatives which must be faced if the species is to steer, and not blunder, its way into the future.

From the fourth panel point of view delinquent performance is *failure to use religious energy in such a way as to secure, protect, and guide the bio-*

logical future of the species. Of the two principal manifestations of religious delinquency the Dionysian or waster manifestation is an old and familiar concept in Christian literature, but the hebephrenic or theological manifestation has not in that particular literature been recognized as a delinquency, since the Christian ratiocination is itself an antibiological construct and is therefore, by our definition, a hebephrenic delinquency.

Possibly the main delinquency of our culture has been Christian theology. This is not the place to review the history of that particular supernaturalism, or to trace the steps by which what seems at one time to have been a comparatively healthy breed of human stock grew so degenerate or so confused as to rest a desperate hope on an otherworldly, supernatural dualism. This story has been told many times. For a sympathetic account of it turn to a scholarly little book by Professor Herschel Baker called *The Dignity of Man.*[4] For a less sympathetic but highly realistic account, read Volume Two of Spengler's *Decline of the West.*

It would seem that until we as a breed, or until some powerful segment of us as a breed, can face up to the starkly fatal hebephrenic nature of all supernatural theologies, and of all supplication addressed to God, we are beaten. I have for a long time listened to men talk, and have come to the conclusion that whenever the term God is uttered, something comparable only to mental masturbation is achieved. It is not a question of whether or not there *is* a Mr. G. It would be arrogant enough of any human being to think he could answer that question, either way, but the really unmitigated impudence lies in the anthropocentric—sometimes even anthropomorphic—assumption that Mr. G, if there is such a Fellow, should entertain a violent partiality for so degenerate and noisy a biped as this one that we are.

That was what dumbfounded me when as a high school boy I first heard such a suggestion made. I had been reared as a naturalist and hunter, mainly in the deep woods, in close contact with a mind that had pondered biological and theological problems more than most minds do. My father was as deeply religious a man as I have met, according to my definition of religion. He had a sense of responsibility for the biological future of the species. To him the Mr. G business and the Church business were psychiatric considerations— symptoms of pathology, as they are to me. Yet he looked upon the Church as potentially a principal hope of the human breed. His view was that the natural role of a religious institution would be, instead of preaching about the religious function, to implement it by setting up and running the machinery for keeping longitudinal genetic records. His idea was that your religion is not only your concern for the future but how hard and how effectively you work at the problem of directing such a concern to useful enterprise. Our Christian Church has played a role of dog-in-the-manger to the development of the fourth panel, both by teaching hebephrenic theology to immature

[4] Harvard University Press, 1947.

minds and by making constant war on the efforts of older ones to advance biological science.

Yet my father felt that the individuals in the Church are for the most part carrying the germinal hope of the species. For they are, by and large, the religious people, however miseducated; and only when the religious people "come to" and in place of expending their energies on heavy mouthings about Mr. G and on the childish business of saving their own "souls," when instead of that they begin to think about saving the biological bacon, the real battle for humanity will begin. My father felt that a great tragedy of human life lay in the harm that good men are permitted to do. He felt that the Church could be rescued from itself and could be rendered useful if civil authority could somehow prevent the vicious business of exposing minors to theology. He believed that the crime of awesomely mouthing the word God in the presence of a child ranked along with the crime of murder—certainly far above that of sexual assault—for fourth panel perversion of the young is more difficult to correct in later life than third panel perversion, difficult as that may be. A famous Cardinal once said, in effect, "Give me a child until he is six, and I will defy you to correct the fourth panel perversion which I shall have inflicted upon him."

I should say that the principal delinquency of our European civilization— of our life for the past sixty or seventy generations—has been more hebephrenic than Dionysian and has been expressed admirably well in Christian theology. Immediately before the Christian period Dionysian delinquency was in the ascendancy, as it is now. We do not know our history well enough to have caught the rhythm of the pendulum swing of fourth panel fashion, if there is such a rhythm, but at any rate there is today a springlike expectancy in the air in some quarters. We may have about reached the end of one dark period. The hebephrenic pall of Christian theology seems to be lifting. We may be about to get over the bad dream of the supernatural delusion, and to escape presently from the most painful monkey trap yet encountered by man. This has been the monkey trap of confusing religion with theology, and it cuts off the best mentality from constructive participation in the institutions of the fourth panel, thus rendering the best mentality delinquent.

If we *are* emerging from this general delinquency the problem of individual delinquency in personalities not mentally insufficient may solve itself with the suddenness of the appearance of a precipitate when the proper reagent is applied to an unknown. But we shall then be confronted with an opportunity for a social delinquency of consequence potentially even graver than that of any of the misanthropies of the known past. This will be the Dionysian misdemeanor of throwing away the religious baby with the theological diaper.

There are many problems in the human near future but the central problem is to recover the respectability of religion and to restore health and strength to the fourth panel. If a human recovery from the ideological confusion of the present society is possible, it would seem most likely to occur under the leadership of a professional class charged with a religious praxis in somewhat the same way that the medical profession is charged with a therapeutic praxis. Any who are gravely doubtful of such a possibility and look askance at the professional crowd who at the moment profess a religious praxis, may perhaps take heart from a fragment of the history of the profession of medicine. A dozen or so generations back this profession was made up of a rabble of "medicine men" who had neither a common basic training nor generally sound operational ideas on the functioning of the human body. Four centuries ago the practice of medicine was so entangled in theological and supernatural flypaper that to have predicted its present degree of extrication from that mess would have required courageous optimism indeed. Throughout the sixteenth and seventeenth centuries, and even into the eighteenth century, the medical profession distinguished itself all over Europe by assisting the professional Christians in torturing and burning to death many hundreds of thousands of "heretics," "witches," and other men and women who laid down their lives in the attempt to lead a break-through against the deadly grip of a fourth panel monkey trap that had teeth in it.[5]

One of the blackest pages in our history is that on witch hunting, a pastime still carried on over back fences, but the public burnings at the stake— really the most exciting part of the sport—have been for the time being discontinued. In this sport the medical profession was as gleefully active as were the professional religionists. A Jesuit priest, Father Spee, published a book anonymously in 1631 in which he dwells on the efficacy of the medical collaboration in the conducting of the more exciting and more productive tortures. After accompanying 200 victims to the stake in Würtzburg, Father Spee's stomach turned a little and in his anonymous book he declared his belief that all were "innocent"; that they had made the usual confessions because they preferred to die (even at the stake) rather than be tortured again. He added his belief that the torturers themselves, both the "Doctors and the Bishops of the Church could all be made to confess to sorcery by the tortures used."[6]

Witch hunting was just the other day so popular a sport that James I, King of England and an outstanding Christian, wrote a book vigorously

[5] If anybody entertains doubt as to the far-reaching consequences of a fourth panel delinquency he would do well to read *Malleus Maleficarum*, in the English translation by Montague Summers, London, 1928. This is a fifteenth-century textbook for Christian inquisitors. Any means of obtaining a "confession" are authorized. One reads that both before and after torture the judge should promise mercy to the accused without mentioning that the accused will be imprisoned. The promise should be kept "for a time" but then the accused should be burned to death. The judge should promise to be merciful but "with the mental reservation that he means he will be merciful to himself and to the State, etc."—not to the accused.

[6] Quoted by Sir William Dampier, in *A History of Science* (Cambridge, 1942), p. 157.

reprobating the few "miserable heretics" and reformers who had dared raise a voice of protest, presumably at the torturing and burning of their wives and suchlike.

One function of this chapter is to ponder the nature of delinquency, and to reflect on the criminality of 200 delinquent boys. We are trying to fix in our minds just what delinquency is. Would it be a delinquency, now, to accuse some woman you don't like of traffic with the wrong kind of spooks; therefore stretch her on the rack until she confesses, crushing off a finger now and then with a pair of pliers and burning off her breasts a little at a time with hot irons? You will of course meanwhile press her feet against a stove handily prepared for the purpose and will otherwise "hasten the confession" in every way, thus showing your essentially kind and merciful disposition. Having promised the mutilated and now condemned woman that you would let her go, in order to hasten the confession, you are naturally released from the promise by the confession. So for the good of her soul you let her lie in physical agony for awhile, then you burn her at the stake as "slowly and painfully as may be."

Would this be delinquency? Just the other day it was being done wholesale, in the name of God, by professional religionists with the enthusiastic aid and abetment of doctors. During the sixteenth and seventeenth centuries hundreds of thousands of us were murdered by the Christians more or less in the manner just now indicated. That was in civilized Europe. There was also a touch of it in the United States.

Led by a handful of men of science and in particular, I am glad to say, by men of medical science, a movement of nearly revolutionary proportions has taken place. In most quarters it would now be considered a delinquency to treat a fellow citizen as the Christian heresy hunters treated those of us who did not mouth exactly the right superstitious jargon on the subject of Mr. G. In a measure we have emerged from the horrible grip of one of the worst fourth panel monkey traps imaginable, for although murder is possibly as prevalent as ever it was, I think that in the twentieth century we have been doing it more humanely than the Christians did in the days when they, as religious professionals, held a license to murder.

For cruelty the Christians may have achieved an all-time high and in that sense Christianity may have represented the high-water mark in human delinquency. It is true that the tortures they employed so freely were in themselves no more than adaptations of devices in use long before the time of Christian theology, but so far as I am aware the systematic, wholesale torturing and burning to death of *women,* as well as men, is a uniquely Christian page in history.

If we could answer the question of *why* that should have been we might achieve some understanding of the psychology of delinquency. What was there in that particular fourth panel monkey trap that instilled so deadly a ferocity into the human mind? Was it the supernaturally rationalized hebephrenic urge to jettison the problem of biological life—to give up, and thus somehow to escape from the "burden of the flesh"? No, it could not have been that alone, for hebephrenics are not killers *of others*. Hebephrenia is suicide, not murder. Was it the *bad mixture* of a hebephrenic philosophy of life in the minds of—and especially in the muscles of—men whose main psychopathy pointed in another direction? Perhaps to the northwest or to the northeast, or both? We must remember that the individuals who get into power in any society, and in any institution within a society, are always the vigorous individuals; that is to say, those nearly or entirely free from the third psychiatric component. It is the northwesterners and the northeasterners who run things on this Pellet, never the southerners. But in Christianity these inevitable leaders, these natural executors of human destiny, were inheriting a hebephrenic, antibiological hierarchy of values. It was a theology of antibiological humanics, a mysticism.

Now a mysticism rampant in the minds of the muscle men of a society is not merely dangerous. It can become hell on wheels. It is the muscle men who are most suggestible and therefore most susceptible to mysticisms, *once the latter are born*. We had mysticisms before the days of the Roman Empire. The East was full of them, then as now, and so was Europe in all probability. (Archeological remains in the island of Britain point strongly to a "culture" at one time infested with mysticism and with associated sacrificial rites.) As a species we may have been more or less caught for a million years in the monkey trap of *leakage of mysticisms from hebephrenic minds over into somatotonic bodies*. That may be the almost fatal weakness that must be overcome before man can live at ease with his new and troublesome gadget, the forebrain. Or it may be fatal.

7. The Specific Delinquency of Theologizing

Religion has to do with the problem of orientation in time. From the standpoint of the first primary component, or affectively, it is emotional concern over the relatively remote implications of behavior. Viscerotonically, religion might be defined as compassion for the future. There may also be some spillover of compassion for present and past institutions or even for individuals, but I think this is secondary to the essential meaning of the concept. Compassion easily turns into worship (as in worship of one's offspring), and religion becomes worship of something such as God, the holy family, motherhood, the phallus, or even the Brooklyn Dodgers. But worship is a religious monkey trap. Although a most pleasant habit, it is one of the emotional pitfalls in which human minds get stuck. To worship is to lose perspective, to go viscerotic, to surrender critical intelligence. Exploiters or practitioners in the name of religion are well aware of this, have long labeled all brands of worship *except the one they sell* idolatry.

In order to maintain the perspective to time it is necessary to guard against all sorts of worship as against any other bad habit. For the worship habit is like the masturbation habit. It produces a sense of relaxation and satisfaction without first requiring of a mind its best achievement. To worship is to relinquish the struggle to understand, in effect to say, Here I stop and dump my load. This is religious jettisoning and in that sense is religious hebephrenia. It is a viscerotic failure, but viscerosis is infrequently recognized as pathology because it does not throw the individual into immediate trouble. Indeed it may solve the individual's immediate problem through social conformity to an emotional hysteria which is in fashion, achieving this goal by selling out the future. This psychiatric problem, then, is one for *social* psychiatry, not for individual psychiatry. That is really to say it is a problem for whose handling a professional group is needed that has not yet come into being. The profession of social psychiatry will be, I should think, primarily a religious profession, and one of its major functions will be to guard mental development (education) against the principal religious monkey traps of the past. The role of such a social discipline will thus be institutionally correctional, in contrast with the opportunistic and adaptational role of individual psychiatry. Its concern will be mainly with correction of pathological influences exerted by established religious institutions.

From the standpoint of the second primary component, or conatively, religion is activity. It is the application of energy—power or force—to the problem of finding the way in the time dimension. Undoubtedly the most conspicuous activity of institutions of religion has always been that of re-enforcing ideas of right and wrong behavior. Ask the average person you meet what is the essential job of the priest or preacher and you will often be told that the job is to teach the difference between right and wrong. Thus religion gets tangled up in social control and in morality, which may be defined as the pattern of current fashion in social behavior. Now social control of morality is a function of urgency and importance. It is of an immediate urgency second only to that of maintenance and distribution of the food supply. But from a religious point of view it plants a second panel monkey trap. The monkey trap arises from too vigorous or too quick participation in the moral controversies, which in the nature of things are both continuous and innumerable. The central job, or the operational function of religion, is to keep the time perspective; to so direct feeling, thought, and action that long-term goals take precedence over immediate goals. To accomplish this, some somatotonia needs to be expressed. It is not enough to feel and to be aware. Achievement in this world also involves action and this is as true in the fourth panel of achievement as in the first three. The religious function therefore has to do with the direction of behavior, in the overt or actional sense, as well as with direction of thought and feeling; and it is as impossible for religionists to avoid participation in moral controversy as to avoid the kind of emotional welling up from within that so easily becomes the habit of worship. Then in the same way that the first component fourth panel monkey trap lies in the waste of this noble viscerotonia on symbols which fail to call forth the best biological responses, the second component fourth panel monkey trap lies in the waste of good somatotonia on action not in the long run contributive to biological achievement.

Religious energy tends to get itself entangled both in moral issues that do not matter and in those that cancel one another. We then see a spectacle that can be described most simply as fourth panel somatorosis, and the religious mind boils over with morality just like an oatmeal kettle. This morality may be mainly of first panel orientation, as when religionists get excited about economic reforms; mainly second panel, when the hue and cry is over democracy or some other second panel red herring of short-run import; or mainly third panel, when religionists intrude their front paws into private sexuality, which has long been a favorite hunting ground for the religious bird dog with a compulsion to point sparrows.

In any of these events the upshot is a religious losing of the way, and a loud din of barking (preaching) where no worthy game has taken cover. Potentially splendid fourth panel somatotonia goes down the drain of an irrelevant morality squabble and the hope of perspective in the fourth panel is lost in oratorical chaos.

From the standpoint of the *third* primary component, or cognitively, religion is an attempt to map a course, to set up a system of orientational signposts for a journey through time. In this sense religion is not "belief" but an effort to see a way, presumably a way toward biological betterment. That is to say, it is the effort to make sense, pattern, meaning, or system from what gets projected on the screen of consciousness. The truly religious cerebrotonic is a seer. He sees future implications. In the effort to find a way through time the third component seems to play a part comparable to that of the navigator on a ship. The job is to read and to interpret the signs and with a goal in mind to lay a course. It seems reasonable to suppose that the goal, for a biological organism, must be biological.

The great third component fourth panel monkey trap of our recent past —of the past few hundred generations—has been theological mysticism, and this monkey trap seems to arise from a simple act of forgetting that we are biological, that our goals therefore are biological. The bad habit of inventing gods may yet destroy the species. Gods or God in general may be defined as nonbiological causation postulated as interfering in a biological sequence of events. When such a postulation is made *by a biological organism* it would seem that the likelihood of its being an act of hebephrenic delinquency ought to be obvious enough. Theologizing has almost certainly been the deadliest third component monkey trap in history. In practice it has been a process of discouraging religious thought by lulling the religious thinker to oneirophrenic sleep. More bad biology has been committed in the names of gods of all sorts than under any other aegis of which we have record. Indeed the very term God has come to be identified with "otherworldliness," and therefore with contempt of biology.

In emphasizing the point that theology is a poison to biological health in the fourth panel it cannot be too strongly stated that I mean theology in general; not Christian or Freudian or Buddhistic theology in particular, but the theological principle of investiture and invocation. Investiture of a word with such potency that it becomes a magic word, then promiscuous invocation of the Word, either in support of particular answers to particular problems, or worse, in support of the choice of not answering or recognizing certain problems at all. The harm of theologizing lies less in the resulting failure to solve fourth panel problems than in the arrogant and false sense of power associated with the exercise of word magic. This is what sells out the future and it becomes an integral element in all three component manifestations of the great fourth panel monkey traps just delineated.

The viscerotic ecstasy of worship is in itself perhaps no more harmful than any other sublime gloating, which is one of the natural pleasures of life, but in the case of theological worship the gloating individual may never come out of it. He tends in the end to take his own gloating seriously and then from a fourth panel point of view he is a spent cartridge, a wasted charge. There is no humor in him. His worshipful contemplation of Mr. G, or of Libido or of his children, as the case may be, becomes not only a purblinding viscerotonia from which he does not recover but such a disease is in some constitutional patterns contagious, and the virus may be passed on to the future. Consider, for example, the suffering and frustration that have resulted from the perpetuation of the Mr. G disease. For scores of generations untold millions have been infected, while throughout all these generations there have been men alive who well understood the nature and the pathology of the disease. But their voices when not stifled by faggots were lost in such an arrogant bellowing of the Word that this once pleasant and harmless word became one of the most delinquent indulgences in history.

8. The Epimethean Delinquency, or the Harm that Good Men Do

The drama of warfare in human consciousness between Prometheus and his brother Epimetheus is a projection of the sometimes puzzling incompatibility between adaptive and corrective achievement. Prometheus restrains present success or eschews present rewards which by the exercise of forethought (Prometheus in Greek *means* forethought) can be seen to be incompatible with long-run objectives. Prometheus thus exercises cerebrotonic inhibition over present adaptational desire, in favor of a presumedly greater future good which from the Promethean point of view will constitute (it is hoped) a corrective against an institutional delinquency. Biologically, this inhibitory role is a principal function of the forebrain. The forebrain harnesses and holds back both viscerotonic and somatotonic expression in a manner somewhat analogous to that in which a team of horses is harnessed and controlled by a human driver.

Epimetheus exercises a contrary function. He is vital, representative primarily of the immediate adaptive need and of the practical direct desire of the organism. To him the Promethean outlook is utopian, impractical, even perverse. Epimetheus loves not the cerebrotonic function of inhibition. Such philosophizing as he may do is short-run and is usually rationalized as "conservative." He tends to trust to Instinct or to God (Zeus) and in so far as possible to let the pattern of the future be determined by the fulfillment of present conventional desire. For him wisdom lies in bringing the underlying instinctive impulses up into the full light of conscious day and in "making an adaptation." Prometheus controls, harnesses, represses elemental impulses. He keeps those horses in the barn or in the mental backyard—the backmind.

Freudian theology refers to the backmind as the unconscious or as unconscious consciousness, and Freudians, not often rural in outlook, have little use for mental barns and backyards. Their religion is one of abolition of the backmind and they prefer to stable the horses of instinctive impulse in the parlor, abandoning the Promethean idea of harnessment, and in short abolishing Prometheus. This is a Dionysian resolution of fourth panel conflict which in our generation has been subtly commended to Epimethean minds. The Freudians have sold the Epimetheans a bill of goods, illustrating one of Dean Inge's favorite observations that the devil rarely bothers to change the flag of a conquered bastion.

Resolution of the Promethean conflict defines what may be the ultimate monkey trap in human life. The bait lies in the temptation to trust the first awareness of instinctive desire, which throughout the millions of generations of the past *appears* to have been a safe guide to higher biological estate. Whether this first awareness of instinctive desire is named Instinct, Zeus, God, or Libido, it always means the same thing. *It always means what is first exhilaratively felt when the grip of the forebrain is broken,* i.e., when the cerebrotonic harness is relaxed. How the exhilarative sense of freedom from the restraint of the third component (cerebrotonia) is achieved matters little. One of the commonest ways of achieving it is by the use of alcohol. For those who are suggestible, i.e., for those who by nature are comparatively weak in the third component, it can be done also by preaching, by hypnosis, by invocation of words previously charged with emotional magic, by any sort of social manifestation of group stampede.

Group singing is one of the traditional implementations of cerebrotoxis, since feeling has always asserted its priority over reason through intonation of the human voice. For most people the conversion experience—that is an old name for the exhilaration of the cerebrotoxic release—can be readily achieved within the usual routines of social life. A few, burdened with too much money power and therefore susceptible to the bad habit of becoming dependent upon special attentions, require conversional transference to some solicitous priest, psychoanalyst, or other professional hypnotizer before they can thus be saved. Transference, in this sense, is sometimes achieved as an instance of that kind of final emotional yielding which pampered or specially privileged people (like women who take satisfaction from being hard to get) reserve for those who have sedulously and convincingly paid court. A psychoanalyst or priest may finally win a transference, in the case of such a person, after some hundreds of hours of masterful browbeating judicially blended with subtle suggestion. The transference is then a sort of "love" which (the analyst usually hopes) will remain at an abstract level. In general, the harder to get a person is, the more urgent the need for a transference. Operationally defined, the conversional transference is an emotional embracement of some priestly praxis or institutionalized outlook. It is a violent resolution of the Promethean conflict and is thereby an *ipse facto* delinquency of humor, or an offense against the humor principle.

We see how institutionalized practice growing out of the fourth primary need is permitted to defeat its own long-run objectives. The Promethean function of forethought is a primary fourth panel function. This is the function that seems to give rise to the need for orientation in time—the need for a religious philosophy. With awareness of time there comes into being a need for some pattern of feeling, of action, and of thought about time. The Epimethean function is that of trying to *settle* the profoundly disturbing questions that arise from these needs, by institutionalizing a set of answers.

Institutions are Epimethean. They amount to the codification of a set of rules of the game, together with such reenforcement of the rules as a system of social rewards and penalties may provide. Their function and their necessity in the first three biological panels is obvious enough. Without economic, sociopolitical, and to some extent reproductive institutions collective living would be impossible and human society would be chaos. But the fourth panel presents the necessity of gearing consciousness to time and change, and institutions are a human artifact constructed like a dyke against the consequences (to consciousness) of time and change. They represent a feeble and perhaps a suicidal attempt to hold our universe in *statu quo,* but they also provide the skeletal structure upon which social life is arranged. We need such skeletal structure. Without it there is no purchase, no leverage, no implementation for further attack on problems. Yet we are aware of the deadly danger inherent in skeletal structure for it gets out of hand, becomes the prison, and ultimately encompasses the destruction of any species investing too heavily in it. The history of life on the earth is a chronicle of tragedies in which countless species, like the great saurians, have wrought their own organic destruction through this monkey trap. An increment of skeletal structure is in general purchased at the cost of a decrement in adaptability, and this is probably as true of institutional structure.

Institutions considered as refuge against change offer a purchase to consciousness which seems as necessary for social life as is the purchase offered to muscles by the organic skeleton. But change is so closely of the essence of time that the one concept is usually defined in terms of the other, and the fourth primary need in human life is for adaptation to time—not for a refuge against it.

Social psychology is almost a new conception. Its brief history to date has consisted mainly in a descriptive exploration of the first three panels, together with some fervent effort to assign the causes of human frustration to one or more of these basic biological panels. Those who have attended college within the past quarter century are only too familiar with the proposition that the major ills of society are to be laid by the heels through some economic manipulation, or through a sociopolitical plan or formula, or through a change in sexual attitude or practice. Social psychology has had little to say about the fourth panel, has in fact often avoided that territory of consciousness as if it were in bad taste even to think about it. Meanwhile the religious institutions—the churches and all of the vested educational power associated with the idea of religion—have been freely expending human energy on the Epimethean disaster of repressing the fourth panel. That is to say, the energies of churches have been channeled toward deadening the human sense of responsibility for finding the way in time. The implementation of the process of unloading the responsibility has been theologizing. When God, an abstraction of all theological postulations, was in effect defined as a 7–7–7 and thus *all* compassionate, *all* powerful, and *all* knowing, it was a stroke of Epimethean genius. One could then utterly ignore the fourth panel, could (thank God) altogether dissociate the Promethean voice and could leave everything in the hands of God.

It is natural enough to want to find such a refuge. Most human beings spend their life energies seeking respite from responsibility and forgetfulness of time. They usually do it by trying to unload themselves on other people, so to speak, and then the victimized or parasitized one has an even more urgent need to lay *his* burden on still broader shoulders. It is nice if he can "believe in" Mr. 7–7–7 for then he in turn can unload on the latter or on one of His surrogates and can relax.

Thus institutions of religion defeat the function of religion and play a mainly "salvational" role, comforting and reassuring individuals *against* the fourth panel, perpetuating and emotionalizing every sort of delusional ratiocination against change in a world which *is* change. It is as if parents, touched by the pathos in the physical growing up of children, were to take measures preventing it, and were to hold the children forever in a state of helplessness. That is the way our fourth panel institutions have been working. The biological urge to find the way in time has been strong enough in human life to precipitate institutions, *but not strong enough to survive the suffocational power of these same institutions.* Now a question of crucial significance is this: Have institutions of religion *always* been delinquent in the sense of being destructive of the hope of fulfillment of the need which gave them birth, or is this seemingly fatal delinquency only a concomitant of theology and therefore the consequence of a minor, almost contemporary monkey trap?

If the answer to this question favors the second alternative, as I hope, we can perhaps recover from the Mr. G nightmare to a state of better religious health, and can rechannel religious energy in the direction of as vigorous a development of biological humanics as was seen just the other day in the direction of building cathedrals and hunting down unbelievers. But for the present our institutions of religion, and with them our "good people," will stand not only as a vast embodiment of almost pure delinquency but very possibly as the deepest root cause of delinquency. It is the weight of all those good people on the wrong side of the balance that sets the teeth in the monkey trap.

9. Freudianity Has Been a Religion of Delinquency

For those having a mind for contemporary religious history no aspect of the HGI study can be of greater interest than the reflection of the progress of the Freudian sect. That thread reappears in every fold of the fabric. The cases offer almost a quantitative indication of the remarkable waxing of this tide in a population in symbiotic collaboration with the profession of social service in an American east coast city during the nineteen forties. Certainly more than half of the boys, possibly two thirds, had picked up some fragments of the Freudian exculpative word magic.

Phrases born of psychoanalytic jargon were found in the mouths of our 200 almost as frequently as were similar fragments of the Christian jargon. By far the commonest of these fragments of word magic were those centering around the word "complex." More than 95 per cent of the boys had been consulted, caseworked, cajoled by social workers or psychiatrists or both. The upshot of all this caseworking had been in many if not in most instances the verbal beginnings of an exculpative exorcism not unlike that of making the sign of the cross and muttering a saint's name or a Latin phrase. Inferiority complexes, castration (or fear) complexes, and intrafamilial complexes of all kinds and degrees were invoked *in seriousness* by our youngsters perhaps twice as frequently as were the parallel Christian formulae. However, the *names* of Mr. G and of Mr. JC were still used freely in casual or profane conversation while that of Freud was often strange or unknown.

To read through the 200 cases is to be aware that the period under review —the nineteen forties—was one in which a religious tide was in some quarters running strongly. These "psychiatric social work" youngsters were living in an outwardly Christian society but the religious indoctrination to which they were most exposed was Freudian psychoanalysis. Great pressure was being brought to bear on them *further* to suppress the inhibiting component and *further* to develop the quality of Dionysian irresponsibility. When one of them was caught at criminality the treatment was almost invariably consultation with psychiatrists or with psychiatric social workers. The upshot of the consultations was with equal invariability a development in the boy's mind of the idea that it was *not his fault;* that he was somehow a victim of fears, doubts, insecurities, inhibitions—all born of a failure (usually on the part of the mother) to be sufficiently Dionysian (emotionally expressive) in early associations with him. The mother had not showered enough "untrammeled affection" on the child. There had been misanthropic effort at discipline or control. The mother–child relationship had lacked warmth and so the child had felt rejected. There had been jealousies of the father and so on. In short the whole situation had been insufficiently Dionysian and complexes had arisen. Complexes are a consequence of failure to extirpate the cerebrotonic component. That is to say, they result from inhibition and conflict, and are to be treated by opening up a broad highway of Dionysian expression of affect and of conation.

The possibility may be worth considering that Freudianity *is* delinquency. I do not advance that idea as a hypothesis but it is (for the moment) permissible to play with possibilities. It does not seem impossible that the psychoanalytic influence is simply a rampant wave of delinquency. Its philosophy is openly Dionysian. It is highly predatory, but more Dionysian than predatory. I have known many psychoanalysts. As an average they have been greedy people, very much concerned with their gettings, but that has not been their predominant characteristic. The predominant thing has been the Dionysian mysticism. Like every successful priesthood they are unquestionably sincere, with the religious light of conversional resolution often shining in their faces.

If a mine-run of 200 psychoanalysts were to be described in constitutional terms they might show a mean somatotype and a mean psychiatric index corresponding closely with those presented by the HGI population. There would certainly be the same lack of the third component morphologically, with predominance of the second, and the same lack of the third psychiatric component, with predominance of the first. This may mean nothing or much. It may mean only that when the whole structure of crime control in our great urban centers permitted itself to be heavily infiltrated by a psychoanalytically dominated priesthood it was really following a program of appeasement, and perhaps was thereby in step with the times. Yet if the psychoanalytic outlook and the motivation of delinquency are related in the manner speculatively indicated, the whole trend of the present generation's academic as well as criminological thinking can be viewed as a precipitous and headlong rout toward Dionysian chaos.

The predominant view in psychiatric social work is based on a supposition that delinquency is mainly an expression of difficulties born of conflict, and that conflict is in turn a product of the Freudian story of socially induced fears, frustrations, and repressions. In Freudian theology the devil, or sin, is personified as cerebrotonia—the repressive inhibitory component. Freudian treatment is almost wholly an attempt to extirpate this factor and Freudian theology goes so far as to explain even hebephrenia as the consequence of failure of such extirpation. Achievement of a mildly Dionysian cerebropenia is for the Freudian communicant simply a good adjustment or the chosen way of life. Such a view seems to find support in the undeniable fact that the mental hospital populations are mainly hebephrenic and only secondarily Dionysian or paranoid (see p. 72).

But the delinquent boys reverse this psychiatric ratio. Among them the Dionysian component predominates. It may follow therefore that any influence tending *further* to encourage this component is precisely the wrong influence from the point of view of preventing further delinquency. It may be then that the upshot of the Freudian influence on social work is to pour gasoline on the fires of delinquency. Some of the cases seem to reflect such a possibility only too eloquently. It could of course be argued that our 200 boys, taken as a group, are found to reflect the Dionysian outlook not because of any constitutional predisposition but because the social work profession has successfully instilled that religious outlook upon their young and malleable minds and that in so doing the profession has on the whole saved these youngsters from graver delinquency, such as hebephrenia and fatally crippling psychoneurotic patterns. These are not very far-fetched assumptions, as modern thinking goes in what has been called social science, and they have been advanced in earnest good faith by one psychiatrist who has been good enough to read some of this manuscript.

He takes the view that the 200 perhaps present the very best patterns of personality that their (fatally crippling) early environments permit. He is in a religious sense committed to the idea that it must have been the postnatal environment that caused all the mischief. With that commitment as anchorage he has to rest the entire burden of personality formation on one very small fragment of time. (It is a small fragment if you take the broader biological view that personality is also determined by the germ plasm, which has been developing its pattern for millions of generations through an immeasurable stretch of time.)

I do not know how much of a personality pattern is contributed by the backlog of past experience that is abstracted and carried in the germ plasm, and how much by what happens in the way of parental reactions and affections and the like that transpire during the opening months and years of postnatal life. It ought to be thought impossible to answer a question like that until we have adequately balanced those two main sets of variables in a century or two of disinterested longitudinal studies of the human personality. It is precisely such studies that must somehow get initiated before the delights of war and sex and rapid transportation altogether transport us out of the notion, and the principal delinquency of Freudianity lies in the dog-in-the-manger role it has been playing toward that kind of project. In our present complex culture there may well be an optimal and a potentially successful adaptive pattern for almost every possible temperamental pattern. Yet few find, or at any rate few employ their most effective personality. The fashion of blaming this mainly on the environment—and thus of seeking an explanation of personality in "something that happened"—is not only bad psychology but in the long run damaging to morale. That kind of psychology, by offering an easy substitute for biological self-insight, and an easy external excuse for failure, cuts people off from the chance to grow up. It blocks the development of a kind of simple and equally sympathetic observation of one's self and of one another that might in the end lead both to individual happiness and to a rational biological humanics.

10. The Disturbing Relationship Between Delinquency and Heroism

There is in human beings a heroic quality which repeatedly and continuously has saved our bacon. It is no small thing to have conquered an earth with the relatively light muscular power that we carry, and finally to have circumvented the great cats, wolves, bears, and the rest of the carnivores who have liked the savor of human meat as we like the meat of those fellow animals on whom we continue to prey. It was done by heroes, and one of the major (and recently most neglected) problems of social life is that of the nurture of heroism. We are always in trouble, always under the power of dragons or monkey traps. Heroes always have to get us out.

When the trouble came mainly from dragons and such, the problem of hero nurture was a comparatively simple one. Heroes were easy to recognize. They were large, courageous mesomorphs, very adept at mortal combat, full of strength and ready for battle. They joyously killed dragons, saurians, sabre-toothed tigers, and the fighting men of rival clans. But the heroes who do battle against the deadly fourth panel monkey traps that lurk in delinquent institutions are not so easy to recognize, *for by the criteria of these very monkey traps the heroes are themselves delinquent and so to survive must also do battle against the society they so heroically serve.*

There in a word is what appears to be the most puzzling complication of the social phenomenon of delinquency. So vexing is this difficulty that the legend of the *necessitous* sacrifice of the Promethean Hero has become interwoven with our institutionalized religious myths. We teach children in our churches that Prometheus (Jesus is the Christian instance) must take on the burden of delinquency and must be sacrificed with thieves in order to carry out the heroic role of saving the rest of us imbeciles from the institutionalized monkey traps in which our tails are caught.

Delinquency and heroism have thus become a continuum in our institutionalized life, and the problem of defining a sharp boundary between the two estates is so difficult that institutional religion, at least, long ago pronounced it impossible. The Christian Church got around the difficulty quite neatly, so far as its own practice is concerned, by the simple expedient of having Mr. G sanction the dilemma and sacrifice a son to it. But that sort of palliation is only a vicarious instance of the legendary offering of the fairest children to the beast-dragons of old. It leaves us still confronted with the dilemma, still in urgent need of further heroism, and still without a talisman for distinguishing heroism from delinquency.

Perhaps no sharply defining boundary can ever be drawn between these two estates. Certainly that impression grew stronger with all of us as the study of delinquency at the HGI progressed. I again and again experienced the feeling, on interviewing certain of the boys, that I was in the presence of what could at least be called a heroic component—and this feeling is not common in the ordinary routine of social contact with people in general. In a hero there is a quality of unstrained defiance which gives a constitutional psychologist a mediastinal tingle. You don't get that tingle from people like my razor blade major and you don't get it from those who are delinquent through physical or mental inadequacy. But read cases 126, 134, and 143. There you should get a touch of it unless the biographies have failed even beyond expectation to express what apparently was there.

In this study we became increasingly aware that a crucial problem in the consideration of delinquency is to detect the presence of the heroic component. Behind the mask of the outlaw the shining countenance of Robin Hood *sometimes* is seen, and a principal purpose of the schema of classification within which the 200 cases are presented was to try to analyze for the heroic component. We tried to approach the problem as an unknown is approached in chemistry. The chemist first precipitates out one element and removes it, so far as possible, then another, until he is left with a residue which is as free from complexity as his skill can render it.

Delinquent youths proved more complex than chemical unknowns in the laboratory and I am afraid that the analogy with a chemical analysis breaks down after the first two or three steps. But sometimes even one short step in the right direction is worth taking. That first step, in the present study, was to precipitate out the cases of predominant insufficiency, mental and medical, and the first-order psychopaths. This left about half of the original group of 200 and did not appear to remove much of the heroic potential, although we were aware that some elements of heroism occur in conjunction with all three of the insufficiencies just indicated. There seemed to be little sign of *competent* heroism, at any rate, among the 100 who marched in Company A. In the Chaplain's Unit of Company B there was competence but no conspicuous sign of heroism.

But throughout the first four sections of Platoon 1 of Company B, among cases 106 through 164, there are individuals with traces of both competence and heroism. There may be a few who have the makings of competent heroism, and present patterns of personality which under favorable circumstances would be heroic. Most of these youths could never have been heroes. Most of them were what army sergeants in the last war called foul-ups—that doesn't seem to be quite the right word but it seems to be close—and there is nothing in the world so fouled up as a foul-up. Yet the haunting likelihood persists that scattered among this 30 per cent of the delinquent youngsters who are presented under the general and noncommittal heading of second-order psychopathy, there are more potential heroes than would be found among the same number of "normal" or nondelinquent youths.

This is a disturbing consideration, and perhaps there is disappointment in it, for we did not succeed in putting a finger on any one objective test or criterion by which a heroic delinquent can be distinguished from a non-heroic one. By reading the biographies it is easy enough to make out which individuals among these 60 or so seemed to the HGI staff to present potential heroism in their make-up. There are about a dozen of them. As the descriptions unfold the heroic component also unfolds, like a pattern in a weave, but if there is a way of indicating such a characteristic except by presenting the whole picture of the individual, I have not found it. Nothing simple and easy like the somatotype or the date of weaning, or the response to ink blots, seems to help much when used alone—out of context. Perhaps this is only to say that psychology as I know it seems not yet to merit much status as a purely analytic or purely statistical discipline, but still requires also, for its viability, an integrative (constitutional) frame of reference and a biographical perspective.

For the present the hard acceptance must stand as one of the conclusions of the study that within the narrow straits of human mentality the bond between heroism and delinquency is still too strong to be altogether broken down—even diagnostically—by the social science reagents at our command. Even yet, and it may be more than ever, I think we are failing to conserve the heroic strands in the human fabric, and when the hero does return to our scene he must perforce lurk in the deep woods with Robin Hood, or haunt the cross—that is, unless he is only partly heroic.

Enough traces of heroism were to be seen and felt at the HGI that the delinquency encountered there—especially when considered in the light of our economic, political, reproductive, and religious delinquency as a species

—was not in itself much to be exercised about. That delinquency may have been about comparable to the pain symptoms of cancer. Doctors treasure symptoms and they know that treating the symptoms will have no effect on the cancer, except possibly to mislead physician and patient alike as to the true state of affairs. At the HGI we were not at grips therapeutically with the underlying problems of delinquency but only with the superficial and secondary symptoms, and the same can very likely be said of every other criminological study yet published.

In the delinquency of the HGI there seemed to be three components of sufficiently general manifestation to raise the question as to whether they may not be primary to all delinquency, and each component has its own heroic overtone. First there was Dionysian delinquency, which appears to stem from pathological lack of the cerebrotonic component, or from a disproportionate predominance of the tensions arising from soma and gut. The religious outlook which has been rightly or wrongly associated with the late stages of the Roman civilization is a good example of Dionysian delinquency. The religion of the Freudian psychoanalysts is a revival of the same thing. Both are expressivistic, antidisciplinary religions. The outlook of the average American businessman is, in the middle of the twentieth century, essentially Dionysian. The boys at the HGI were predominantly Dionysian in their manifest patterns of expression. But also there is *heroic* Dionysian delinquency. Franklin Roosevelt as a personality was a good example of Dionysianism wedded to ambitious power. His career offers a fine study in what will probably have to be called almost pure delinquency. Yet even to many whom he infuriated (and I was one) his heroic qualities were sufficiently manifest and he was a charming, courageous, and delightful man. How splendidly he drew the hate of the kind of people who would prefer a stuffed shirt in the White House to a Dionysian delinquent, and how he loved that! Even now the sight of a Roosevelt dime is heartwarming, if you have just a trace of the Dionysian delinquency in your blood. That man had a good enough time almost to justify his cost to the future. And the cost will be high for Roosevelt probably tipped the scales toward selling out what hope there was in our English-speaking breed. This he did by trading on first panel inflation and on second panel (melting pot) inflation for votes—two inflations that are perhaps among the most obvious and direct of the Dionysian delinquencies.

Babe Ruth, another good example of Dionysian delinquency, was a hero to millions. "Son of a Baltimore saloonkeeper, he was brought up in a Baltimore School for delinquents and he never quite grew up. . . . He scoffed at training rules, took his drinks where he found them, abused umpires. . . . His emotions were always out on the surface. . . . When the late Jimmy Walker gave him a talking to before a banquet, the Babe gulped, and with enormous tears rolling down his enormous face, promised the kids of America he would reform. He tried to. But nothing could stop him from living handsomely. He made more than $2,000,000 and spent most of it." [7] The *New York Times* [8] said of him: "Affable, boisterous and good natured to a fault . . . he made friends by the thousands and rarely, if ever, lost any of them. . . . He could scarcely recall a name, even of intimates with whom he came in contact, but this at no time interfered with the sincerity of his greeting. . . . Single-handed, he tore the final game of the 1928 world's series in St. Louis to shreds with his mighty bat by hitting three home runs. That night, returning to New York, he went on a boisterous rampage and no one on the train got any sleep, including his employer. . . . Of such phenomenal strength, there seemed to be no limits to his vitality or stamina. It was no trick at all for him to spend an evening roistering with convivial companions right through sun-up and until game time the next afternoon and then pound a home run. . . . Money meant nothing to the Babe, except as a convenient means for lavish entertainment. He gambled recklessly, lost and laughed uproariously."

Babe Ruth was a medical delinquent, [9] of remarkably burgeoned northwestern somatotype, and a Dionysian hero of almost Rooseveltian proportions. What if there had been no commercialized baseball and if he had turned up at the HGI as a wandering youth in 1939? What would his ID have been?

Second, there is paranoid delinquency, stemming apparently from pathological lack or disengagement of the viscerotonic component; thus from disproportionate predominance and bad integration of tensions from the soma and forebrain. Lack of viscerotonic participation in a personality is lack of sweet reasonableness, of a sense of fair play, and of the capacity for give and take. When paranoia is wedded to ambitious power ruthless hate and cunning are at play wherever power can reach. For our time Hitler will doubtless stand as the symbol of paranoid delinquency, with the Prussian ruling caste drawn up behind him in arrogant array. Yet to many discriminating minds, and to some who lived blameless and dedicated lives, this man was a hero of high magnitude. One of our great problems of the future will involve the relationship between the paranoid component of delinquency and the guardianship and administration of power. Is it possible for any nuclear group on this earth to win to such an exercise of power as is patently necessary for world order without first selling itself over irretrievably to a religion of paranoid delinquency? This is not intended as a leading question for I do not know the answer. Our own British history seems *almost* to suggest a favorable answer. Britain almost achieved a functional world dominance, while as a breed apparently maintaining the humor balance. Yet

[7] *Time* magazine, August 23, 1948.
[8] August 17, 1948.
[9] He was subject to overwhelming infections, had high blood pressure, died of cancer in the early fifties.

Britain failed, and had turned far enough toward hebephrenia in the eighteenth century to slough away her future along with the American colonies,
thereby opening the floodgates to paranoid ambition in many quarters, and
to the world war deluges of which we as yet have felt only the first few rain-
drops. The cynical view can be defended—was advanced by Hitler—that
Britain was bound to fail because of lack of that very component of "iron
ruthlessness" which Hitler knew well in his Prussian compatriots. That
Hitler misjudged the strength of deadly catatonic resistance still lurking
in the now also hebephrenic British breed may be irrelevant to the correct-
ness of his main hypothesis that we were degenerate. It may be that the
principal reason for the debacle of our abortive bid for world power, and our
degeneration presently into a breed of English shopkeepers and American
businessmen, was lack of *enough* of the second psychiatric component—lack
of paranoid ruthlessness. Perhaps that component *must be predominant* before an agglutination of people can fight their (heroic) way through to the
world power-for-order that the human breed needs to achieve. If this is so
the human outlook is almost certainly dark, but there may be another way.
Perhaps it can be done by maintaining all of the primary components of
temperament at a high level.

Third, there is hebephrenic delinquency, stemming from pathological
lack or disengagement of the somatotonic component (and thus, at least before general deterioration sets in, with disproportionate predominance and
bad integration of tensions from the viscera and forebrain). All three delinquencies express ways of failure of the humor balance. We dwell on a
promontory that seems to slope off to the northwest, to the northeast, and to
the south. At the top is strength in all the primary components of temperament—affective strength, conative strength, cognitive strength. Integration
of all three components is health and humor. Failure in any direction is
disaster. (Small wonder that theologians endow Mr. G with the trinitarian
quality of supreme strength in all three directions.) If Franklin Roosevelt
and Babe Ruth personify Dionysian delinquency, and Hitler paranoid delinquency, perhaps we can take as a fair contemporary example of hebephrenic delinquency the Anglo-American appeasement-and-pacifism group
that played so fatal a part in the dreary political prologue to World War II.
Probably Neville Chamberlain, the British prime minister whose policy of
appeasement finally turned Europe over to Hitler, will go down in history
as a symbol for hebephrenic delinquency. This may not be quite fair, for
Chamberlain was a professional politician who as such was very like an actor
on a stage. He rose to power by playing consistently a role. His biographer
(Feiling) indicates that beneath the pacifist exterior he was something of a
man, and that at times he felt cast in the wrong part. This may also have
been true of Hitler—for Hitler too the role he played may have proved a
monkey trap—but both men *chose* their roles and posterity will know them

for the parts they played, not for their stage asides nor for the unsuccessful rebellions within their own consciousness. For posterity Chamberlain will go down as spokesman for the delinquency of a hebephrenic slide-off to the south, Hitler for the delinquency of an unsuccessful thrust to the northeast, Roosevelt to the northwest. Each of these three was a thousand times more delinquent than any boy in the HGI series, for each wielded enormously more power in a delinquent direction.

Such is the heroic background of the world in which our 200 boys were living. That they were as a group delinquent to that world is certified by the records of all sorts of social and civil agencies. These boys were not playing the game as most of their contemporaries were playing it. Probably the majority of them would have failed to play the game in any society, and by the criteria of almost all cultures would have fallen short of reasonable expectation. But among them are a few who seem to have been delinquent to their society not through manifest shortcomings but because of the presence of qualities which in a "right" society (right for them) might have made them heroes, along with Roosevelt, Babe Ruth, and Hitler. The presence in the series of even a few of whom this may be true raises the vital question as to whether our current conception of delinquency is even on the right track. One criterion of a good society would be the effectiveness with which it discriminates its potentially most creative personalities from those who on the one hand are insufficient or criminal and on the other should be classed as only normal. If we are bailing out some of our best blood along with the delinquency bilge, we may be throwing away the future. That is to say, we are then as a society delinquent in the fourth panel. As the present study has progressed that has become the central theme and really the main point of the report.

11. An HGI Antitoxin to Delinquency

At the HGI we lived rather intimately with our 200 boys and for a sufficient length of time to find out in some measure what was going on in their heads. An impression grew steadily that, with the possible exception of the platoons presenting gross insufficiency, one thing most wrong with these youngsters was that they *felt* the fourth panel pathology of the society in which they were living. They needed a religious outlook acceptable to their intelligence, and they needed it just about as badly as they needed food. Yet many of them were in their vague way aware of the hebephrenic pathology in the Christian and other supernaturalisms to which their elders had more or less perfunctorily (and in some instances with obvious insincerity) been exposing them. A few were intelligent enough to be aware too that the prevailing psychoanalytic mysticism of the social work profession did not answer any questions that mattered but only provided a palliative to the Christian sickness.

For decades now I have watched wave after wave of not-yet-wholly-disillusioned young human beings break against the great monuments of sand and cement that we call colleges. These youngsters too were looking for sustenance and orientation in the fourth panel. After a while each potentially splendid wave of them has fallen back broken up and dissipated into paltry little skullfuls of economics and sex, with at best a few grains here and there of medicine and "science."

These college youngsters too, compared to the standard of what they seemingly ought to have been—and here and there a solitary and usually unknown individual has become—have been nearly all delinquent. That is, they have been disappointing beyond reasonable expectation, as were the HGI boys. *All* of them, all the youngsters I have ever known from the colleges, from the HGI, and from everywhere have felt urgent need for a philosophy of the time dimension of consciousness that would whet their intelligence and would square with their experience. This is only to say that everybody has a powerful religious drive and need. In our present society that need finds expression mainly in early youth not because the need is naturally greater in youth but because most human personalities are beaten, frustrated, and bewildered in the fourth panel long before they reach even their full physical stature. This is religious delinquency.

Therefore what I hope the 200 biographies will have revealed beyond all possible misinterpretation is (a) the manifest *religious hunger* of those boys who were not by birthright already too far out in the back eddies of the biological stream to feel time at all; and (b) the evident narcotic quality of both of the institutionalized mysticisms on which those youngsters had been fed. They had asked for bread and had been given narcotics.

This is why the point can be so reasonably defended that the HGI boys were not particularly delinquent in the sense of personal culpability. That as a group they represent a population bred down and promiscuously mongrelized to a shocking level of biological insufficiency is apparent. They resemble the Arkansas dogs in that respect. But that delinquency is not theirs. It stems directly from the failure of the religious values of their culture to jibe with biological reality. It stems from leaving the dead carcass of a theological misanthropy unburied, where morons can roll in it.

The HGI boys *reflect* delinquency. As a group they reflect it in such blinding brilliancy as to make you blink. But I had not lived among them for long before I began to realize that they also reflected some light of another color. Among those boys there were more than a handful, perhaps a score or 10 per cent of the lot, who by their own effort had won through to achieve the habit of radical questioning. That habit may save the species. I do not mean that radical skepticism is enough. Beyond that must lie hard work, and an honest, humble struggle to answer the questions raised. But the habit of radical questioning is a first essential to the mental growth we must soon achieve if we are to avoid self-destruction. College students do not as a rule achieve that habit. Not 2 per cent of them. They tend rather to absorb the indoctrinations to which they are exposed and thereby to "adapt," as have their teachers before them. They tend to "let sleeping dogs lie." That is to say, the colleges find it convenient to their own immediate ends to avoid the fourth panel of consciousness and to hurry the students into little compartments of specialized techniques.

I believe that per capita among the HGI population there was five times as much sincerely radical questing into the underlying fourth panel fabric of human life—questing for long-term answers to whence-and-whither-and-why—as on the average campus. The HGI boys reflected not only delinquency but also what may be the only effective antidote to delinquency, which is the capacity to go to the roots of social questions. There were about a score of those HGI boys who pressed me harder, more searchingly and realistically and objectively, for substance and fabric of a fourth panel nature than I have ever been pressed (in a quarter-century of teaching) on college campuses. When one of those youngsters looked me in the eye and started a sentence with "Now exactly why . . . ?" I occasionally had the feeling of being civilization itself on trial for its life, and with the outcome far from certain. I learned a certain respect for delinquency, and it was a little like the respect a layman feels for the antitoxin to a deadly disease.

12. The Delinquent Predicament of Psychiatry

Psychiatry may become the salvation of social science. When psychiatry frees itself from the mysticism of "psychoanalytic dynamics" and emerges from the acute episode of autistic thinking that has been given character by Freudian theology, psychiatrists will find themselves confronted by the job of developing an operational attack on the *institutional* problems underlying delinquency. But human institutions both in health and in pathology are expressions of human temperament and an attack on the study of institutions must be first an attack on the study of temperament. This task appears to be basic to any approach to life laying claim to the prefix *psych-*. To invoke that prefix is to undertake the responsibility of comprehending the components of temperament.

Psychiatrists are in better position than any other professional group to cope with such an undertaking, for they watch a continuous parade of the variations of temperament with its clothes off; that is to say, with much of the culturally superimposed habit pattern removed. There is no place like a mental hospital for picking up the main watersheds in the operation of mapping human temperament. But psychiatrists, confronted as they are, constantly with patients in trouble and with relatives who *want something done,* have been tempted to seize too eagerly upon the implied environmental determinism which has been read into the magic word *dynamic.* The psychoanalytic approach is called by psychoanalysts a dynamic one, and the literature of this group has appropriated the term psychodynamics to refer to the process by which the patient got the way he is. This process is nearly always reviewed in such a way as to place virtually the entire burden of causation on those factors with which the psychoanalysts have elected to concern themselves. They have selected their causative factors in such a way as to overemphasize grossly certain external agencies for which neither the patient nor his heredity can be blamed, and to underemphasize grossly not only the rest of the environmental story but the whole of the story of constitutional and temperamental differences.

One may be sympathetic with the Freudian motivation and may assume that the predicament which psychoanalysis has brought to psychiatry has come about through the best of motives—that of "serving" or of helping individuals solve their problems. From the point of view of the individual in trouble it is obvious enough that the psychiatric outlook bound to be easiest to sell would be one which (a) views the difficulty as relatively superficial, and (b) blames it on an external agent, such as the malice or stupidity of a parent. Psychiatrists after all are people with something to sell. They have to live, and theirs would not be the only profession to rationalize the shoddiness of what it sells on the ground that "that is what the people want." But the long-run consequence of such a point of view is moral, mental, and physical chaos. Psychiatrists as individuals are sometimes aware of this, but so are some politicians and businessmen. They still have to live, or so they say, and the way to live is to give the people not what you think is good for them but what they think they want. To question that is to question democracy, I have been told.

It is possible to be sympathetic with a predicament without forgetting the nature of it. The psychiatrist F. A. Freyhan has written what I think is a most cogent analysis of the psychiatric predicament.[10] In reading the excerpts from Dr. Freyhan that follow it should be borne in mind that I have selected such sentences as support his main theme dealing with the nature of the predicament, and have necessarily omitted his excellent interstitial expressions of sympathy and of a sense of fraternity with his fellow psychiatrists in the predicament. In these quotations the italics are mine:

The future of psychiatric research depends on the scientific orientation of those who are students today. . . . If [the student] is exclusively trained to be an alert historian of patients' life stories in search of intrapersonal dynamisms, *he will fail to recognize . . . the fundamental disturbances which are primarily responsible for the constellation of dynamic factors.* . . . Analysis of the psychogenetic mechanisms is a prerequisite for the understanding of the behavior of the individual but it must not block the road which leads to recognition of the more fundamental biologic disturbances.

[10] *Psychiatric Realities, An Analysis of Autistic Trends in Psychiatric Thinking,* J. Nerve & Ment. Dis. 106: no. 4 (October, 1947).

Positivistic [dynamic] ideologies have . . . produced a tendency to underestimate or even to ignore the necessity of appraising constitutional and hereditary aspects of psychiatry. *It is hardly an exaggeration to state that these factors are actually taboo in general psychiatric discussions.*

Researches in biology, neurophysiology and genetics provide today a wealth of valid information on correlations between constitution and personality characteristics. Genetic investigations . . . have established . . . predisposition to major psychoses. The reluctance and resistance in psychiatric circles which interfere with the acceptance and assimilation of these scientific data are rather remarkable. The fact that constitutional evaluations are hardly admitted to discussions of causality indicates a distorted sense of . . . dynamic principles. *This situation must be traced to the fear of therapeutic paralysis.*

Hereditary tainting and constitutional inferiorities are clinical realities, not inventions of "organic-minded" reactionaries. The population of state hospitals and institutions offers enormous material for genetic studies. . . . [At the Delaware State Hospital] one finds multiple families represented by 3 to 5 siblings suffering from major psychiatric diseases, great numbers of families with high incidence of mental, neurologic and various degenerative disorders. . . . There are, for instance, in one family 5 dysplastic schizophrenic siblings. . . . Here, then, is convincing proof of the existence of constitutional inferiorities. . . . It is rather surprising that in spite of these scientific data, the term "constitutional inferiority" *evokes emotional indignation in psychiatric quarters.*

Masserman's recent book on *dynamic psychiatry* . . . devotes less than a page to the problem of heredity, which is simply dismissed as an approach that lacks reliable evidence. Statements of this kind tempt one to believe that it is scientifically legitimate to accept "penis envy" as a cardinal symptom of the order of a negative T-wave while, at the same time, it is unscientific to consider genetic data.

Myerson realistically states: ". . . It is obvious that if there is a constitutional basis to a good deal of the ills of mankind, mere cure of the individual case *only pushes the problem of diseases on to the next generation in increasing measure.*"[11] Lewis states: "Many psychiatrists still show no tendency to distinguish between the problems of mechanism and of psychic content, or of *fundamental* etiology and psychogenesis. These workers are so exclusively concerned with the determinants of the psychic content that it is apparently impossible for them to see below the anecdotal level."[12]

The mere mentioning of constitutional factors often arouses suspicion of backwardness *and reference to heredity is actually taboo.*

Phases of psychiatric thinking have been compared to a swinging pendulum. At present the pendulum appears to have swung to the extreme pole of panenvironmentalism. . . . Insight is necessary in order to avoid the *note of intolerance* which creeps into discussions as soon as dynamic concepts are critically approached.

The uncontrolled expansion of hypothetical psychiatric concepts into numerous nonpsychiatric fields has had a boomerang effect on psychiatry. . . . Formulations have been widely abused and have consequently outgrown their scientific usefulness. . . . Liberal applications of such concepts as "repression," "anxiety," "regression," and last but not least "unconscious" to psychopathology, religion, politics and philosophy is not representative of scientific thinking but of intellectual mediocrity.

[11] Myerson, Abraham: *Some Trends of Psychiatry.* Am. J. Psychiat., 102:571, 1946.
[12] Lewis, Nolan D. C.: *A Short History of Psychiatric Achievement.* New York, 1941.

. . . The assumed omnipotence of certain concepts constitutes the real difficulty. . . .

There now exists a type of psychiatrist who looks at the world through psychiatric spectacles . . . ever ready to pick out symbolic meanings and hidden significances in pursuit of manifestations of the unconscious. A large sector of the public has become accustomed to misidentify this phenomenon of psychiatrism with scientific psychiatry. Psychiatrism is characterized by an ill-founded sense of intellectual security based on imagined omnipotence of concepts. . . . It tends to . . . oversimplify complex problems of relationship and causality. Such tendencies, for example, can now be noted in psychosomatic medicine. Already concepts like "upper gastrointestinal disturbance personality" [peptic ulcer] and "lower gastrointestinal disturbance personality" [colitis] have emerged. The crucial problem of vascular hypertension is being attacked in terms of "repressed hostility" etiology. . . . It remains to be investigated whether pathophysiological disturbances and personality characteristics [may not be] parallel developments, both depending on constitutional dispositions. . . .

It is quite true that among practicing psychiatrists there is often an emotional hostility to any consideration of the constitutional factor in the psychiatric picture. I think that Dr. Freyhan has correctly interpreted the root of the trouble as arising from a "fear of therapeutic paralysis." The psychiatrist earns his fee by doing something, or by seeming to do something. He is hired by the patient or by the patient's representatives, and he seems to become in a sense the patient's advocate before the bar of social justice. Most nonpsychotic patients who come to psychiatric attention do so in consequence of social delinquencies of one kind or another and the psychiatrist finds himself in large measure in the role of lawyer hired to win a case for his client. To win the case is to fix successfully the blame for the delinquency *somewhere else*. The psychiatrist is constrained to prove that *it is not my client's fault* and therefore to admit the presence of any constitutional or predisposing factor in the client seems to concede the case at the outset. In such a practice, a psychiatrist not one-minded on that score would be in the position of a lawyer unsure of his client's innocence.

The patient almost always thinks he has a case against society, or against certain individuals. That is only tantamount to saying that some second psychiatric component is present. "Paranoid" means, almost literally, to be convinced that one has a case against. The immediate task of the psychiatrist in order to achieve a transference of the patient's confidence and affection to himself, is somehow to gear with the patient's established mental set and to help the patient make out his case. If he can do that, the patient is bound to feel better, for a time. He feels vindicated, has a sense of getting somewhere in the right direction, i.e., in the direction in which he was already going, and the psychiatrist has good medicine. For practical purposes, and for the rewards attendant upon precipitating in the patient that happy feeling of being understood and helped, the psychiatrist's opportunism lies in helping the patient unload the blame on somebody else, or on something outside himself.

The Christian formula for doing this by postulating original sin, with a supernatural sacrifice or scapegoat for the sin and an in-the-flesh priestly intermediator for the official forgiving, worked fine so long as the patient's mind could be held in a state of mysticism or supernatural awe. But in just the last few generations the fog of supernatural mysticism has been lifting at an alarming rate, and unfortunately the second psychiatric component has not lifted with it. The result has been a psychiatric harvest.

The priestly function remains always the same. According to your sophistication it can be expressed as the urge to bring succor and reassurance to those who cry out most loudly for it, or the urge to garner as fat a living as possible from other people's psychiatric difficulties. Psychiatry has been rapidly taking over the priestly function and psychiatrists have not only been getting into an ancient theological monkey trap but have been stampeding the whole ovine band of us into it. The Freudian theology was made to order for that level of priestly praxis more concerned with immediate exculpative results than with remote or moral consequences. It is a perfectly straightforward blame-unloading formula and psychoanalytic psychology is dynamic psychology in the sense that it goes straight and forcefully to the heart of the problem of exculpation. Dynamics means an explanation of cause. Psychodynamics for the psychoanalytically indoctrinated means a particular kind of explanation of cause, always in terms of specific external influences which are assumed to be responsible for such "shaping of the psyche" as has eventuated in the present state of affairs with the patient. In practice, psychoanalytic psychology is the promiscuous application of a philosophy of exculpative environmental determinism to all problems. This amounts to anarchy, although it is often a kind of slap-happy, Dionysian anarchy which is not without a certain charm. For some personalities it is undoubtedly the answer, but when applied promiscuously it is a monkey trap, and this kind of religion is an outgrowth of a parasitical outlook on human society. It is an outlook which contemplates the social arrangement as a field for exploitation, not as a field for the exercise of a biological responsibility for the future. The philosophy of eugenics and the philosophy of psychoanalytic dynamics define almost perfectly opposed antitheses.

This predicament of psychiatry is an old dilemma arising whenever a priesthood comes into power. Whoever exercises a priestly function takes upon himself the priestly responsibility, which amounts to advocacy of the future (the fourth panel function). Priesthoods come into power only when older priesthoods fail. The psychiatric priesthood, now doubtless in a position of greater religious power than was ever before exercised by a medical group, owes both its opportunity and its danger to the collapse of Christian supernaturalism. The psychiatrist "can help"; he can establish a transference, can strike a chord of understanding and can win conversion where the old supernaturalism falls upon deaf ears and is like the droning of insects in August. But the psychiatrist has been elected to power on the Freudian ticket, and the Freudian platform calls for both Dionysian disregard and paranoid defiance of the future. That is the predicament of psychiatry.

There has been within our own time a violent religious indigestion—so violent that the supernatural vehicle of religion has been expelled with *projectile force,* and the mental stomach will not again for a long time tolerate the supernatural odor. That is true, at any rate, for such as will have read thus far in the present book. Yet the fourth hunger—for orientation in time—remains, and has indeed become the more acute for the enormous emetic loss. The rejection of supernatural religion has in no sense lessened the human appetite and need for religious sustenance and it is still the job of the priest in power to lead the way to such a coping with the thought of the future that by day men shall work with joy and by night shall sleep in peace. The priest continues to be man's duly invested professional advocate of the future but the professional group upon whose shoulders has fallen willy nilly the mantle of the priestly function in this odd chaos is committed *against* the case of the future. The psychiatrist came into power on the wave of revolution that washed away the power of the old religious priesthood. So far as most psychiatrists are concerned, they are still fighting a battle against religion in general and therefore they are fighting against responsibility for the future in general. They are on the other side in that war, and it is by being on the other side—by committing themselves to find the dynamics of personality formation in postconceptional events—that they have struck the sympathetic chord for the Dionysian mood of the day and have come into power.

By failing to differentiate between religion and theology our culture has failed to maintain a religious profession except for its morons, and has thereby placed the psychiatrist in the position of being the only available priest who is acceptable to what may be called the intellectually sophisticated class. This gives the psychiatrist a monopoly but puts him in a predicament. There are enough advantages and amenities attached to the priestly position that no priesthood ever gives them up voluntarily. Psychiatrists will therefore try to maintain the position, and they are in for trouble. For if they do maintain the priestly function they must necessarily betray their own contingency which swept them into power. Politicians have got into that predicament too. Psychiatrists cannot for long hold the priestly position with no more solid foothold under them than the crest of a revolutionary wave. Their job is to dig in, to consolidate, to fabricate a rational structure that will support the weight of the fourth panel of consciousness. This is to say that psychiatry must commit itself to a philosophy of social control which in the light of our present knowledge of life—our biology—can be sold to the public as an effective device for serving the interests of the future. Priestly advocate of the future the psychiatrist must become in fact, or lose his priestly advantage.

But the Freudian priesthood came into power through vigorous implementation of a philosophy which discredits not only the supernatural and otherworldly future that was the Christian ratiocination but also the biological future, which is squarely dependent upon selective reproduction—either upon a rigorous natural selection or upon a consciously controlled eugenic selection. The medical profession has just about destroyed the operation of natural selection. At the same time the Freudian gorge is roused to fever heat by the very word eugenic. Mention problems of eugenics in any psychoanalytically dominated atmosphere and you are right back in a Fundamentalist camp meeting trying to persuade the deacons to endorse atheism. To be faithful to the contingency which gave rise to the psychoanalytic sect your psychiatrist must *despise* the future, *and in both senses;* in the spiritual-supernatural and in the eugenic-biological sense. But to hold the advantage that (in a society of economic competitiveness) he is now almost fatally constrained to hold, he must convince and must continue to convince the public that he is the very advocate of the future in some sense which will seem to satisfy the general need for fourth panel fulfillment. The most important problem in psychiatry, I suppose, is to reach a decision as to which way to jump. The day of the validity of the Freudian position of religious revolution-for-its-own-sake is already gone. That position is never tenable far beyond the span of the generation of its birth. Psychiatrists must jump.

There are two possible directions in which the jump can be made:

1. Psychiatry might "get religion" in the supernatural sense and might attempt a still further intellectualization or sophistication of the Christian position along Thomistic lines with Dr. Robert Hutchins and his University of Chicago associates. The Church already boasts a few psychoanalytically trained priests. A variant of this same move would be to try to merge the Christian supernaturalism with a vague oriental mysticism. Some of the more articulate of our religious apologists are already writing hard to that end. It is a point of view easily geared to the political drift toward "tolerance." Call it fourth panel compromise, or perhaps just religious jettisoning.

2. Psychiatry might go all out for biological humanics; which is to say, for the development of eugenics in so far as eugenics is "the science which deals with influences that improve inborn or hereditary qualities of a race or breed" (Webster). I do not mean that biological humanics and eugenics are quite identical concepts, but the latter is a branch and possibly the main trunk of the former. Psychiatry might take that jump. I think it must jump one way or the other. Until it does jump, and until a generation of human beings in our culture is reared under the fourth panel aegis of a dominant

priesthood whose orientational position is thus rendered articulate, it will continue to be difficult to define delinquency—let alone do much about it.

So long as the psychoanalytic priesthood holds its power and dominates the mentality of the social work profession, which is mainly charged with liaison with the kind of families presented in this book, it will be almost impossible to get at the problem of delinquency. For whatever else may be true of the delinquency I saw in Boston, it is mainly in the germ plasm. Efforts to treat the individuals, even if successful, would as Dr. Myerson says, only push the problems on to the next generation in increasing measure.

13. What of It? A Possible Answer

The Greek outlook on life, from about the fifth to the second century B.C. at any rate, was predominantly humanistic. That short period may represent a rift in the clouds. That may have been a brief oasis of hope and promise between two long nights of darkness, and we may now be approaching another such oasis. Some of the Greeks answered their fourth panel hunger with a humanics, but for those who have been conditioned against that term it is important to remember that the Greeks did not have a *biological* humanics. They had no biological praxis, or science, on which to rest a humanistic effort to do something about the biological future. They had a philosophical humanics and they practiced a rudimentary eugenics—in the dark as it were. Our practice is far from eugenic, especially in the dark, but we have been developing some biological foundations *which might serve* a humanics, and to the extent that we have done that have freed ourselves from any necessarily pessimistic implications of the failure of the Greek gesture toward a humanics. I think that a ray of hope can be retained within the enclosure of five propositions:

1. That the boys in the HGI series, delinquent as they are with respect to first, second, and third panel *minutiae,* may be innocent as lambs when their guilt is compared with that of men and women who are responsible for the perpetuation of mysticisms and theologies; for it is these that block the development of biological humanics. The delinquency seen at the HGI may be so secondary and so insignificant as to reflect practically no pessimism at all on the long-run outlook. There may be available a medicine for that kind of delinquency, and one beside which penicillin would be a bland cough syrup.

2. That the basic delinquency in human life appears to be of the fourth panel, religious.

3. That the Mr. G business symbolizes the principal fourth panel delinquency of our era. The operational function of the fourth panel is to direct present energy toward the provision of an improving biological future. Supernaturalism directly and specifically blocks that. (There are professional religionists, obsessed with this monkey trap, who have gone so far as to fight openly against eugenic research and experimentation. Leave that to Mr. G,

they indicate. I even heard one say out loud once, in a pulpit, "Leave birth control to God.") The religious profession as we know it is so hopelessly entangled in the Mr. G superstition that of its own accord it will not and cannot come out of it. Our whole institutional investment in the fourth panel —the Church in all of its relations—will remain a delinquency so long as the Church rests its case on the Mr. G concept, and this cannot be remedied from *within* the religious profession at the present time.

4. That this difficulty is, however, being remedied. The profession of medicine, notably with its psychiatric shock troops, is already competing successfully for the religious soul-saving concessions. It is true that the medical profession, lured by profit, has in a measure made itself sticky with the same kind of flypaper as that which the religionists adorn. In the competition for this business the medical profession has not wholly resisted the temptation to employ Freudian mysticism. The latter is antitheological, in the Christian sense, but psychoanalysis and the psychosomaticisms are basically as mystical as the Mr. G idea and in the end they would therefore be as dangerous to the hope of the human future. They represent merely a pendulum swing from a mystically hebephrenic to a mystically Dionysian religious outlook. However, psychiatry is serving one good purpose and has brought the medical profession and the religious profession into such close relationship that the former is in fact in the process of taking over the latter. There may be few members of either profession who as yet will altogether relish the idea but the process is patently going on. It is the psychiatric "new growth" that is playing the role of amboceptor between the two bodies. Psychiatry is getting involved in the fourth panel institutions, and the latter are not only delinquent but bankrupt. On *their* mysticism they cannot backtrack. They cannot "demonstrate the inadequacy of the hypothesis," publish a monograph to that effect, and go on with the experiment, as scientists do. That is to say, they cannot goodhumoredly confess the Mr. G business as a monkey trap, for they have built their edifice too solidly on that mysticism and have even written it into all the dictionaries. But the psychiatrists are not so deeply involved with *their* mysticism. Some of them can even laugh about the castration complex, whereas if a professional religionist should laugh out loud about the Mr. G complex, even in our day, he would not for long draw his pay check. Even at the Riverside Church in New York, stronghold for "religious liberalism" that it is, the name of Mr. G rolls out without a smile. (This once more raises the question that possibly the mechanism of fourth panel delinquency is failure of humor, and it may be that humor could be defined operationally as *the power of lightening the grip of monkey traps— especially fourth panel ones.*)

5. Since delinquency is almost certainly a fourth panel problem at bottom; since the roots of delinquency lie therefore in failure of the religious profession to avoid monkey traps and to maintain humor; since those drawn

toward that profession are nevertheless the men and women who feel most strongly what may be called a sense of responsibility for the future; and since the medical profession through its psychiatric pseudopod is actually in the process of taking over the presently bankrupt profession of religion—at least two optimisms pertinent to the problem of delinquency may be in order.

One, the medical influence may pull the religious chestnuts out of the theological fire. Dominated by a religion of scientific operationality as medicine is—except for the minor psychoanalytic indiscretion which after all offers a sort of bridge across to the mystically Dionysian mind and may therefore serve a strategic purpose—medicine in gradually taking over the *institutions* of religion will possibly redirect religious energy through scientific rather than theological channels. This would attack the problem of delinquency at its roots.

Two, the religious influence may in turn pull the medical institutions out of *their* monkey trap, which is myopic environmental determinism. With the discovery of micro-organisms a sharp thrust toward the Dionysian outlook was given to the medical profession. For since it was demonstrable that these minute organisms are associated with disease it was easy to assume that they might constitute the cause of disease. Such a possibility was wonderful grist for the Dionysian mill. There was then justification for a *vast* irresponsibility. If disease is caused by specific exogenous influences, why then we can forget the matter of endogenous or constitutional differences, in the study of medicine, and with that we can dismiss all human concern for the biological future. The job of medicine is then to deal with exogenous factors. Let the endogenous ones take care of themselves, and let's have a drink. Environmental determinism is a perfectly natural Dionysian answer to the fourth panel, although from a religious point of view it is a deadly pathology and one reflecting the *essential* delinquency of our present human society.

As the medical profession takes over religion it must of course also take over religionists. More and more of the latter will be trained in medicine. A movement in this direction is already afoot, and quite rightly, for there is really no other training available for professional religionists except reiterative indoctrination in their theological monkey trap. From such a movement there may emerge a fraternity of medically trained religionists who will in time bring a strong fourth panel influence to bear on the medical profession. That profession may then concern itself not less with the treatment of disease but more with responsibility for the quality of the life stream.

Religion means *responsibility*. The religious mind is the (morally and biologically) responsible mind. There is at present in medical training and in medical practice almost no trace of an influence toward religious responsibility. The medics still confuse religion with theology and they throw religious responsibility into the garbage can along with the holy Mumbo Jumbo of the Christians. The Freudian psychosomaticists preside over the disposal of the garbage and the average medic is well enough pleased with that concessional arrangement.

Medicine means an operational approach to some of the problems of biology, although as yet not to the important problems. By its lack of *rapprochement* with religion medicine cuts itself off from important problems.

Delinquency means the failure of society to bring an operational approach to bear effectively on the problems that matter. This is to say that the formula for delinquency when reduced to its simplest terms appears to be expressible as a failure to bring about coordination between our best problem-solving methodology and those educational undertakings whose function it is to direct the conditioning of religious emotion. (By religious emotion is meant simply those emotional exaltations which are universal in the human breed and are inevitably associated with—conditioned upon—the thought of one's relationship to what lies far out beyond the self.) These emotional exaltations, loyalties, reverences—or whatever you may care to call them—undoubtedly constitute the ecstasy and the beauty of human life. They can be harnessed to the real problems confronting us as biological organisms on this planet, or they can be thrown away on delusional word symbols (mysticisms) and thereby jettisoned. Hebephrenia is, I think, only an extreme example of the same kind of dissociative pathology that is manifest in greater or less degree whenever these splendid religious feelings are masturbated away on some abstract word which does not represent or gear with an operational praxis associated with responsibility for the biological future. Thus when you teach a child to feel and express "reverence" for the word God, it may be that you are not merely committing a careless and conventional delinquency but *the* delinquency. This may be (at the moment) the central delinquency of human life.

Religion has to do with an emotional yearning for something quite definite and specific—for an identification with something bigger and better than the present organism that *I am.* This is a perfectly natural yearning. Nothing is more manifest to consciousness than the littleness of one's biological self, in comparison to what is outside and beyond, and the littleness of one's fragment of time in comparison to what has been and will be. One feels a religious urge to spend the little penny that is me to buy a share in this greater and more permanent thing that in every atom of me I somehow know is also me—and is my birthright. In a sense, then, the religious urge is the urge to *get back home.*

The easy thing to do is simply to be overwhelmed with religious awe, to give the Overwhelming Vastness a name and to surrender to the Name. I thus give myself to "God" and so I have the sense of at-one-ment with God— *without doing another damn thing about it.* This is hebephrenia. I have lost my little penny in a semantic monkey trap.

That is what happens at best. If now in addition to having thrown away

the most precious jewel of human life—the religious impulse—I happen also
to have got tangled up with a church which has fabricated an otherworldly
and therefore antibiological theology, and is thus playing an actively delinquent role, then the situation is more serious. I have then not only thrown
away myself but am poisoning and harming the greater thing beyond. This
is more than hebephrenia, for militant self-righteousness is now added to the
simple delinquency of failure. From this it is only a step to the kind of delinquency indicated on page 845 (heresy hunting).

We begin to see that the *rapprochement* between religion and medicine
may be of greater importance and of greater future consequence than appears on the surface. Both disciplines are delinquent. Each retains and is perpetuating an element vital to our life despite the delinquency. In such a
rapprochement a primary objective of the medical influence will be to rescue
religionists from their obsession with the Mr. G business. A primary objective of the religious influence will be to rescue the medical profession from
its fear of applying its operational methodology to human problems that
matter. Such problems have to do mainly (just now) with the general question of biological quality and with the extremely difficult problem of selective reproduction. Without the forebrain we never should have had to face
such problems. With the forebrain, we have not only the problems but an
instrument which, if we can use it, may be of value in meeting them. The underlying job of any crime-control commission is to harness the forebrain to
the reproductive business. However delinquency may be defined, there is
where its roots are. Having occupied the forebrain for quite a while now
with some of the inconsequentia of sexuality, we need to contemplate the
central implication of the subject.

After finishing the biographical summaries of the 200 boys of the HGI
series I left them for a time with a friend whose opinion I respect, and later
asked him to tell me what still needed to be said—in the final section of this
book. "Very little," he answered. "It would be impossible to read those cases
without seeing the nature of the problem. The boys tell their own story with
such eloquence that I am afraid your elaboration of the theme could be only
an anticlimax. You might just tell us what to try to do about it. How can we
get the forebrain to take hold of the problem of selective reproduction?" If
there is an answer to that one, I suspect that it lies in catalyzing the *rapprochement* between the institutions of medicine and those of religion.

14. Can Psychology Catalyze the "Rapprochement" Between Medicine and Religion?

Nearly half a century ago Shaw pointed out in his *Back to Methuselah*
that the possibilities for development of human personality may have
reached and passed their high-water mark *for our present degree of biological longevity.* When the maximal span of vigorous adult life is not more

than four or at the very best five decades, it is difficult to find a way of moti-
vating young personalities to invest a major portion of this span in "education," or in what amounts to mere preparation for the "more important"
activities and achievements of a short and problematic future. Shaw diagnosed the central delinquency of human life as biological, not "socio-en-
vironmental," and he wrote a cleverly conceived play around some of the
probable psychological concomitants of a radical extension of the life span.
However, Shaw did not write as a biologist, and his method for remedying
the "central delinquency" consisted only in the prescription of an "act of
will."

Yet the shrewd Irish philosopher was possibly right in the prescription as
well as in the diagnosis. The biological difficulty upon which we seem to
have impaled ourselves may be more of the order of an elephant trap than a
monkey trap—that is to say, a really grave dilemma—and to get out of it
may require, as a first step at any rate, something very like what Shaw would
call an act of will. In other words, before much can be done it will be necessary to find the mental and emotional integrity to *want badly* to solve the
problem and to make major sacrifices (acts of self-control) to that end. I suppose that is about what Shaw would mean by an act of will, and I have spec-
ulated on some of the implications of such an idea in an earlier book, *The
Promethean Will.*

Diagnosis of the far-advanced medical delinquency into which we have
fallen is easy enough to make, and the exculpative din raised by environmental determinists is easy enough to condone. The first thought of the normal child, when he falls into the flower bed, is to blame the stone over which
he stumbled. But as Shaw says, the next step, that of starting to *do* something
about it, is an undertaking of another order of difficulty, and one calling for
an unprecedentedly new kind of outlook on life.

In this case we know well enough *what* to do. We know that it is necessary
to replace a sentimental and supernatural religious outlook with a biological
humanics. Among the biologically well read that is almost a unanimous
opinion. And we know in a general way how to begin such an undertaking.
We know that the important thing in human life lies in the quality of the
germ plasm, and that therefore a first need is to gauge it. Not many will deny
that. It is clear enough that in order to effect a controllable or scientific approach to the germ plasm it is necessary to establish a descriptive science
dealing with its external consequences—the morphogenotype. That step in
the logic is more radical, but I think that most biologists have *in the abstract*
long since taken it. The genetic influence can be defined only in terms of its
manifested consequences, and in practice there is no genetics except a con-
sequential genetics. Finally, it should be clear that since in any particular
person many environmental factors have been at work more or less modify-
ing and obscuring the morphogenotype, to arrive at a descriptive science of

morphogenotypes is an undertaking calling for great patience and for a co-ordination of effort extending across generations. It is because of this long time element that the only hope for biological humanics seems to lie in a *rapprochement* between medical and religious institutions. Whatever else religion means, it always involves an advocacy and some institutional protection of the time element in consciousness.

The problem is to stir up the energy to plan and to implement a start toward the kind of record keeping that will in time bring the morphogenotype and then the whole story of personality up into the full light of day. For this problem Shaw saw no solution except through what he called an act of will. Perhaps such an enterprise must always be carried on abortively by individuals for a long time before the "act of will" can extend to sufficient masses of the population to set off the ultimately necessary institutional implementation. The difficulty may be one of inadequate communication between the pioneering contingent and the institutional contingent, or it may be deeper and may be inherent in the Promethean conflict.

In the present circumstances it may be a fatal difficulty. For it is quite possible that no imaginable amount of individual effort can assemble sufficient material to get the constitutional study of human personality adequately started. Methodologically the subject may be more simple than we have had the courage to imagine it, but it is all-inclusively vast in scope and before the constitutional method can work it must embrace every aspect of behavior, from morphological growth to consciousness. It must catch on as a whole before it can catch on usefully at all. The problem is not unlike that of kindling hard coal, and application of individual matches singly, even in unlimited succession, will not do the job. There must be intermediate kindling, which is to say, some degree of institutional or professional intervention. One practical question centers on whether the kindling for a biological humanics can be found in a professional nucleus already in existence. The problem is really to unite medicine with religion. Psychiatry we have considered as a possibility, and have recognized that the pressure on psychiatrists for individual therapy, like that on doctors, militates against too sanguine a hope in that quarter. Psychiatry is a little too close to medicine, and the institutions of medicine—taken by themselves—are perhaps as delinquent as those of religion. Medicine during its recent period of divorcement from religion has in fact taken long strides toward our ultimate destruction.

The upshot of the recent surge of medical effort has already been a lessening of human longevity in the sense that really matters. A child born in the United States in 1840 stood a slightly better statistical chance of living to the age of 90 than did a child born in 1740. The percentage of nonagenarians in our population was a little greater in the mid-nineteenth century than it had been in the eighteenth. But in the mid-twentieth century this percentage has begun to drop. Although the *average* length of life is now greater than a century ago, the life expectancy of the biologically best—i.e., the longest lived—has begun to fall back. The principal reason for this seems to be that we have begun to forget *who are* the biologically best. That is another way of saying that the religious enzyme has been missing from the medical formula.

It would not be difficult to find out who are the biologically best. If standardized photographic records of even a few hundred thousands of a well-sampled population were to be kept for so short a time as half a dozen generations, together with biographical summaries embracing the physiological, psychiatric, and social adventures of this sample population, it might be possible to define both medical delinquency and biological superiority in one operational frame of reference. The standard photographs of such a sample population would not need to be taken every year. Possibly such photographs would serve their purpose if taken every five years, as the census is recorded in some countries.

It is a shameful thing for a biological scientist to have to admit, in the middle of the twentieth century in the "most progressive" of nations, but it is a fact that we know next to nothing about even the simple morphological variation of our own population. We have a few tables of measurements, taken chiefly on such anatomical parts as are most easy to get at, but when you are dealing with a three-dimensional organism about the only thing that linear measurements are good for is—if you have enough of them—to try to reconstruct in its three dimensions what the organism might look like. We have had photography available for about a century now, but have not yet begun to keep photographic records of human organisms in any standardized way. That too is delinquency.

For a fraction of the cost of maintaining the rearguard palliation that we do against cancer, which may be only one kind of hereditary constitutional disease, we could keep central files of standardized photographs of the entire population. Such photographs taken periodically for a half-dozen generations, and accompanied by concise medical and social histories, might accomplish more against the remediable ills that beset human life (including cancer) than would even a first-rate semifinal war against Russia. One thing that such a set of photographic and medical records would accomplish would be clarification of the question of what is the *nature* of the massing to the northwest seen slightly in our delinquent youths, more pronouncedly (perhaps) in their mothers, dramatically in the expressive psychoses, and still more dramatically in certain disease entities, particularly cancer.

The practical problem really comes down to this: Is it possible to provide social agencies with an outlook and a procedure which will render them useful to the state as well as useful to the individuals they serve? Useful to the state, that is, in such a specific sense as that of collecting biographical and correlated medical data pertinent to the needs of the state. Such data might find many uses. Their need in times of military crisis is obvious enough. But there are other, ultimately more important purposes that might be served. It grows clearer every day, for instance, that if our state and our civilization are to survive for many more generations it has become incumbent upon the state to solve the problem of implementing a differential encouragement and discouragement of reproduction. This is a tough job and one calling for quite a new kind of professional outlook.

If social agencies are to play a useful part in the solution of this most difficult and most immediately important of social problems, they must find a way of becoming expert in the art and science of describing people. It is a *psychology* that is needed. But psychologists have failed timorously to live up to this implied responsibility of psychology and in consequence we have what amounts to a sort of academic lost generation of psychologists—men and women who are bright enough as individuals but are trained either in nonoperational jargons or in disciplines that fail to take hold of the real problem. Yet for their own bread-and-butter purposes these particular men and women need to continue to be called psychologists, and therefore the practicing social agencies look in vain to academic psychology for real help. They may have to develop their own biographical praxis. Meanwhile, if wars will serve the function of stimulating them to do it, and if nothing short of a series of survive-or-perish struggles can serve such a function, then war is in all likelihood man's best friend. War may in the end help save psychology from its unhappy impasse, and psychology may then serve its function of catalyzing the *rapprochement* between medicine and religion.

15. But We Still Have to Face the Music for the Delinquency of the Recent Past

In any case it will be necessary to foot the bill for the delinquency of the recent past. Part of the price will be a series of what may be rather dreadful wars. But this is earned punishment for recent third panel delinquency. We have explosively quadrupled the load of human soma and gut on a planet that was already groaning with that commodity. Human life has thus been so cheapened and so inflated that in many quarters of the earth it already has negative value. That is to say, it is as ready for war as steam is ready to escape from an overheated boiler. Meanwhile we have failed to solve such elementary and common sense problems as respect for the earth, equitable economics, political organization, and the specialization of reproduction. We know well enough that the inheritance of large sums of money is a (first panel) monkey trap; that the political power for world control must be headed up somewhere (second panel); that the recently conventional notion of the family as the functional reproductive unit of society is indefensible on the ground that it spells reproductive chaos (third panel). But instead of facing up to elemental problems like these we have dissociatively gone on breeding promiscuously, rationalizing it always on the ground that *food* could be produced for a *still heavier* population load, as if food were the only consideration involved, and as if human life dwelt only in that first corner of the first panel.

We may need to adopt the view that war is the cheapest way out of the mess we have got into. Grim, decimative war carried to the point of settling on a power basis the question of political organization of the planetary population. This question may have to be met head on before planning of any other nature can be more than preliminary wishful phantasy. What could the idea "control of reproduction" amount to, for example, except when enforced simultaneously throughout the planet? Surely nothing except suicidal self-effacement of one group from the scene, and that will always be a group advanced in the very qualities they themselves desire by their sacrifice to preserve. Birth control movements, except when universally enforced by political power, constitute only another monkey trap. Since as yet a central political power has not been established for our time, any talk of birth control now is like pacifism. This is to build the second story of the house before the first.

The price we have to pay for the delinquency of the recent past will be either war carried to its full decimative fury or the achievement almost by magic of a universal *voluntary* moratorium on reproduction. I say almost by magic because so far as my knowledge goes there is little more hope of such a planet-wide voluntary agreement on this question (except through the power of a planet-wide military conquest) than there is that all the dogs and fleas will similarly decide to call a moratorium on their reproduction. This is religious realism. It discounts any beneficent power of supernaturalisms, theologies, all notions that the human organism has or is going to have any more "outside help" in its fourth panel navigation than fleas have. It is simply a facing of the fact that at present the vast majority of the individual human beings on this earth *are resolved to continue to breed*—to produce as many offspring as they think they can secure food for. There are many who do not even think as far ahead as the question of future food. They just breed, as did most of the parents of the HGI series.

Statisticians motivated toward what I think is the same kind of hebephrenic complacency that paralyzed the Anglo-American powers in the nightmarish decade of the thirties write books on "population trends." They point out that the *rate of increase* of population is slowing down. They suggest that after two centuries, or after some other period of time, population in general on the earth will reach a "state of equilibrium" at, say, three and a half billions. This is just the kind of reasoning that the fleas would advance could you converse in their language. Here now is our dog, with say about three pints of blood—a fine, juicy dog. That is enough blood, if we make full flea use of every drop of it, to support six thousand fleas. The present number is say about four thousand. All right boys and girls, carry on. We are still underpopulated and will reach a state of equilibrium at about six thousand.

There is no more reason to believe that the present earth population of about two and a quarter billions is *good,* as compared with the half billion population of just the other day, than to suppose that the fleas on the dog (and the dog) are better off at a four-thousand level than at a four-hundred level. But there is *every* reason to believe that our present level of two and a quarter billions means incessant, inescapable, and horribly painful war. How long can we stand that?

We might stand it for quite a while. With the hebephrenic outlook already dominant in many quarters of the earth—perhaps before long in all the more civilized quarters—we might stand it for centuries, just as a hebephrenic patient in a mental hospital lasts sometimes for many years, even into old age. In these coming wars the softened and pacifistic (hebephrenic) elements of society will gradually be wiped out, trampled under, enslaved, and destroyed, a little at a time, and the process probably *can* go on for many centuries. What human flesh that retains some catatonic resistance can stand before finally dying is beyond ordinary belief.

The question is, do we want this future of blind hebephrenic drifting on the part of the presently more conscious elements in society, with incessant predatory war waged with increasing cruelty, always from less conscious and less hebephrenic quarters? Read Winston Churchill's books on the Second World War. Thoughtfully consider the British and American policies of the nineteen thirties toward the war that everybody knew was coming but that many of our old men and pacifists hoped could be postponed "until the next generation." It may not be possible to continue for long to turn a hebephrenic cheek to the prospect of war, and we may not have to suffer for long the lot of a vermin species that has overbred and so must make ready to fight with itself until only the more ferocious are left. One alternative would be realistic acceptance of responsibility in the second panel, which is the police responsibility for social order. In some quarters there has been an idea that world order can be established without the prior establishment of world power. Such an idea is of the same vintage, I am afraid, as the notion that heaven can be attained by wishing for it, by praying for it, by "accepting" Jesus. There is, I suppose, the same chance of persuading Russians, Americans, Chinese, and Japanese to call a simultaneous voluntary moratorium on reproduction as to persuade the fleas. Probably that problem has to be settled head on, on a power basis. If we (as a nation) lack the resolution to undertake the second panel responsibility, there remain only two remoter alternatives. One is to attach ourselves if possible to a powerful human nucleus not yet sufficiently confused or degenerate or mongrelized to have lost such a resolution, and to try to ride through as a satellite of that stronger agglutination.

In the nineteen thirties there were some Americans who, regarding our own English-speaking nucleus as a moribund organism, looked to Germany for that sort of hope. Now, less than a generation later, there are Americans who look still further away from our own native blood and language for their hope: to Russia, and to the Orient. For my part, I think it will be more satisfactory to find extinction and sleep even in a catatonic cause than to pay so much for the continuation of a particular strain of stock that will have failed. *If we ourselves lack the resolution to rule,* it is probably better, having been rulers, to die defiantly.

The second and only remaining alternative that I can see to our own resolute establishment of police power is the hebephrenic way. To try to pretend. To dissociate from reality. To pray that the evil day can be put off for a little and to hope for peace in our time. But that is a pitiful hope. Being now a fat, overly nourished catatonic nation, the United States cannot hope for long to escape earnest attention from *some* strong and realistic quarter. Weak, asthenic hebephrenes who are well jettisoned are usually allowed to crouch in their corner and to die in their own comparatively pleasant manner. But the *catatonic* hebephrenes, well nourished and resistive, catch hell. They are not permitted to die in peace. Men are not yet that civilized. Perhaps the worst fate on earth today is to be a *wealthy* catatonic, and unless we face the music that is what as a nation we are.

Epilogue

EPILOGUE

Delinquency may be defined epigrammatically as a measure of the difference between what human beings are, biologically, and their prevailing notions of themselves. The field of delinquency, then, lies mainly in the realm of social rather than individual psychiatry, and the problems presented by delinquency are inseparable from the underlying defections of social institutions.

Since medical and social practices are in the long run no more than translations of prevailing beliefs into procedures, delinquency is in a practical sense a reflection of the shortcomings of men's institutionalized notions, and the most compact summary of delinquency would be the most compact summary of these institutionalized idea structures. Such a summary has been attempted in *The Promethean Will*, under four headings or four panels. In that frame of reference, four constructive proposals may offer the nucleus for a broad synchronic attack on delinquency in all its mogrifications. These proposals are:

1. FIRST PANEL (ECONOMIC). Extract the teeth from the basic economic monkey trap. Perhaps if it were made illegal to transmit by inheritance more than enough wealth for an education, the motive to waste the best human energies on a struggle for surplus gettings would be destroyed. That might eliminate the desire for private surplus wealth, an arrogant desire stemming mainly from the institution of the family. Arrogance based on money might then dry up at its source, for then a man devoting his life to the business of getting would only be taking on an embarrassment—he himself would be faced with the job of unloading the gettings. Only in a society prohibiting hereditary transmission of wealth could the basic arguments in support of economic delinquency advanced by the brighter HGI boys be answered honestly.

2. SECOND PANEL (SOCIOPOLITICAL). Look war in the face. Establishment of a central world government is now of such pressing importance that any further postponement could be fatal to the life wish of the species as a whole. We English-speaking people have long realized a vague intention of retaining this responsibility—have recently felt the intention strongly enough to muster up a stubborn catatonic-like resistance to efforts in that same direction from other quarters—yet we have not as a group brought the matter resolutely to full consciousness. We have to do so, and we have to decide whether to assume the full responsibility of world-wide military and police

879

maintenance, or whether by our submission to encourage another agglutination of people to do it. If this decision cannot be made, the only alternative remaining to us may be the kind of treatment that catatonic *individuals* receive. That is to say, shock therapy, mutilation, imprisonment, continuous physical and mental frustration until the release of death.

3. THIRD PANEL (SEXUAL-REPRODUCTIVE).   Prepare for drastically reduced, and for selective reproduction. We are caught in a rat race of promiscuous overpopulation which has already gone so far that there is probably no way out except through crescendic war. We have to face the problem of curbing and qualifying reproduction but cannot attack it until an attack is made simultaneously all around the earth, for a local attack on this problem is but self-destruction. Local birth control movements are only hebephrenic gestures, like pacifism. Not much of a practical nature can be done about the third panel until a central political power is secured, but meanwhile we can get ready for an unprecedented shift in third panel values and for corresponding changes in third panel institutions. The basic change will no doubt rest on recognition of reproduction as a kind of licensed and subsidized specialty instead of a *laissez-faire* competition. This could bring relief from the delinquency of "the family," which in its monogamous form is already disappearing. As the paranoid obsession with monogamy lifts, vast resources of human energy and affect may be released. The growing separation between reproduction and individual sexuality (to which Dr. Kinsey has effectively called attention) will continue until production and rearing of children are delegated to a relative few adapted and trained to these specialties. This may put an end to sexual possessiveness, with its frustrations and delinquencies, and to the sense of tragedy associated with death—family-borne tragedy growing out of unnecessary interdependencies and consequent failures of maturation.

4. FOURTH PANEL (RELIGIOUS, ORIENTATION IN TIME).   Rescue the religious mind from its fatal habit of intoxicating itself with theology. Dissociation of the fourth panel from common sense is the acute tragedy of our age. Theology is the cause of that tragedy. Theology plays dog in the manger to biological humanics, alienates the institutions of religion from their function of serving the biological future, turns the mind and hand of man against himself. Atheism, however, is no effective antidote to theism. Atheism is, in effect, acceptance of an unnecessary quarrel. To labor the question of *whether or not* there is such a thing (or person) as Mr. 7–7–7 is not to allay the harm of theism. The God question is almost irrelevant. If a Mr. Benevolent Omnipotent Omniscience is looking in on the human show, it should be an honor to have so distinguished an audience. Then the last thing we want to do is muff the show. If Mr. B O O is *owner* of the show, as the theologists proclaim, then the more reason for making good our biological humanics which *is* the show. Meanwhile we dare not, we who have climbed

but to the stature of 4–4–4 dare not, and need not intrude our petty affairs upon the attention of Mr. G.

Atheists are often as humorless as theists. Both would do well to take a leaf from the book of Santa Claus—about a 7–5–3 who should be addressed on formal occasions as Dr. Benevolent Polypotent Pluriscience. Santa Claus is a relative of Mr. G, even if only a jolly old pensioner. Traffic with Santa Claus never did anybody harm. However much you may love Santa Claus you always take him *lightly*. There, possibly, is an answer to the Mr. G problem. The religious mind may need to be rescued only from its *heavy* theological fog. Light mysticism may be harmless if there is humor to support it. Heavy mysticism swamps our 4–4–4 endowment and the religious mind sinks into a theologic quagmire. But the religious mind is the time-conscious mind, as necessary to the plan of biological humanics as life itself. The immediate problem in biological humanics is to ferry the religious mind across that fatal quagmire.

INDEX

INDEX

Adler, Dr. Alfred, somatotype of, 551
Adlerian overcompensation, mechanism of, 551
Adlerian psychology, 739
Alcoholism, an adapted case, 555
  an advanced case, 614
  as expression of cerebrophobia, 198
  as preservative, 303, 613
  in relation to IQ, 210
  one kind of background for, 140
  parental, 777
  possible therapeutic uses of, 595, 706
  progressing cases, 570, 599, 608
  relationship to psychosis, 176, 372
  treatment of, by support of the first component, 500
  with DAMP RATism, 619
American Red Cross, 9, 104
AMI (Appeal to the Maternal Instinct), 103
Anal-erotic, as cerebrotonic, 50
Analytic therapy, mechanism of, 625
Anima and *animus* as expressions of gynandrophrenia, 106
Aplasia, aplastic structure, 23
  example of, in case of hebephrenic psychosis, 80
Aquinas, Thomas, 64
Aristocracy, mesomorphic, example of, 476
  of the poor, 420
Arkansas dogs, 790
Arson a bad early sign, 213
Artiness without DAMP RATism, 282
Asthenia, asthenic structure, 24
  not to be confused with ectomorphy, 354
Asthenic, 23
Asthenic constitutions, 125
Asthenic estate, pathology of, 764, 773
Athletic, in Kretschmer sense, 51
Aviation cadets, somatotype distribution for, 789

Baker, Herschel, 835
Balanced endomorph, mesomorph, ectomorph, 17
Barton, Bruce, 64
Big shot complex, 469
Biological counterfeiting, 812

Biological humanics, as affected by Freudian religion, 849
  consequences of disregarding, 780
  five constructive propositions, 864
  moral philosophy of, 9
  radical premise of, 3
  relation to religion, 833
Bleeding as therapy in northwesternism, 261
Bleuler, 44, 88
BM-PH (Boston Mothers-Presbyterian Hospital) syndrome, 785
Boston Dispensary, 12
Boston Psychopathic Hospital, 12
Britain now a catatonic nation, 854
Burgeoned estate, pathology of, 764, 772, 773
Burgeoned northwesterners, 784
Burgeoning, defined, 805
  of children, fad for, 810

Cancer, as counterbalance to hebephrenia, 794
  as "paranoia on the cellular level," 792
  in relation to delinquency, 773
Catatonic, difficulty in defining, 58
Catatonic hyperphrenia, 96
Cell, in relation to delinquency, 792
Central file of constitutional records, need of, for military purposes, 119, 285, 454
Centrotonia, 29
Cerebropenia, cerebropenic, 28
Cerebrosis, cerebrotic, 28
Cerebrotonia, defined, 27
Chamberlain, Neville, 854
Character analysis, systems of, 800
Chicago Study, the, 75
Christian psychopathology, speculation on, 838
Christian renunciation vs. hebephrenia, 90, 93
Christus, in relation to hebephrenic archetype, 64
Church, relation to religion, 835
Churchill, Winston, 874
Coarse-heavy mother, frequent appearance of, 782

from the brink of generalized social psychosis and human chaos now seems
unlikely.